HOW TO KEEP HEALTHY FOR DIABETICS

JUDY CHEN

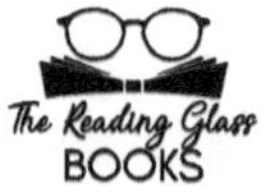

The Reading Glass Books
1-888-420-3050
www. readingglassbooks. com
fulfillment@readingglassbooks. com

TABLE OF CONTENTS

Chapter 1

Health Got Trouble

Over Eating Produced Hyperlipidemia

It is common for modern people to have high blood lipids. Look at your eating habits to know if you are suffering from hyperlipidemia. I told others that my blood lipids were very high and I couldn't socialize anymore. However, people around me say it's okay, we all have high blood lipids.

I used to work in the sales department. Although it was foreign trade, it was still sales in the final analysis. Our company is a large state-owned enterprise with customers all over the country and some countries in the world. We receive many customers every day. It is part of our work to make customers happy and eat well.

In the Chinese-style free economic market, the eating and drinking habits between supply and marketing are becoming more and more serious. It seems that it is not the case to invite others to do errands without eating or drinking. Similarly, customers come, in order to keep customers, try to entertain and satisfy customers. Because there are customers to buy, the product can be sold. The more products sold, the better the company's benefits. Therefore, the main task of the sales department is to satisfy customers as much as possible and sell more products.

In the 1990s, the awareness of universal health care in society was still dormant. The era of relying on the state to distribute tickets was just over. People had just struggled out of poverty. How could they stop their hands and mouths when they saw so much delicious food.

Therefore, eating and drinking have become an indispensable part of life and work. Such a bad eating habit, even an iron stomach can't stand it. At first, the blood flowed happily in the clear blood vessels, and was slowly blocked by the garbage of wine and meat. The rotten stench filled the blood vessels, and the blood became turbid. As a result, hyperlipidemia breeds various diseases.

Heart disease, diabetes, fatty liver, high blood pressure, pancreatitis… So one by one appeared.

Trembling Hands When Feeling Hungry

During the few days in Beijing, work and family issues were crowded together and it was stressful. A year before going abroad, I always felt hungry, as if I couldn't get enough to eat. Every day at noon, I started to feel hungry before I even had lunch, very hungry. When I was hungry, my hands will tremble involuntarily, and my heart was particularly flustered. I heard that people with low blood sugar will have this symptom like this, and they must eat immediately when they are hungry, otherwise there will be very bad consequences. So, I prepared some snacks to eat before lunch. This is a really good trick, as soon as I eat, my hands stop shaking. At this point, I didn't realize there was something wrong with my blood sugar level. I was so careless to even think about it, let alone go to the hospital to see a doctor.

In the early stages of type 2 diabetes, most people experience periods of low blood sugar. Due to eating too much food, the insulin in the body is stimulated to secrete excess insulin, causing the body to accelerate the metabolism of sugar, so it is easy to be hungry. When the sugar is low, the human body feels weak, and the human consciousness is also very vague. I can feel the energy in my body disappearing, not only the whole body is weak and weak, but also the hands are constantly shaking, the feeling of prostration.

Stay Up Late

Since there are usually many customers in the evening, the banquet usually ends at 10:00 to 11:00 pm. It was almost 11:00 or 11:30 pm when I got home and washed up. I couldn't fall asleep immediately when I lay on the bed. I woke up at 6:00 in the morning, and the whole sleep time was at most 5 or 6 hours. In the long run, sleep is seriously lacking. Day after day, month after month, in a vicious circle, the body is constantly overdrawn and worn out.

The liver works from 12 am to 3 am, on detoxification and hematopoiesis, and provides fresh blood to the body. Long-term binge eating has caused severe overload and insufficient blood supply to the liver, and frequent numbness in the hands. At that time, I thought my hand numbness was due to poor peripheral nerve circulation, and I never thought that the liver used hand numbness to warn me that the hematopoiesis of the liver was not enough, the body was not nutritious, and there was a lack of fresh blood to replace it.

Going Abroad for Medical Examination

In the winter before leaving the country, a C-shaped wound appeared on my ankle inexplicably, and would not heal. It lasted for a long time, until the wounds healed in the late spring/early summer the next year. I have been very tired during that time, I didn't have any strength all over, and I wanted to lie down when I was tired. I went to the Beijing Second Artillery Hospital for an examination. The doctor said that I have mild liver fat, which is not in the way. People who don't drink alcohol can also get fatty liver, which is caused by high blood lipids. It's all the fault of a greedy mouth.

I went abroad for a physical examination at the United Family Hospital in Beijing. The examination list said that my urine sugar exceeded the standard, and I was suspected of diabetes. So I was told to have a second medical examination, and if I passed, I could go abroad on time. The doctor asked me not to take medicine, so as not to affect the judgment of whether I really have diabetes or not enough glucose tolerance. At that time, the itinerary for going abroad had already been arranged. In order not to affect the plan, I bought Xiaoke Pills, a proprietary Chinese medicine for treating diabetes, which lowered my blood sugar in a short period of time. In the end, the doctor diagnosed me with insufficient glucose tolerance and allowed me to go abroad on time.

Obese People are Divided into Two Types: Body Obesity and Blood Lipid Obesity

People around me were shocked when they found out that I had diabetes, and they always thought it was incredible, because I was of a moderate body, neither too fat nor too thin. I had standard body weight in the eyes of my friend, no one thought I would get diabetes. The person who gets sick should be fat. I'm not overweight at all, and I did not carry any extra fat. Why did diabetes find me? Not only did others wonder how I got this problem, but I myself couldn't figure out what diabetes was all about and what caused it.

Generally speaking, the amount of fat in the human body can be seen from the shape of a person. People who are obese basically have a round body, and a big belly. The excessive fat was not only on the muscles, but on the internal organs as well. The beer belly is a sign. Thin people are inherently not full of muscles, and fat is not to be mentioned. How can thin people have excessive body fat? With this question, I started to pay attention to my body.

People judge a person's fatness and thinness mainly from the appearance, which is divided by the amount of fat stored in the muscles. The content of fat in the human body actually only accounts for 5%. Most of the fat is the increase of water in the body, so the appearance of fat is not terrible. Although I am not fat and look very standard in appearance, the fat in my body has been stored in the blood, which has caused high blood lipids in the blood vessels which seriously damages the internal metabolism of the human body. Because the high fat in the blood is not easy to be found, this hidden danger is extremely harmful. Once people find the harm, the human body has already developed a certain disease, even to a very serious point. From this point of view, I am actually a fat woman, a fat woman with high level of fat in the blood.

There are two types of obese, one is physical obesity, and the other is blood fat obesity. Generally, people who are obese are more likely to be alert to themselves or their family and friends, actively control their diet, exercise, lose weight, and take some measures that are conducive to health to prevent the development of high fat in the body. And thin people with hyperlipidemia who are not obese in appearance are worse than those with obesity, because thin people do not need to lose weight and do not need to eat moderately. Under that illusion, hyperlipidemia quietly spreads, until it causes harm. The disease began to alert.

Taking Health Products for the First Time

I didn't know anything about health care products before, and I always thought that as long as the diet is of high quality and the body does not lack nutrition, what can I do if I eat those health care products. In the first few years after I came to Canada, my blood sugar level was unstable, I didn't sleep well, and became sick easily. I would catch a cold when I saw the wind, and my face was swelling with puffiness. Once I went to work in the Chinese Culture Center in the city and saw an American health care company organizing an event there, so I was attracted to listen. Those who market health supplements advertise their products heavily, and I'm starting to pay attention. Mainly because of my poor health, I desperately need to find a remedy. So, I started to pay attention to the products of this health supplement company.

This health products company is headquartered in Utah, USA, and the main person in charge of the company is a Taiwanese American. The raw materials for manufacturing health products are various dehydrated fruits, vegetables and Chinese medicinal materials. They are all foods to be eaten, and I thought that there are no side effects anyway, so just give it a try. The product that the company promotes to the public is to use natural ingredients to make health care products needed by the human body to enhance the body's immunity and improve the quality of life. This statement fits my mind. I originally wanted to strengthen the immune system in my body without taking medicine.

I ordered the most expensive kind of full-body health care, and I took one packet every morning. There are other conditioning liver, kidney and stomach. Because it is made of fruits and vegetables and Chinese medicine, it is much more comfortable than taking medicine. After eating for a few months, it cost about 1, 000 Canadian dollars. With daily physical exercise, my body gradually improved. First of all, I stopped catching a cold when I saw the wind, and my sleep was also improved. Since then, I have become interested in diet therapy, and I have also carefully prepared my own side dishes according to the food attributes introduced on the Internet.

Dinner with Meat for Hypoglycemic

As the saying goes, go to the doctor in a hurry. At first, I didn't know how to control blood sugar in my body, and I didn't know where to start. Others say East, it makes sense, others say West, it also makes sense. Because rice contains sugar, you can't eat more, and it's limited to rice at noon. In the morning, milk, fruit juice, and health care products will be dealt with, but for dinner, what can I eat to prevent the blood sugar level from rising at night? I checked the food sugar content table, only the meat has no sugar, so I started the hypoglycemic method of using meat as the main food for dinner.

For a period of time, I mainly eat meat and some vegetables for dinner every day. Braised pork ribs and stewed pork ribs are almost a must-eat every night. In this way, the blood sugar level has remained stable, but the blood lipids have risen. I often feel dizzy and confused. The blood pressure also rises. It seems that I am wearing a hoop curse on my head, which is often tight and uncomfortable.

Many people, including many people with diabetes, think that meat is protein and rice is sugar. I also thought so at first. It's okay to eat meat. As long as you eat less food with high sugar content, your blood sugar will not rise. In fact, meat can also be converted into sugar when it enters the human body. The total daily intake of cholesterol in diabetic patients should be less than 200mg, in addition, it is necessary to limit the intake of animal fats and fats high in saturated fatty acids, and try not to eat fried foods and animal offal foods, so as not to cause thick blood viscosity, high fat, arteriosclerosis, and cause harm to the heart.

If high-fat and high-protein food is used in the long-term diet, it will appear to suppress the rise of blood sugar levels in the short term, but it will be more harmful to the human body in the long run, and it will cause serious internal dysfunction of the human body. In particular, the water control in the body is out of balance, and once the body edema occurs, it is difficult to control. Therefore, a long-term low-carbohydrate, high-fat, high-protein diet is harmful to diabetic patients.

Eating Vegetables to Lower Blood Sugar

Since eating meat does not work to lower blood sugar, let's eat vegetables instead. The sugar content in vegetables is very low and will not increase blood sugar levels. Therefore, in the morning, the vegetable juice is symbolically eaten with a little meat and rice at noon, mostly vegetables, and in the evening it is mainly vegetables. The daily total amount of carbon compounds is very small, so the blood sugar level is maintained very well. But after eating for a while, I felt that I had no strength, my whole body was soft and slack, and the sour water in my mouth seemed to increase, and I felt lazy and could not lift my spirits.

Eating a lot of meat will not work, it will cause high blood lipids and high blood pressure, and not eating meat will not work, people do not have enough high protein and fat to nourish the body, and it will lead to malnutrition over time. Diabetics themselves are not well absorbed. In addition to controlling their diets and focusing on vegetables, the body will be severely deficient in nutrients, resulting in a decline in the immune system in the body and accelerating the degradation of systemic functions, which is not conducive to comprehensive treatment of diabetes.

If I eat too much, my blood sugar will rise. If I eat too little, I'm running out of energy. How can I lower my blood sugar level and satisfy the happiness of eating and the needs of the body? At that time, I really didn't have any experience in self-help. I'm really new to diabetes and don't know my friend at all.

Work Out at the Gym

During the period of eating low-carbon compounds, the blood sugar level remained stable, but the body was always weak. I always loved colds and my body's resistance was very poor. I coughed and caught a cold immediately when the wind blew. Because my body is often ill, I didn't go to work and stay at home to do nothing, so I went to the gym to exercise. Since I exercised, my body slowly began to improve. The carbohydrates I ate at first no longer raise blood sugar levels, and I also feel empowered. I have developed a habit of exercising every day. If I don't go there someday, my body will not improve comfortable. After exercise, the body obviously feels relaxed.

During that time, I drank a large bowl of Chinese herbal medicine every morning and then had breakfast. After eating breakfast, tidy up the house, bring some fruits and dried fruit snacks, and set off to the gym. Usually, I spend two or three hours in the gym. My routine procedure is to warm up and run slowly on the treadmill for half an hour, then go cycling, play with exercise equipment such as arm pull, exercise each part of the body separately, when I go to the sauna, I'm sweating. I like the feeling of sweating profusely, and my whole body is relaxed. Then, rinse off and walk briskly home.

After exercise, the heat energy is dissipated, the physical energy reaches the exercise, the meal is more delicious, the carbohydrates are more than before, the overall food intake is also increased, and the blood sugar level is stable.

Gyms often organize some activities, such as teaching yoga, endurance running and jumping, etc. Participating in a yoga class is a quiet exercise, and the mind is greatly relaxed. Listening to the soothing and beautiful music is as fresh as the old forest in the deep mountains, and it is like lying on the windy blue sea floating freely, feeling relaxed and happy. Participating in endurance running and jumping, sweating profusely and exhausted, after taking a shower, I was relaxed on the way home, and my legs were extraordinarily strong.

Just exercise in the gym for a whole year. During this year, I did not take any western medicine, except for some homemade Chinese medicine tea. The blood sugar level has been kept below 6. The doctor said that I was keeping well. My hands and feet are not damaged, my feet are smooth, and my eyes are no problem. I also feel energetic and flexible in walking.

Hypoglycemic with Bitter Melon Tea

For a period of time, my teeth were often on fire, and the inside of my ear was swollen and painful. I checked the book and said that the Sanjiao was blocked, which is a characteristic of diabetes. That is, the waterways that run in the body are not functioning well.

All kinds of information are publicizing that bitter melon has special effects in lowering blood sugar and is the nemesis of diabetes. So, I bought a lot of bitter gourd tea from the traditional Chinese medicine store and brewed several large cups of tea every day. However, after drinking for a period of time, there is still a lot of internal fire, and the Sanjiao nerve is still swollen and painful, and because of the large fire in the body, it is impossible to take supplements, the throat is often swollen and sore, and lymphatic inflammation is common. Moreover, drinking bitter gourd tea not only did not lower the stomach fire, but instead had an unpleasant taste in the mouth.

Later, after reading some knowledge of Chinese medicine, I realized that the fire in the body belongs to the virtual fire, not the real fire. Otherwise, the more I drink bitter gourd water, the worse my health will be. I have to conquer the virtual fire first, and wait until the body reaches a balance before I can supplement with nutritious ingredients.

Taking Sanhuang Tablets to Reduce Blood Sugar and Eliminate Fire

Instead of drinking Chinese herbal soup and bitter gourd tea, take Sanhuang tablets instead. At that time, there was a Chinese patent medicine Sanhuang Pian in China to lower blood sugar in diabetic patients, and the effect was good. My dad bought me two big boxes for a year's supply.

According to the data, the main components of Sanhuang Tablet are: rhubarb, berberine hydrochloride, and Scutellaria baicalensis extract. Contains heat-clearing and detoxifying, purging fire and laxative effects, used for symptoms such as heat in the triple burner, red eyes and sore eyes, sore mouth and nose, sore throat, bleeding gums, upset and thirst. Sanhuang tablet is bitter and cold in nature, and can clear away heat and dry dampness. It is used to deal with dampness and heat, and the effect is very good. My stomach often feels hot, isn't it just the time to clear the fire? Besides, Sanjiao often gets angry and needs to be cleared. That's it, it's easy to take, no need to boil soup, no need to drink bitter gourd tea. Those large packets of Sanhuang tablets have been taken for more than a year, and they really work. The blood sugar level has remained stable for more than a year.

At that time, I often got irritated with triple focus, and the inside of my ears, teeth, and eyes became red and swollen every few days. Especially in the teeth and ears, and from the jaw to the neck. The stomach is often full and congested. After taking Sanhuang Pian, the condition improved greatly. Not only did the blood sugar drop, but the facial features were no longer red and swollen.

Diabetes is a triple-joule disorder in Chinese medicine. The ancients classified the heart and lungs as upper jiao, spleen, stomach, liver and gallbladder, small intestine as middle jiao, and kidney, large intestine, and bladder as lower jiao. The Meridian Triple Jiao is the channel of the entire body cavity. If the channel is blocked, people will naturally get sick. The ears, teeth, eyes, etc, are all on the channel of the triple jiao meridian. The three Sanhuang Pian has a function of clearing heat and dampness, extinguishing the fire on the triple jiao meridian, and the channel is opened.

Sanhuang Tablet has the functions of clearing away heat and detoxifying, purging fire and laxative. This means that there is heat poison in my body, and the pancreas cannot produce the normal amount of insulin and pancreatic juice. By clearing the heat toxin, the islets get a chance to breathe, and the blood sugar reaches a steady state.

After all, Sanhuang Tablet is a medicine, and if it is a medicine, it has three points of poison. Besides, rhubarb is cold in nature. Long-term use will definitely have a destructive effect on the body. The cold constitution will increase the cold. One contradiction was resolved, and another contradiction reappeared.

During the treatment of diabetes with Sanhuang Tablet, I was wondering how to avoid fire in my body without taking Sanhuang Tablet? Where does the fire in our body come from?

Blood Sugar Levels Soared After Returning Home

The biggest temptation to return to China to visit relatives is food. There are too many delicious foods in China, and it feels like I am sorry to refuse to eat good food. Relatives and friends, classmates, and former colleagues are rare to get together, everyone is so enthusiastic, how can I go on a diet alone? Besides, the gluttonous bugs in my stomach have already jumped in my throat, and the tempting delicacy is really irresistible.

The banquets outside cannot be avoided, and I cannot eat less. I should eat less of the meals at home. Every time I eat, my dad keeps saying, eat more, you like this, you like that. I said, Dad, my blood sugar level has risen a lot since I returned to China, and it has already exceeded the warning line, so I can't be greedy anymore. Dad said, it's rare for you to come back, and you can't eat hometown food in Canada, so you should eat more. Now that the blood sugar level is high, go back and find a way to lower it. There is no way, who told me to be greedy, my ears are soft, I have to continue to complete the daily sumptuous meal obediently, let the high blood sugar in my body run rampant.

It is very nervous to measure blood sugar every morning, and the blood sugar level is very high, hovering between 13 and 18 moles. Every time I see the blood sugar level displayed on the instrument, I think I must eat less food and less meat today. But sitting at the dinner table couldn't help it. As a result, the poor stomach was still full of high-fat and high-protein food.

If my mouth is greedy, my body will be hurt. High blood sugar is corroding and hurting my body, but I don't care. I always comfort myself, and I will lower my sugar after returning to Canada.

Itchy Face, Numb Hands, Taking Vitamins and Propolis

After returning to China for the first time to visit relatives, not only the blood sugar remained high, but even the face was itchy, like little ants crawling on the face. My hands are numb, and my fingers are numb, so it's better to use hot water bubble. Itchy face is really embarrassing sometimes. Sometimes when talking to others, the face suddenly itches, like there are many little ants crawling around on the face. It's really scratching. Sometimes I just can't bear it anymore, and I just scratched it without being polite. This ant sensation is different from the itchy skin, as if there are really many small ants crawling on the face, it is extremely itchy.

At that time, I didn't know why the body appeared in this state. Later, I checked the information and found that this is one of the characteristics of diabetes. It is the result of the harm of high blood sugar in the body. It has already invaded the peripheral nerves. This phenomenon is peripheral nerve inflammation. Peripheral neuritis belongs to peripheral neuropathy. Although it is not as severe as diabetic foot that will cause amputation, the abnormal sensation brought by this peripheral neuritis to diabetic patients is very painful. You don't know when this type of peripheral neuritis will get sick, and it often embarrass you suddenly in public.

This kind of ant feeling on the face and hand numbness has lasted for a long time, and there is no way to eliminate it. Later, it was reported that it seemed to be caused by the lack of vitamin B family in the body. So, I started to eat B1, B6, B12 and other B-type multi-vitamin mixed health products. Later, it was introduced on the Internet that propolis can lower blood sugar. For diabetic patients, taking propolis is better than taking medicine, at least with less side effects.

Since taking B vitamins and propolis, the ant feeling on the face has not reappeared, and the blood sugar level hasstabilized a lot.

Why does propolis have such an obvious effect? Follow the instructions on the manual as follows:

Propolis and royal jelly are rich in amino acids, trace elements and vitamins necessary for the human body, espe-cially the B vitamins are very rich. These effective ingredients have a good function of nourishing nerves. Among them, the B family vitamins can become the raw material for the manufacture of insulin, which has obvious effects on patients with type II diabetes.

The flavonoids and flavonols in propolis have the effects of expanding and softening blood vessels, which improves blood circulation. After blood circulation is improved, nerve nutrition is also supplemented.

Propolis has the functions of activating blood and removing blood stasis and promoting blood circulation, thereby providing more nutrients to the nerves.

In addition, propolis and royal jelly also have anti-free radicals, regulate blood sugar, blood pressure, lower blood lipids, blood viscosity, etc, and prevent further damage to nerves. In other words, propolis and royal jelly are fundamentally repairing and nourishing nerves, which are not only effective, but also not lightly reture back.

Since then, I have been taking the vitamin B family for all these years to protect my nervous system from being damaged by diabetes and forming complications of diabetes.

First Time Taking the Hypoglycemic Drug Glyburide

After visiting relatives, the blood sugar level remained high for a long time, even if I was a vegetarian diet, it didn't work. The blood sugar level used to be as high as 18 moles. I'm really a little anxious, I blame myself for being too greedy, and I don't have the willpower to control my gluttony. Before returning to China, all the efforts I had made were in vain. Now my condition has not alleviated but has worsened. It seemed that I had to ask my family doctor for help. The blood sugar level that couldn't drop made me start to take the western medicine.

After the laboratory test, not only the blood glucose level exceeded the warning line, but the blood lipids were also higher than the normal range. So my family doctor prescribed the western medicine glibenclamide three times a day, one capsule each time. The doctor told me that this medicine will cause stomach discomfort, and its effect is to reduce blood sugar by reducing appetite.

After taking it for a period of time, the blood sugar level and blood lipids really dropped and fell within the normal range. The problem of blood sugar level has been solved, and new problems have emerged. Since I took glibenclamide, I felt sick in my stomach, anorexia, and sometimes nausea, and my interest in food was not so strong. I often feel full after eating a little bit. At first, I was very proud that I could strictly control my blood sugar because my body automatically refused to eat more. After a while, I found something was wrong. As my blood sugar level dropped, my weight plummeted. During that time, I was noticeably thinner. My originally round thigh muscles became lax and slack. The tight pants I used to wear became much looser, and my colleagues said that I was thinner. When I went to the clinic for a review, I measured my weight by the way, which shocked me. My weight dropped to the lowest level since an adult. If I lose weight at this rate, I will soon become dry wood. I want to talk to my family doctor and stop taking glibenclamide immediately.

Taking the Hypoglycemic Drug Gliclazide

A colleague of mine has diabetes and his wife is a doctor. I think he usually eats the same food as ordinary people, and he eats rice and fruit at night. I asked him what kind of medicine he was taking. Isn't he afraid of higher blood sugar levels if he eats rice and fruit at night? He said that his diabetes condition is not very serious, and taking half a capsule of hypoglycemic drugs before each meal can keep the blood sugar level stable. I said that I was taking Glycine, although the effect was good, but I didn't want to eat after taking it. The mechanism of this medicine is to prevent eating to control the increase in blood sugar level, so the weight will drop a lot. He said that the hypoglycemic medicine he was taking was prescribed by his wife, and the name of the medicine was Gliclazide. Since then, I have changed to gliclazide, which is called Dameikang in Chinese. It is a small pill with 80mg each. At the beginning, I took two pills a day, one in the morning and one in the evening. The effect is the same as that of Glycine, the difference is that my appetite has started to recover, and I feel delicious when I eat. In this way, my weight does not continue to drop, but it is really not easy to return to the original level, because I cannot eat more, and there is no excess nutrition in my body to provide for muscle growth.

I have been taking Gliclazide now, but instead of taking two capsules a day, I take it based on my body's blood sugar level. Since I found an effective way to control blood sugar level naturally, western medicine has become a supportingrole in controlling blood sugar level, and it is only occasional and special circumstances that I take half a pill. For a long time, I didn't take medication, I ate a normal diet every day, and my blood sugar was normal. Bad Eating Habits Cause Internal Fire in the Liver.

Liver fire is a kind of sickness.

The main reasons for the irritability are irregular life, often staying up late, feeling stagnant, depressed, stressed, hot weather, unreasonable diet, such as eating too much salty food, eating spicy food, etc.

I used to be a person with heavy taste. I like to put salt in cooking, and I can't satisfy my cravings without spicy food. Every time it is me who is in charge of cooking, it must be a heavy taste. According to the common people, if the taste of the dish is heavy, you can eat more. I like to eat fried pork with pickled vegetables and some red peppers. I also like to eat braised pork, especially the pork knuckle, which is soft and fat. This eating habit has caused a large amount of internal heat in my body to accumulate, which needs to be excreted urgently.

The liver is the human body's hematopoietic factory, and the spleen is the body's blood supply minister. There is a problem with the blood supply of the human body's internal organs. Insufficient blood supply to the spleen, insuf-ficient food for the organs, resulting in increased deficiency of fire.. This is because there are too many harmful substances and tox-ins in the human body, and the blood gas in the body is insufficient, and there is no ability to remove these harmful substances in time. Therefore, the dry heat of the liver and the fire of the heart can only rise upwards and vent out by means of anger.

As long as you adjust your eating habits, actively invigorate the spleen and replenish qi and blood. After detoxif- ication and dampness, these hot phenomena will automatically disappear. However, at the time, I and the people around me mistakenly believed that this was a character and temperament problem, mainly looking for the reason from the ideology, but sometimes there was no reason, well, suddenly an unnamed fire burst from my chest, even I was inexplicable, and I didn't know where the fire came from.

Now my taste has faded, and I have eaten some light foods, and my mood remains calm, so my anger is gone.

Anger Can Cause Many Diseases

People generally get angry with the people closest to them, and rarely get angry with colleagues and unfamiliar people, and the two main subjects of friction in the family are husband and wife. No one is perfect, everyone has one kind or another of shortcomings, and when two people live together, they rely on mutual understanding and tolerance. If the husband and wife often bicker, disagree with each other, and neither will let the other, the relatio-nship will become indifferent after a long time. Home is no longer a peaceful harbor, but a battlefield filled with gunpowder smoke.

When I lived with my ex-husband, the two of us didn't let anyone else, and we argued more together than when we were calm. When I came to Canada, I stayed at home except for work, which created a lot of opportunities for the two people who were originally discordant to argue. After often bickering, I was so angry that my chest was blocked. In fact, it was all small things, as long as there was one aspect take a step back and we won't create a quarrel deadlock. But both sides are not convinced, and neither is willing to speak softly.

For a long time, I often feel chest tightness, and I always want to sigh, as if sighing can make my chest more comfortable. The head is also very uncomfortable, from the forehead to the back of the head as if there is a curse, tight all day long. Check the blood pressure, the highest high pressure reaches 160. I often suffer from insomnia, and I can't sleep with my eyes closed at night. Opening my eyes and staring at the ceiling, my brain went blank. I don't think about anything, how can I not fall asleep. I have insomnia at night and can't sleep during the day. The vicious circle made me almost collapsed.

I have a bad stomach, I have no appetite for eating, I have diarrhea or dry stool every day. Going out in the summer can cause a cold and cough. My throat is itchy all day long, and I can't cough up phlegm. My blood sugar level is very unstable. I know in my heart that this situation is very unfavorable for my diabetes treatment. If it doesn't change, not only will my physical condition not improve, on the contrary, it will get worse.

Life is an art. To form a family, this art depends on the husband and wife nurturing each other. If two people are unwilling to tolerate each other, conflicts will accumulate, the family will not be harmonious, and living together will not be happy. Quarreling every day not only hurts feelings, but also hurts the body. After arguing for more than ten years, we broke up. In exchange for quiet days, days without quarrels.

Since the divorce, my heart has calmed down and my mental condition has improved greatly. As soon as the mind calmed down, the body really began to be well taken care of, and the originally damaged body parts were slowly recovering on their own.

It is very important to maintain a good mood. The mood directly affects the body and directly affects the disease. As the saying goes:three parts of the disease, seven parts of nourishment. Sickness mainly depends on nourishment. This nourishment depends not only on food and medicine, but also on spiritual nourishment. Sometimes the role of spirit is more important than food and medicine. In the process of self-medicating diabetes later, I gradually learned how to maintain a good mood, learned to be tolerant, and had a better understanding of people, things, and myself.

Chapter 2

Comprehensive Ways
Cure Diabetes

In Western medicine, diabetes is a disease of endocrine disorders, that is, a problem with metabolism. However, Chinese medicine considers that it is a disorder of the spleen and stomach, and internal heat damages the yin, so it is called Diabetes.

Although diabetes is due to insufficient insulin secretion, it involves the whole body. Insulin is a hormone secreted by the pancreas. It adjusts the blood glucose level in the blood vessels. The whole body has only insulin, a hypoglycemic hormone. There is no other hormone to replace it. This shows its importance and uniqueness.

It only takes about 20 seconds for blood to circulate in the body. 180 laps can be circulated in one hour, 1, 576 800 laps in a year. If a person lives for 80 years, then the blood circulates 126, 144, 000 times in the body.

If the hyperglycemia in the blood vessels of diabetic patients is not controlled, it will travel around the body along the blood vessels and capillaries all the time. Wherever the blood containing high sugar flows to the damage, wherever the body part is weak, it is prone to disease. Therefore, the treatment of diabetes must be comprehensive.

Since I have diabetes for more than 20 years, I have gone from being ignorant of diabetes to becoming a good friend with diabetes. I can accurately grasp the pulse of diabetes and use a variety of therapies to communicate with diabetes, so that I can successfully control blood sugar levels. Normal blood sugar levels can be kept within the normal range for a long period of time even without medication.

Diet Therapy

Diet therapy is the most basic and direct way to control the blood sugar level. The sugar content of the food we eat will be faithfully shown on the blood sugar level. When the blood sugar control is not ideal, eating more will cause the blood sugar level to change. It's that accurate. I have tried many times, and I have to admire the strict teacher of diabetes. The supervision is very tight, and the diet is not sloppy at all. However, when the blood sugar level tends to be stable, all aspects of the body's indicators are very good, and the blood sugar level will not rise if you eat a little more, which indicates that the body's sugar tolerance has been strengthened. The treatment of diabetes is not just to maintain the stability of the diabetes value, but to improve the glucose tolerance in the body. Only in this way can the necessary nutrients be added to the body, the immunity of the body can be improved, and the health of the body can be restored.

As the saying goes, illness comes from the mouth. Controlling gluttony makes it easier to control the blood sugar level of diabetes. The stability of blood sugar level is directly related to the effect of treating diabetes. Only by keeping the blood sugar level stable for a long time can the body's sugar tolerance be improved and the body has the opportunity to maintain health and repair. Therefore, diet therapy is the most important part for diabetic patients, and it is also the homework we have to face every day.

I mainly grasp three points in diet therapy, one, comprehensive nutrition, two, control the staple food, three, reasonably configure meals according to the sugar content of various foods.

1. Balanced Food and Adequate Nutrition

People take food as their heaven. People do not necessarily exercise every day, but they must eat every day. When it comes to eating, everyone will say that who else can't eat. Since I got diabetes, I have gradually realized that it is really not an easy task to eat a healthy body. Generally speaking, many delicious foods are unhealthy, and many healthy foods are not very tasty.

Especially when the needs of the body and appetite are in conflict, whether it is the satisfaction of choosing good food to taste or eating moderately in order to maintain the health of the body is a topic that tests us repeatedly every day. Because human desires and needs are always antagonistic. To put it bluntly, as long as diabetic patients can actively control their diet and eat healthy food scientifically, they can seize the initiative in the process of treating diabetes and gain time for physical recovery.

The nutrients the human body needs are diversified, so I try to focus on my diet and eat omnivores.

Carbohydrates, protein, and fat are the three basic substances needed by humans to maintain life, and provide the main energy for the growth, movement and reproduction of organisms. It is one of the important substances necessary for human survival and development.

I must include these three main foods in my diet every day, and add some other nutritional s upplements, such as fruits and vegetables.

The source of staple food is carbohydrates. Rice, noodles, steamed buns. Although carbohydrates are the main contributor to the increase in blood sugar, carbohydrates are inseparable from the human body. Carbohydrates not only increase the body's energy, but are also an important source of various vitamins and minerals in the body. Without carbohydrates, the body's nutrition is not complete, and it also brings hidden dangers to the body's metabolism.

Diet has the most direct impact on the induction and treatment of diabetes, so diet control is very important for diabetes treatment. The level of blood sugar is closely related to the amount and type of food intake due to the secretion of insulin. Diet therapy is the basis of various diabetes treatments. Regardless of the severity of the disease or whether there are complications, whether or not to use drug treatment, diabetic patients should strictly abide by and adhere to dietary control for life.

Adhering to diet control does not mean resolutely not eating carbohydrates, and eating carbohydrates does not mean giving up control. There is no contradiction between the two. The key is to strictly control the amount of daily carbohydrates.

The ratio of staple food to non-staple food for each meal is usually three to seven, with three servings of staple food and seven servings of non-staple food. The staple food is increased to four at most, and the non-staple food's reduced to six, but it will never be half of the non-staple food and half of the staple food. There are always more non-staple foods than staple foods. This is my control standard for carbohydrate diet. A portion of protein and fat, vegetables and fruits account for half of the diet. One egg every morning, with protein, and some meat， when cooking, put some meat, sometimes shrimp or fish, but the portion is not much, which has changed the eating habit of big fish and big meat in the past.

According to some data, the human body generally consumes no less than 150 grams of carbohydrates per day to maintain the body's daily activities. Eating more carbohydrates will not help the body much, and it will also cause the blood sugar level to rise linearly. The sugar content in carbohydrates is very high. It will be converted into glucose immediately after eating, and enter the human blood. Excess carbohydrates will also be converted intofat through the action of enzymes and stored in the human body, making people fat.

I used to think that diabetes is caused by eating too much sugar, and it doesn't matter if I eat more other foods. There is no concept of the attributes of various foods. With the increasing popularity of modern health care, people are beginning to pay attention to how to eat healthy. The research on food began to be more detailed. Carbohydrates are actually members of the sugar family.

In the past, refined white rice and white noodles were always eaten. It was believed that white rice and white noodles were nutritious and not only delicious, but also good taste, while brown rice and whole wheat noodles were rough and not tasty. Later, I saw some information that excessive consumption of polished rice is one of the main factors that cause diabetes, so I began to pay attention to the properties of food. My family doctor also suggested that my staple food should not be too refined. White polished rice has a high sugar content. It is best to eat yellow rice, which contains less sugar.

The health preservation of whole grains is a staple food trend advocated in recent years.

Brown rice

Brown rice has a good curative effect on patients with obesity and gastrointestinal dysfunction, and can effectively regulate metabolism in the body.

Brown rice can treat anemia, and brown rice can treat constipation and purify the blood, so it has the effect of strengthening the physique. The vitamin E rich in germ can promote blood circulation and effectively maintain body functions.

Brown rice can normalize cell function and maintain endocrine balance. Brown rice has the effect of connecting and decomposing radioactive substances such as pesticides, thereby effectively preventing the absorption of harmful substances in the body and achieving the effect of cancer prevention. Brown rice can also improve human immune function, promote blood circulation, eliminate depression and irritability, and prevent cardiovascular disease, anemia, constipation, and bowel cancer.

The nutritional value of brown rice is high, but brown rice contains too much phosphorus and is an acidic food. Human body fluids are close to neutral. It is necessary to maintain a balance between acid and alkali. If brown rice is simply eaten for a long time, it is not good for health. The taste of brown rice is not very good, so brown rice should be paired with polished rice to not only neutralize the properties of the food, but also neutralize the taste of the food, achieving the best of both worlds.

Diabetes patients eat brown rice not only to lower blood sugar levels, brown rice also regulates the body's endocrine abnormalities, and promotes and protects the secretion of the pancreas.

Millet

Millet is sweet, salty and cool in nature. Entering the kidney, spleen, and stomach meridians, it has the effects of harmonizing the middle and benefiting the kidney, removing heat and detoxifying.

Millet stops vomiting and eliminates belching, nourishes the stomach, clears the bowels, stops diarrhea, nourishes blood and replenishes qi, strengthens the spleen, lowers blood sugar and quenches thirst, nourishes yin and invigorates deficiency.

Millet is rich in phosphorus, which can form bones and teeth, promote growth and repair of body tissues and organs, supply energy and vitality, and participate in the regulation of acid-base balance.

Millet is rich in magnesium, which helps to regulate a person's heart activity, lower blood pressure, prevent heart disease, regulate nerve and muscle activity, and enhance endurance.

Millet is rich in potassium, which helps maintain nerve health, a regular heartbeat, prevents strokes, and assists in normal muscle contraction.

Eating millet has many benefits. It has the effect of lowering blood sugar, promoting the decomposition of sugar, converting excess sugar into heat, and improving the balance of fat in the body. It can be used as a dietary supplement to treat diabetes.

Millet has the effect of invigorating the spleen and stomach. Cooking porridge with millet and taking it before going to bed can easily make people fall asleep peacefully. When cooking millet porridge, after the porridge is cooked, it cools down for a while. We can see that there is a layer of fine viscous material floating on the top layer of the porridge. This is porridge oil, which has the effect of protecting the gastric mucous and nourishing the spleen and stomach. It is most suitable for patients with chronic gastritis and gastric ulcer. Most of the spleen and stomach of diabetic patients are not good and their function is decreased. Eating millet can help strengthen the spleen and protect the stomach, thereby increasing insulin secretion and lowering blood sugar.

Buckwheat

Traditional Chinese medicine believes that buckwheat is sweet and flat in nature, has the effects of invigorating the spleen and replenishing qi, appetizing and widening the intestines, eliminating food and resolving stagnation.

Buckwheat protein is rich in lysine, iron, manganese, zinc and other trace elements are richer than general grains, and it is rich in dietary fiber, which is 10 times that of general refined rice. So buckwheat has very good nutrition and health effects.

Certain flavonoid in buckwheat also have antibacterial, anti-inflammatory, anti-tussive, anti-asthmatic and expectorant effects. Therefore, buckwheat also has the reputation of "anti-inflammatory food"

In addition, buckwheat has the effect of removing gastrointestinal garbage. It can lower the gas and widen the intestines, remove the five internal organs garbage out of the body, reduce the retention and absorption of "intestinal toxins", and make the body healthier.

Buckwheat also has the effect of lowering blood sugar. Often mixed with other staple foods is beneficial for our diabetic patients to stabilize blood sugar.

Mung bean

Traditional Chinese medicine believes that mung bean is sweet and cold in nature, enters the heart and stomach meridian, has the effects of clearing heat and detoxification, relieving heat and diuresis.

Mung bean powder detoxifies, treats sores and swelling, and treats burns. Mung bean hulls detoxify fever and improve eyesight. Mung bean sprouts can detoxify.

Patients with hypertension and hyperlipidemia often eat mung beans, which can help lower blood pressure and prevent blood lipids from rising.

Diabetics who often consume mung beans can help clean up toxins in the body, and food detoxification does not have any side effects.

Soya bean

The lecithin in soybeans can prevent excessive fat accumulation in the liver, thereby effectively preventing fatty liver caused by obesity.

Soybeans contain a variety of minerals, supplement calcium, prevent osteoporosis caused by calcium deficiency, promote bone development, and are extremely beneficial to the bone growth of children and the elderly.

The soluble fiber contained in soybeans can both laxative and reduce cholesterol.

The iron in soybeans is not only high in content, but also easily absorbed by the body, which has a certain effect on iron deficiency anemia.

Soybean contains a substance that inhibits pancreatin, which has a therapeutic effect on diabetes.

Soy oligosaccharides can promote the proliferation of bifidobacteria that are beneficial to the human body, inhibit pathogenic bacteria, prevent constipation and diarrhea, protect the liver and anti-cancer. Soy isoflavones can prevent cardiovascular disease, anti-cancer, anti-oxidative damage, and strengthen cells Immune Function.

Soy isoflavone is a kind of phytoestrogens with estrogen activity similar in structure to estrogen. It can delay female cell aging, keep skin elastic, nourish the skin, reduce bone loss, promote bone production, lower blood fat, and reduce female menopause syndrome, etc.

Soybean has the effects of preventing and treating diabetes, regulating and improving immune function. Soybeans for diabetic patients can reduce fat, help clear blood vessels, and help the recovery of diabetes.

Wheat bran

Wheat bran is rich in dietary fiber and is an essential nutrient element for the human body. It contains a large amount of insoluble cellulose which can expand and accelerate excretion in the large intestine, improve constipation, and promote the excretion of fat. It can also reduce estrogen in the blood. The content of hormones can prevent breast cancer. The B vitamins contained in wheat bran play many functions in the body, and also have nutrients that are indispensable in the normal metabolism of food. They can improve constipation, prevent colon cancer, rectal cancer, and reduce serum cholesterol, efficacy in slowing the formation of atherosclerosis.

Because wheat bran is the outer skin of wheat, it is difficult to swallow when eaten alone, so it can be mixed with other foods, such as sprinkling a few handfuls when cooking rice, mixing it with milk and oats to cook porridge, and mixing it with flour to make noodles, cakes, steamed buns, can also be mixed with flour, vegetables, and meat to make pancakes, which taste very good.

Eating a little wheat bran every day can ensure the smoothness of the intestines and excrete garbage and poison in the body in a timely manner. This is great for diabetics to clean up the intestines and reduce the absorption of toxins in the body.

2. Control Appetite

Eat about 70% full of each meal, which is good for gastrointestinal function

Our body's need for food is not to eat 100% of every meal, we have to eat to the point that we can no longer eat it. The stomach is flexible. If you eat more, the stomach will swell automatically. This is also my own experience. If you eat a lot of food often, your stomach will adapt to eating so much. Such eating habits are very bad. The desire for gluttony is higher than the actual needs of the body. There is no scientific meal, which is not conducive to the functioning of the stomach and intestines.

When the grain is processed in the factory, electricity is consumed, and the food our body eats also consumes various resources in the body to i ntegrate it into the nutrients needed by the body. Excessive food intake not only makes blood sugar out of control, but also wastes unnecessary body resources, which is not beneficial at all. Eat until about 70% full, just so that the body consumes the energy of this part of the food and takes in the nutrients in a balanced way, which is very beneficial to the metabolism of the body.

I used to have to eat very full. My previous diet was to eat rice at noon and at night. If I didn't eat rice at night, I would feel hungry and couldn't sleep. This result brings trouble to the control of blood sugar. Later, some improvements were made. Rice was eaten at noon, and pumpkin or sweet potato and carrot were eaten at night. Gradually, the amount of rice at noon was reduced. Vegetables were the main food, supplemented by staple food and meat. A meal ratio of one serving of staple food and one serving of meat. It not only ensures a certain amount of nutrition, but also reasonably controls the sugar content in the food. If I have lunch at work, eat a bit more than when I am at home, and eat it in two portions, so that the damaged insulin doesn't work so hard.

I was not used to reducing the amount of food at the beginning. I always felt that I was not full, so I liked to eat some snacks to supplement it. In fact, it was not good. The total calories still did not decrease. Later, I figured out a way to limit it. The lunch box I brought to work was changed from a large to a medium one, so the appetite had to be reduced. Do not bring snacks to eat, drink as much as possible every time I rest, and ensure that I drink 8 glasses of water every day.

The human body is inert. If you always eat too much, the stomach is always full, and there is no rest and breathing time, then the delicious food will be tasteless when it comes to the mouth. The cells of the human body also become lazy and don't wan t to work in a saturated state all day long, and the brain's desire for food is greatly reduced. Without hunger, the activity of human cells cannot be well stimulated, and the human body's immunity is also reduced a lot.

We have seen a documentary of African antelopes. On the endless African savanna, antelopes are constantly running to survive. If they move slowly, they will be eaten by lions. In the harsh environment, the antelope has developed the ability to survive with agility and fast movements. The human instinct is also the same. If the body is constantly hungry a little, the functions of all parts of the body will be greatly stimulated, and the metabolic function will work well, and the body's immune capacity will be improved.

Moderate hunger can help control blood sugar better. Maintaining proper hunger can reduce carbohydrate intake and help better control blood sugar levels after meals. Prevent the blood sugar from suddenly rising sharply, causing instant hyperglycemia symptoms.

We can live longer if we eat less and are of high quality. Someone has done an interesting experiment, feeding the old hens with water and anti-hunger plants. After two months of breeding, the old hens regained their feathers, and 81% of the old hens lay eggs again. In fact, human beings are also the same phenomenon. The world's longest life and the best health in old age is Japan. The average life expectancy of Japanese people is over 80 years old. The most important factor is diet. The traditional Japanese diet is small in quantity, high in quality, light and small.

Moderate hunger will make people more sensitive and not sleepy. When a person has a full meal, the brain is easy to feel tired and want to sleep. This is because most of the body's blood runs to take care of the digestive system, ignoring the needs of the brain, and reducing the efficiency of the brain. Don't eat too much for lunch, we can avoid drowsiness in the afternoon and increase work efficiency.

Eating Less Dinner Is Good for Digestion and Lowering Blood Sugar

The night is an excessive time for the handover of dynamic and static. People work and study for a busy day, and they start to calm down, so their body's calorie consumption drops sharply. People's body is almost in a static state and loses calorie consumption. Therefore, it is difficult to digest a rich dinner, especially fat and protein foods. If you eat a lot of dinner, the internal organs will have to work overtime to release the maximum energy. If this happens, the energy will be exhausted and the human body will develop various diseases. There is a scientific basis for eating less dinner, and it meets our human body's food needs.

If you are a diabetic who takes medicine, excessive intake of food during dinner will cause an increase in the amount of medicine to meet the demand for increasing insulin

The effective time of each drug is different. For example, the glyburide (glibenclamide) promotes the secretion of insulin by pancreatic islet B cells. The prerequisite is that the pancreatic islet B cells have a certain function of synthesizing and secreting insulin. Insulin in the portal vein may act directly on the liver, inhibit liver glycogen decomposition and gluconeogenesis, reduce liver production and output of glucose, fast oral absorption, high protein binding rate, 95%, blood medicine 2 to 5 hours after oral administration the concentration reaches the peak value and continues to act for 24 hours. It is metabolized in the liver and excreted by the liver and kidneys each about 50%. The overall effect is to reduce fasting blood sugar and postprandial blood sugar.

After oral administration gliclazide, the gastrointestinal absorption is slow, and the plasma concentration reaches a peak about 8 hours after taking the drug. Its plasma protein binding rate is about 94. 2%, and the average half-life is 12 to 14 hours. Therefore, taking twice a day can be effective. Gliclazide is mainly metabolized in the liver, and its metabolites have no hypoglycemic effect. Through urinary excretion, the content of the prototype drug in the urine is less than 1%.

Comparing with these two kinds of hypoglycemic, glyburide (glibenclamide) is absorbed quickly by oral administration, reaching the highest value of the drug effect in 2-5 hours, while Damekang (gliclazide) only reaches 8 hours after taking the drug the highest value of the drug in the blood. Taking glyburide (glibenclamide) for dinner, the excess food has not been digested in the stomach, the highest peak of the drug has passed, causing the blood sugar level to soar at night. Taking Damekang (Gliclazide) takes 8 hours to reach the peak value.

At this time, excessive food has caused the blood sugar in the body to rise sharply, and it is difficult to drop to the normal value. Therefore, it is not advisable to eat too much food for dinner, it is best to eat less for dinner, try to eat less high-fat, high-protein foods, carbohydrates, and eat more cellulose-containing vegetables.

I have tested it many times, and my blood sugar level is usually normal at night, but in the morning the blood sugar level rises again. If the blood sugar level in the morning should be kept within 6 moles, the blood sugar level before going to bed must be less than 6 moles. Therefore, eating less dinner is not only beneficial to control the blood sugar after dinner in the evening, but also beneficial to control the blood sugar level at night and early in the morning.

Understand the Sugar Content and Properties of Various Foods, and Scientifically Configure the Diet

Our body is a passive receiver. The body accepts whatever food is eaten every day, what it acts on, and what it affects. This is determined by the structure and nature of the human body. To keep our bodies healthy, we must obey our body's preferences and needs. Especially when certain functions of the body are damaged, they must be taken care of carefully to prevent them from getting worse, and to transform to the good ones, as much as possible to restore the original functions and maintain normal body operations.

Therefore, on the premise of determining the staple food, I don't avoid all kinds of seasonal vegetables, soy products, black fungus, mushrooms, all kinds of fish and shrimps, and all kinds of meat. Vegetables also have attributes. Some vegetables are hot, some are warm, and some are cold. Just like the staple food, only by mastering the attributes of vegetables, and then eating according to one's physique and illness, can master more initiative to serve our body.

Because my physique is of a cold nature, I often have cold hands and feet, fear of wind, and love to catch colds, so when I choose vegetables, I will avoid cold ones, and choose hot and warm vegetables as much as possible. I did not like to eat ginger and garlic before. Since

I learned about the properties of vegetables, I began to like ginger and garlic. I can't do without ginger and garlic almost every day. Ginger warms the stomach. For a while, I believed that bitter melon could cure diabetes, so I ate bitter melon and drank bitter melon tea. As a result, my stomach was damaged by eating it, and the more I ate it, the colder my body became. The undigested food in the stomach kept smelling out of the mouth.

After eating ginger, my stomach began to improve slowly, my mouth no longer had any peculiar smell, and my body began to warm up. Garlic is a scavenger of blood vessels. I didn't like it before because garlic has a special taste, which is unpleasant. Now I have developed a habit. Every day garlic does not leave the mouth. I need to add a few cloves to increase the flavor when cooking. Generally, fried garlic has no peculiar smell and its nutritional value will be compromised, but it is still helpful. I also learned from my colleagues to make a side dish of raw garlic, which is to chop raw garlic and green chilies together and stir with salt and sesame oil. After a few days, it can be eaten. The taste is very fresh and refreshing.

Eating hot and warm vegetables is also easy to get angry in the body. You should regularly eat cool vegetables to reduce the fire. Use warm vegetables as the main and hot and cold vegetables as supplements, so that the body is easy to maintain a balance, no yin and yang imbalance, too cold or too hot.

Learn from Western Cooking Techniques

My Western colleagues love to eat raw and cold vegetables. Western food's vegetables are never fried in the pan. Cucumber, tomato, lettuce, cabbage, cauliflower, celery, and broccoli are commonly used vegetables when making Western food. Basically, do not put oil in, but some Western salad dressing is stirred, it tastes crunchy and refreshing. These vegetables are low in calories, some have a diuretic effect, and some contain a lot of insoluble cellulose. The cold vegetable salad fully retains the vitamins and nutrients of the vegetables. In fact, we diabetics can learn from some common methods in western food, such as hot steaming, cold dishes, boiled in water, etc, to cook our meals.

Basically, western food is cooked with little or no oil, which not only keeps the vitamins and nutrients in the food to the maximum, but also conforms to the concept of healthy diet for diabetic patients.

Learn to eat more healthy foods in Western food. In Western food, celery and onions are often used as ingredients. These two kinds of vegetables have the effect of lowering blood pressure and softening blood vessels, while onions have the effect of lowering blood cholesterol and triglycerides. Commonly used in Western food are carrots, asparagus, fresh mushrooms, milk, yogurt, oatmeal, whole wheat bread, etc. , which are all healthy foods.

In Western food, potatoes are used as a staple food, such as mashed potatoes. The calories of potatoes are only rice, 1/5 of noodles, and the carbohydrate content is only 1/4 of rice noodles, and the glycemic index is lower than that of rice and noodles. But I am used to eating rice at noon, so I had to eat potatoes at night. I have a medium potato and a little vegetable in the evening. After testing, eating potatoes for dinner can lower blood sugar levels without feeling hungry.

Lettuce is also a commonly eaten cold salad. It is crispy, raw, green, good-looking and delicious. Both Chinese and Western supermarkets sell it. I will mix lettuce, tomatoes, onions, cucumbers, put some salt and vinegar, a little sesame oil, and pat a few cloves of garlic, it tastes very good. Because carrots are hard in texture, I boil them or fry them with warm fire.

There are thin pancakes sold in supermarkets, ten sheets in a small bag, and each pancake is only 30-50 grams. I wrap my lunch with pancakes and roll them into a tube. The two pancakes are only 60 grams, plus a lot of vegetables and meat are enough to eat, the calories are not large, it is easy to control the meal size and blood sugar level.

Oatmeal not only lowers blood fat, but also cleanses the intestines. There are many ways to eat oats, so you can do whatever you like. Consistently eating a few spoonfuls of oatmeal every day is beneficial to blood vessel maintenance, reduces the toxins in the blood vessels, reduces the risk of heart disease caused by arteriosclerosis, and makes the body lighter. Oatmeal is the most economical and effective supplementary food for lowering blood sugar and lipids for diabetics.

Exercise Therapy

Life is movement.

1. Walking exercise

I always take the city rail and bus to work. After getting off work, I have to buy food and go home to cook. The time is full every day, and I don't have time to go to the gym to exercise. Even on days off, I still have to deal with things like going to the bank, seeing a family doctor, going to the city for shopping, etc.

After I came back from China in 2011, my blood sugar level was a little high due to various reasons, so I started walking to work. It takes more than 40 minutes to walk from home to work. It was summer when I first started walking to work, because my bare legs were often bitten by mosquitoes on the side of the road. The mosquitoes in Canada are surprisingly big. It is unceremonious to bully people. They bite to the death, and the bitten part immediately shows a big red and swollen lump, which is very itchy, and it will not heal for many days. Later, I was fully armed and wrapped myself up tightly, trying to keep mosquitoes nowhere. The feeling of walking is really good. The pace on the way to get off work is easy, and I am exhausted when I get off work. When I walk, I keep shaking my arms, kicking and breathing fresh air to help relieve fatigue.

In this way, I walked from summer to winter. Faced with the cold weather, I, a person who is afraid of the cold, is wondering whether to give up walking in winter. In winter, it is icy and snowy. The temperature here is often minus ten degrees, minus twenty degrees, and the wind is nearly minus thirty degrees. It is no exaggeration that the heat coming out of the mouth will immediately turn into ice flowers. Every day I go out, I always wonder whether to take a car or to walk. When I reach a fork in the road, I don't have to move in the direction of walking. It seems that my body has chosen to exercise. In the freezing winter, white snowflakes are flying all over the skyin the ice and snow. On the side of the road, a woman wrapped like a giant panda walks forward in the silver-white world against the wind and snow. That winter I became a roadside the most beautiful scenery.

One day, the temperature dropped to more than 20 degrees below zero, and the wind was more than 30 degrees below zero. That day, I was fully armed. With a scarf and two pairs of gloves on my hands, I rushed directly into the sky full of snowflakes. At that time, I just wanted to test my cold tolerance. Along the way, I kept waving my arms, doing some stretching exercises, moving my stiff arms away, and gradually my frozen face started to heat up, and my whole body was sweating when I reached the company. Through this test, I feel that my walking to work this year is still very effective, and my ability to withstand the cold has improved. However, it is important for diabetics to keep warm, and it is best not to walk to work in such harsh weather.

In this way, after walking for a few years, I feel that my physical strength is stronger than before, and my body is also stronger. Blood sugar also dropped naturally and remained within normal values. Walking to work and shopping at nearby malls have become my habit. Exercise makes me feel relaxed and improves my physical function.

Some colleagues joked that you are reluctant to buy a ticket to walk. The reason for walking to work is to exercise to reduce blood sugar levels, which invisibly saves not only the cost of monthly passes, but also time and fitness costs. Direct exercise every day for free has many benefits!

2. Exercise at Home Anytime

Housework has become the best way for me to relax myself. Every morning before I get up, I will do acupressure massage on the bed, and then when I go to the bathroom, I massage the acupuncture points on the face, eyes, nose, middle and chin. My eyes are often tired, blurred vision, mild rhinitis, and dry lips. After massaging these acupuncture points, the fatigue of the eyes was significantly improved, the rhinitis was also much better, and the dry lips caused by diabetes were also much better, and I did not feel thirsty anymore.

Then, drink a glass of boiling water to moisten the intestines and start making breakfast. After making breakfast, take ten minutes to do wall-banging exercise, it is to collide the back and shoulders against the wall with force, so that the body can be greatly relaxed. The Governor

Vessel in the back is positive. When hitting it in the morning, it is called Kaiyang, and the front of the human body is negative. I then eat breakfast and go to work.

Kneeling, this is a wonderful way to draw blood down. If the blood is not easy to be drawn to the soles of the feet at once, then first lead to the knees. If the knees have sufficient blood, they will not be far away from the soles of the feet. According to the theory in the book "Seeking a doctor is worse than asking for yourself", the knee is an axis and needs lubricating oil. What is the lube of the knee? It's just fresh blood, if the blood is drawn through, the knee will not wear out, and there will be no swelling and pain. So how to solve it? Kneeling or walking on a not so soft bed or on a carpet, blood will flow continuously to the knees, and the knees are provided with fresh blood, so that the cold can dissipate, the effusion can be eliminated, and the swelling and pain can be eliminated. But at the same time, the book also reminds that if someone has knee pain, they should kneel down on a softer bed and exercise slowly. You will soon adapt, and then the knee will not hurt.

In the past few years, my knee hurts when I go up the stairs because of the wind, and I can't bend it freely. Also, my hands and feet are often cold. So I used kneeling method combined with housework to do exercises. There are special mops and vacuum cleaners for mopping the floors and carpets at home. I gave up these tools and used manual cleaning. After cooking, I squat on the ground, or kneel on the ground to wipe the floor and clean the carpet. First, it can be wiped clean, and second, knees and foot joints have been exercised on the ground. Kneeling on the floor at the beginning is very uncomfortable, even painful, so I need to put some soft towels on it. Gradually my knees became stronger. I didn't feel pain anymore when I knelt on the floor. On the contrary, I felt very comfortable. After the whole leg and foot tendons were stretched, I could stretch naturally and feel relaxed. Now my knee no longer hurts when I go up the stairs. Not stiff anymore. The legs and feet have also become warm.

Take a shower before going to bed at night, and the blood circulates smoothly throughout the body. Then use a dry towel to wipe your back, which will help reduce the blood sugar level of diabetes.

Doing these auxiliary exercises does not need to spend a lot of time, as long as you develop a habit of doing it every day, you can get obvious results.

3. Gym Exercise

Going to the gym is an ideal way to exercise. There are professional coaches in the gym, and there are various exercise methods and equipment to choose from. Exercise on the walking machine must follow the set speed and walk fast. It can be said that it is a little compulsory. The walking machine takes exercisers to exercise. I like this. When I feel a little tired and don't want to walk anymore, but the walking machine can't stop, I have to follow it. After I have passed the tired point, I feel relaxed. I usually spend half an hour on the walking machine. The gym has a variety of stretching equipment, some are stretching arms, some are stretching thighs, some are stretching calves, some are extending chest strength, some are stretching down, and there are manual swing machines to coordinate left and right balance and stretching. In short, all parts of the body can be fully exercised on these sports equipment. I like to stretch on the equipment, it feels very comfortable.

The fitness center usually has various physical exercise classes. Sports exercises, aerobics, yoga, balance exercises, physical exercises and other activities. Every time I finished a section of exercises with my teacher, I sweated profusely and I felt comfortable all over, even though I was tired and wanted to stop during the process. Doing yoga is a static exercise. Each person uses a small blanket and follows the melodious and soothing music to imitate the teacher's movements. Yoga is an elegant way to clean up trash in the body, elegantly adjusting rigid muscles to make them soft, and elegantly stretching unwilling muscles and bones to restore elasticity. The more important thing is the purification of the soul. When doing yoga, any distracting thoughts are excluded from the mind, as if being in the sea, drifting with the waves, as if being in the primeval forest, the ethereal mountains and the fragrance of birds and flowers. Every time I finish yoga, my sleep at night must be very good.

There are many retired elderly people in the gym where I went to come every morning. Because there are few people in the gym from 6 to 8 in the morning, and the elderly are used to getting up early, taking advantage of the absence of people in the swimming pool, they take a morning swim. Swim dozens of back and forth in the swimming pool, and then go to eat breakfast. I can only make a few gestures of dog puddling in the water to experience the gentleness of the water.

Soak in the hot pool for ten minutes and paddle your legs in the clear water. It's a good way to relax.

Then I went to the sauna room. Many people couldn't stand the high humidity and hot air in the sauna room and escaped after a few minutes. I can stay in the sauna for more than 20 minutes, endure the suffocating high humidity and heat, sweat profusely, and there is indescribable comfort and ease in the body. Finally, take a shower and relax the whole body.

This kind of gym has the best effect. I only kept it for a year. Later, because I didn't have a lot of time to go to work. When I retire later, I will return to the gym and exercise daily.

4. Rapid Exercise Between Breaks

On the way to work, it is also a good opportunity to use to do exercises. Along the way, I will rotate the joints of my hands, exercise my legs and my hands. It is mentioned in the health book that a person's hand and foot joints are the intersection of many meridians. Frequent rotation of the hand and foot joints will bring unexpected benefits to the blood vessels and meridians throughout the body.

Every hour of my work I have a 15-minute break. I will use the break to beat my legs and relax my legs that are overworked while standing. When there is no client, I will exchange my legs under the table to do some circular exercises, massage the meridians on my arms, and make them dredge.

My work requires constant use of hands. Hands, arms, and joints are all vulnerable to injury. I am a diabetic and can't do the same repetitive action continuously and quickly. My colleague suffered wrist injury, occupational disease, frequent illness, and wrist pain. I also had wrist pain for a while, so I needed to wear a wrist health protective cover. Ever since I had a meridian massage on my arms and wrists, it dredged the blood vessels and relieved the tension of the muscles, so it didn't get worse. But the damage is permanent and I get pain in my arms and wrists whenever I overwork.

5. Bath Massage Exercise

Taking a bath in North America is a very convenient thing. Every household has showers and bathtubs, and you can choose to take a shower or a bath. My feet are always cold except in summer. Taking a hot bath before going to bed not only keeps the feet warm, but also promotes blood circulation throughout the body. Under the impulse of hot water, rubbing various parts is equivalent to massaging acupuncture points, so that the body after a tiring day can be fully relaxed. When the body relaxes, the muscles and bones also relax. Bend over, keep my legs straight, put my hands on my feet, and let the hot water rush to your back. Then stretch your arms up, turn your waist left and right, and my whole body is liberated. After taking a shower, use a dry towel to pull around my back for a while, I can lie on the bed comfortably and prepare to fall asleep.

Medical Treatment

Usually, the doctor will prescribe some medicines for patients who are diagnosed as diabetes, and they must take the medicines on time to control and prevent the blood sugar from rising. When the initial blood sugar is unstable, it is necessary to take the medicine on time when the patients have no grasp and understanding of their physical condition. At first, I didn't want to take western medicine to lower blood sugar. I mistakenly thought that after taking western medicine, I would not lose it for a lifetime, which delayed the process of treating diabetes and brought trouble to my body. Through the subsequent medication, I realized that it is necessary to take western medicine to lower blood sugar, especially when the blood sugar level remains high, it must be taken immediately without delay. Only when the blood sugar drops, will it not continue to cause harm to the human body. After the blood sugar level is stable for a long time, the drug can be stopped completely. I summarized the rules of taking medicine as follows:

A. Always Take Medicine When You Feel Unwell

When the body feels uncomfortable, there must be a problem in the body, and the immunity will decrease. Taking medicine is to keep the blood sugar stable without adding additional symptoms. So as to make the body return to normal as soon as possible.

B. When Encountering Friends and Family Gatherings, I Must Take Medicine.

People are members of society, no matter what disease you suffer from, you can't break up with friends and family, normal social interaction is still necessary. However, diabetic patients should have regular diet and work and rest habits, and attending banquets will definitely disrupt their living rules. I used to go back to China to socialize too much, which caused my blood sugar level to get out of control, and it couldn't be lowered after a long time. Now, I use the help of hypoglycemic drugs to solve this contradiction. As long as I gather with family and friends, I must take hypoglycemic drugs, and at the same time, I also control the amount of meals properly, do not eat sweets, eat less rice, high-protein, high-fat food, eat more vegetables. In this way, the blood sugar level will not be too high, and even if it is on the warning line, it can be quickly lowered the next day.

C. Taking Medicine While Traveling

When traveling, the daily routine and eating habits of life have been broken. It is very tiring to go out and play, eat very irregularly, and blood sugar levels can easily rise. At this time, I must take hypoglycemic drugs to ensure that my body's metabolism remains normal. With the help of hypoglycemic drugs, the blood sugar level in the body will be well controlled. Diabetic patients can enjoy the beauty of nature happily and enjoy the joy that nature brings us just like normal people.

D. Attempt to Reduce or Stop Medication When Blood Sugar Is Well Controlled

Everything is done in an orderly manner, life is very regular, and blood sugar levels are well controlled. After the blood sugar level remained stable for a period of time, I stopped taking the hypoglycemic drugs appropriately, relying solely on the body to secrete insulin and regulate my metabolism. Moreover, after the drug is stopped, the blood sugar level will not rise and has been maintained within the normal range. I have maintained this situation for almost several years.

Diabetes is an irreversible systemic degenerative disease. With the gradual aging of human body functions, the organs in the body are gradually declining normally. Appropriate use of hypoglycemic drugs is a necessary means of protection. In short, the blood sugar level is controlled within the normal range to ensure that the occurrence of complications can be minimized.

Meridian Massage for Diabetes

Grasp the main contradiction and solve the secondary contradiction incidentally.

The treatment of diabetes mainly starts with nourishing the stomach, nourishing the kidneys, replenishing qi and blood, and strengthening kidney function. The kidney is the foundation of the human body, and the stomach is the source of nourishment.

Western medicine for the treatment of diabetes is nothing more than medicine, supplemented by diet and exercise therapy. These are all methods of treating the symptoms but not the root cause. By chance, I discovered the human body meridian manual, which guides people to actively use it. Use your own meridians to prevent and treat diseases in your body. After reading the manual, I think what the book says makes sense. After a long period of stable blood sugar, I stopped taking medicine and started using acupressure instead of medicine.

The book explains that the occurrence of diseases is mainly because the function of human organs is disordered and the meridians are blocked, and the human body loses the ability to balance and regulate. Massage the meridians is stimulated by various passive manipulations, causing local and systemic reactions, thereby adjusting the body's function, making the meridians unblocked, eliminating pathogenic factors, and achieving the purpose of curing diseases and maintaining health. Massage has the effect of balancing and regulating, and massage can strengthen the body and eliminate pathogenic factors, and enhance physical fitness. During massage, the local skin is often red, and the skin temperature is significantly increased when measured, which is the result of vasodilation, local congestion and improved blood circulation, which is conducive to the repair of damage.

Massage therapy is a natural therapy. Practice has proved that massage has a certain therapeutic effect on diabetes. It can not only improve the symptoms of diabetes, lower blood sugar and urine sugar, but also prevent and treat vascular and nerve complications.

A. Back Impact Appoints to Open Up the Du Meridian

The human body is divided into two major meridians, the Du and Ren vessels. Opening up the small Zhoutian means that the Du and Ren vessels are unobstructed and integrated. In popular terms, the blood vessels and meridians of our body are like rivers and lakes, and the rivers and lakes are blocked by silt. If it is not cleaned for a long time, stagnant water will become rancid, and floods and droughts will occur. The meridians and blood vessels of the human body are the same as in nature. If they are blocked, they will get sick. Over time, the disease will worsen, and even lead to cancer and death. The strength of the Governor Vessel is the most effective main river and main channel to show whether the vitality of the human body is strong. The back is full of internal organs. It can be said that the Governor Vessel protects the internal organs and has an extremely important connection and promotion role. At the same time, it also promotes blood circulation throughout the body, promotes metabolism in the body, and increases resistance and immunity.

I brought a small rubber health hammer from China to beat uncomfortable parts. When I first arrived in Canada, my back, neck and shoulders were very painful for a while, so I used a small rubber hammer to beat my back, but the effect was not very obvious.. One day, my shoulders and back hurt so much that I couldn't stand it, so I hit the hardwood on the door frame with my shoulder, and it felt better, not so painful. So I used the method of hitting the door frame to relieve back and shoulder pain.

After reading the book on the introduction of meridians, I found that hitting the back can not only open up the supervisor channel, but also treat diabetes. It has many benefits. It made me re-recognize the importance of back hitting and insist on doing this exercise every morning.

I usually drink a glass of warm water after I get up in the morning, and I start hitting the wall. The order of hitting the wall is the upper right arm, the upper right back, the middle right back, the lower right back, the upper left arm, the upper left back, the middle left back, and the lower left back, for two minutes for each part. There are Ganshu point, Danshu point, Pishu point, Weishu point, Sanjiao point, Shenshu point and other points in the upper and middle parts of the impact for three minutes. Generally speaking, the intensity of my impact is moderate, and sometimes I increase the intensity of the impact when I feel a heavy back.

I didn't feel any discomfort after the impact, I just felt comfortable all over my body, and my arms and back were a lot easier. Immediately after each impact, I felt a significant difference, and my whole body began to warm up, especially my back was warm and comfortable, just like the feeling of having physiotherapy, my back felt warm after being illuminated by a physiotherapy lamp. Because hitting the back clears the Governor Vessel, increasing the Yang Qi in the body.

Hitting the back can also warm the kidneys and improve kidney function.

B. Single-Leg Independent Bleed Air Return

My hands and feet are often cold. Often in autumn, I wear winter clothes. My body is kept warm by clothing as much as possible. I have always wanted to make my feet warm. Soaking my feet in hot water in winter was very warm. After that, my feet became cold again. Because of the lack of self-heating, external heat can only work for a while, and it cannot be solved. The key issue of not getting warm. For diabetic patients, cold hands and feet are not conducive to the recovery of diabetes, and it also greatly affects the treatment effect.

The "Golden Rooster Independence"(in English, it means standing on one foot) fitness method introduced in the health care book is a balance system that uses thoughts to control the brain, guides the blood in the body to the legs and feet, so that the lower half of the body has sufficient blood flow, thereby fundamentally changing the disease of slow blood circulation. The golden rooster independence method is very simple, just close your eyes, one foot is independent, and both hands are placed on your sides, or your hands are stretched forward, or your arms are stretched out to maintain balance. The key is to close your eyes so that the cranial nerves can be mobilized to adjust the balance of the various organs of the body. Closing the eyes can concentrate the mind and guide the body's qi and blood to the soles of the feet, which has a good effect on hypertension, diabetes and cervical spondylosis. It can also prevent brain dementia, and has a miraculous effect on foot cold syndrome.

Because the golden rooster independence can lead the blood down and return the qi to the origin by itself, it can collect qi and blood in the Taichong point of the liver meridian, the Yongquan point of the kidney meridian and the Taibai point of the spleen meridian, so that the functions of the liver and kidney can be quickly obtained enhanced, this is a good permanent cure.

I remember playing hopscotch and kicking shuttlecock with one foot when I was a kid. I thought to myself, I just closed my eyes and stood on one foot, of course I can. When I closed my eyes and started standing on one foot for the first time, I immediately felt dizzy and the earth was spinning. I couldn't stand before I counted five. When I opened my eyes, the sky stopped spinning and the ground became stable. I remember that it was introduced in health care knowledge. If I can hold on to one foot for ten seconds with my eyes closed, my brain balance function is very good. If I can't hold on for five seconds, my brain balance function is not good, at least it can't reach a healthy brain standard indicators. I don't want to become Alzheimer's in the future, with my mouth open and drooling not understanding anything. So, I started to practice the Golden Rooster Independence Health Exercise, and every morning after the back impact exercise, I did the Golden Rooster Independence. I choose to stand in the corner of the wall, the left and right are the wall, no matter which way I fall, there is support. I stand for one minute on the left and right feet, no matter if I fall down, it is one minute. Gradually I closed my eyes and stood for longer and longer. Sometimes I could stand for a minute at a time. Usually, it was not a problem to stand for more than ten seconds or twenty seconds. The balance function of the brain began to improve, reaching the target.

At the same time, whenever I had the opportunity, I practiced on one foot independently for a few minutes. With my eyes open, the golden rooster could stand independently for a long time. I changed my feet and soon my feet began to warm up, and my feet and legs were warm. Since I practiced Golden Rooster independence, my brain has become less sleepy, and the quality of sleep has improved. I fell asleep on the bed and fell asleep until dawn. A good sleep guarantee is an essential part of the rehabilitation and treatment of diabetes. At the same time, I also found that the dizziness that I had experienced for many years has disappeared, and I no longer have eye pain and headache when I go out to the mall, and my mind has become clearer.

I practiced Golden Rooster independently divided into two types: closed eyes and open eyes. Closing eyes is to exercise the balance function of the brain and strengthen the function of the nervous system; opening eyes is to draw blood to the soles of the feet and strengthen the blood circulation system. These are of great benefit to the rehabilitation of diabetes, reducing and eliminating the complications of diabetes.

Acupressure for Diabetes

The occurrence of everything in the world is regular, and a corresponding and solution can always be found.

Diet therapy and exercise therapy are the most commonly used basic therapies for diabetic patients, and they are also the most effective therapy for blood sugar control. However, these two therapies only control the blood sugar level in a standard range, but they cannot achieve the best effect of improving the body's internal body.

For a period of time, although my blood sugar level was controlled within the ideal range, I was thirsty, blisters on the skin were prone to the sun, and the symptoms of diabetes still existed. The balance of yin and yang in the body has not been well coordinated, so this task of remedying the balance of yin and yang in the body falls on the meridian recommended by Chinese medicine.

The meridians of the human body are invisible to the naked eye, nor can the instruments be seen, only by feeling. It is said that the ancient and profound Chinese medicine practitioners can see with the naked eye, which is what qigong masters did after practicing and opening the eyes of the sky. No matter what, the ancestors left us with the magical meridian theory and practice, which played a role that Western medicine could not do. The mixed treatment of Western medicine and Chinese medicine can achieve the best diabetes treatment effect.

The meridians in our body are like blood vessels extending in all directions. The blood vessels can be seen with medical instruments, and the meridians are invisible, but the meridians and blood vessels exist side by side. The blood vessels are the streets on the ground, and the meridians are the sewers under the ground. The sewers drain properly, and the streets above ground remain clean and tidy. When the sewers are blocked, the stinky water spreads to the ground, and the streets are flooded with sewage and become dirty, which affects the foundation of the house and the beauty of the city. In the same way, in our human body, the first two channels in which the meridians and blood are parallel, the meridians are unobstructed, and the qi is sufficient, and the qi is the only driving force for the blood to flow. When there is qi, the blood can circulate normally. If there is enough qi, the blood will flow smoothly, and if the qi is deficient, the blood will flow slowly. This is the principle of qi stagnation and blood stagnation in traditional Chinese medicine, and the flow of blood will be hindered if qi is insufficient.

In order to maintain the qi in the body, in addition to providing certain nutrition in the diet, exercise more to increase physical strength and immunity, massage is the best way to dredge the meridians. Doing massage on the meridians is equivalent to often dredging the sewers, making the meridians unblocked, especially for people with physical diseases, massage appoints to dredge the meridians is more important.

According to the recommendations of many health professionals, I chose some key acupuncture points to assist in the treatment of diabetes and prevent complications of diabetes.

Lao Gong Point

Laogong Point: heat dissipation and dampness. Cold will replenish it, and heat will relieve it.

Location: Located in the palm of the human hand, when you make a fist, the corresponding position of the middle finger is the Laogong appoint. Lao Gong, as the name suggests, Lao means labor; Gong means palace. The palace to rest when tired is Lao Gong.

Laogong appoint belongs to the pericardium meridian of Hand Jueyin, the heart is the official of the monarch, and the heart is the main god. The pericardium meridian has a protective effect on the heart. Massage Laogong appoint can calm and refresh the brain, clear the heart fire, and relieve the mind. It is used to treat insomnia, neurasthenia and other diseases. It is applied at the same time with other acupuncture points to replenish the body's qi.

Hegu point

Hegu Point: The Large Intestine Meridian of Hand Yangming is an important point for the treatment of fever and various diseases of the head, face and facial features.

Improve immunity, prevent and treat colds, coughs, asthma, sore throat, and acute tonsillitis.

Location: between the first and second metacarpal bones on the back of the hand, approximately at the midpoint of the second metacarpal bone. Inner pass point

Neiguan is a commonly used specific point, it is one of the main points for body strength.

Location: Two cun above the transverse crease of the wrist, between the tendons of the palmar longus and flexor carpi radialis tendons.

In daily health care, you can press this acupoint frequently, which can relieve pain, relieve fatigue, and relieve fever, insomnia, and migraine headaches. It has an adjuvant therapeutic effect on heart, stomach and neurological diseases.

Quchi Point

Quchi Point: He points, belonging to soil. It has the functions of clearing away heat and removing the surface, dredging the meridians and collateral.

Location: The Quchi point of the human body is located at the lateral end of the elbow transverse lines, flexing the elbow, when the Chize point is at the midpoint of the line connecting the lateral epicondyle of the humerus.

Quchi point is mainly used for hypertension, fever, headache, dizziness, joint pain, shoulder and back pain, toothache, stomach pain, red eyes, swelling and pain, eczema and other diseases.

YangChi Point

Location of Yangchi Point: On the wrist, that is, on the horizontal stripes on the back of the wrist, facing the middle finger and ring finger. (Or in the transverse stripes of the back of the wrist, when the depression of the ulnar edge of the extensor tendon.)

The effect of Yangchi Point is on tinnitus, deafness, red and swollen eyes, wrist pain, hair loss and other diseases.

This point is one of the important Shu points on the Shaoyang Sanjiao meridian of the human hand.

Daling point

Daling, which means "Datushan", means that this acupuncture point produces the most soil. The soil in the five elements refers to the spleen. Daling point is the main point for strengthening the spleen

Location: Da Ling is in the middle of the wrist stripes.

Daling point is good for treating bad breath, which is caused by the accumulation of heat in the pericardium for a long time, damage to the blood network, or the spleen deficiency and dampness. Daling point is the most effective way to relieve fire and dampness.

Xuehai Point

Blood Sea: It is the key point for blood production and blood circulation.

Location: Located on the inside of the thigh, from the upper corner of the inside of the kneecap, there are about three finger-wide muscle grooves on it. When you press it, you can feel the pain. There are acupuncture points called "blood sea".

This acupoint is one of the important acupoints on the spleen meridian of the Taiyin of the human foot. In ancient times, people inadvertently discovered that puncturing this place could get rid of blood congestion in the body, and used it to treat the disease of blood congestion in the body. It can not only remove congestion, but also promote the production of new blood, so it is named "blood sea".

This acupoint nourishes the liver and nourishes blood.

Lieque Point

Position: The two hands are crossed between the tiger's mouth. At this time, the left index finger is on the back of the right wrist, and under the tip of the index finger is the Lieque acupoint.

This point is located at the intersection of the three meridians, so it has a regulating effect not only on the lung meridian, but also on the meridians of the large intestine meridian and the Ren meridian. In many cases, we will cause indescribable headaches due to occasional cold. At this time, we can press and rub the missing points to relieve the table, and we can also use a hot towel to apply the forehead.

The effect of Lieque points to nourish the lung and kidney also comes from its connection with the Ren Vessel, which itself is the "sea of Yang Vessel", which can invigorate the yin deficiency of the lung and kidney. Therefore, Lieque points also followed the role of Ren Channel. Frequently massaging this health acupuncture point has a good regulatory effect on diabetes, tinnitus, dry eyes and other symptoms caused by insufficient kidney yin.

Xiaohai Point

The acupuncture points belonging to the meridians of the small intestine are on the inside of the elbow, the depression between the olecranon of the ulna and the inner epicondyle of the humerus. This acupoint is like the sea of the small intestine. The scope of the qi and blood field is huge, hence the name Xiaohai.

It acts on poor absorption of nutrients in the small intestine, hematopoietic dysfunction, and anemia.

When you flick it with your hand, your fingers will numb and you will find this Xiaohai point. No matter how you move your fingers, it doesn't numb, which proves that this meridian is a bit weak, the blood is blocked, and the heart's blood supply is poor. Therefore, the small intestine meridian is also a barometer of the heart. Poor conduction in the small intestine meridian proves that the heart's blood supply is weak. Massaging this little sea, touching it, increasing its conduction power can also increase the strength of the heart.

Xiaohai acupoint is the combined point of the small intestine meridian. Traditional Chinese medicine teaches that it can treat the internal organs of the small intestine. Therefore, massaging the small intestine can regulate the function of the small intestine. The digestive ability is weak, and it will not digest after eating, and it is stuck inside. Rubbing Xiaohai acupoint can enhance the digestive ability of the human body.

Xiaohai acupoint is a combination of acupoints and belongs to the soil. The small intestine meridian itself belongs to fire. Fire can generate soil. It disperses the fire from the small intestine meridian to the spleen meridian, so it can enhance the power of the spleen meridian.

Massaging the small intestine meridian can relieve the body's irritability, and the body's fire syndrome can be dispelled through this meridian.

Diji Point

Earth machine: belongs to the spleen meridian of foot Taiyin.
Location: 3 inches below Yinlingquan Cave.
Function: To invigorate the spleen, soak dampness, regulate menstruation and stop band.

Experiments have shown that acupuncture at Diji and Quchi can cause hypersecretion of pancreatic islets. Yinlingquan Point

Yinlingquan point: the combined point of the spleen meridian of the foot Taiyin, the five elements belong to water. This acupoint is an important point for diuresis and dampness in the spleen meridian of the Taiyin meridian of the human foot. It can be used for treatment of all diseases related to dampness.

Location: On the inner side of the lower leg, when the inner tibia is in the depression behind the malleolus. Opposite Yanglingquan, between the medial edge of the tibia and the gastrocnemius, above the starting point of the soleus muscle.

This point mainly treats the imbalance of spleen water transportation and can assist in the treatment of diabetes. Sanyinjiao Point

Location: Three inches upwards from the inner ankle bone of the ankle is Sanyinjiao.

Efficacy: It has special effects on irregular menstruation, dysmenorrhea, infertility, leucorrhea, and back pain.

Sanyinjiao is the place where the meridians of the three yin meridians-spleen, liver, and kidney intersect. If you continue to massage, blood stasis can be removed. It can improve physical fitness for people who are particularly fat or thin.

Fuliu Point

Fuliu: points on the kidney meridian, nourishing yin and invigorating the kidney.

Location: The inner side of the calf, the upper inner side of the Achilles tendon is in the depression. (Or Taixi point straight up 2 inches, in front of the Achilles tendon.)

Fuliu acupoint is a meridian of the kidney meridian of Foot Shaoyin. The kidney meridian is more abundant here. Therefore, it has the dual functions of nourishing yin and nourishing the kidney and strengthening the surface and benefiting from it.

This point is an important Shu point on the human foot Shaoyin Kidney Meridian.

Targets disease nephritis, neurasthenia, energy decline, memory loss, cold hands and feet, and swelling of hands and feet.

This point can improve kidney function, treat edema, abdominal distension, diarrhea, spontaneous sweating, night sweats, numbness of the fingers and other diseases.

The combined use of this point and Chize point also has the effect of lowering blood pressure. Taixi Point

Taixi: Foot Shaoyin Kidney Meridian points to replenish innate roots.

Location: Inside the foot, the depression between the tip of the medial malleolus and the Achilles tendon.

Taixi point is not only the infusion point of the kidney meridian of Foot Shaoyin, but also the original point of the kidney.

This point is one of the health-preserving points, but it focuses on replenishing congenital roots, and has a good effect on kidney-related diseases, such as renal colic and phoenix pain. Zusanli Point

Location: Zusanli is on the upper part of the outside of the lower leg, between the tibia and fibula. This acupuncture point is not easy to find. Remember to place one inch from the highest point of the tibial tuberosity below the knee and one inch outward.

Zusanli can adjust the digestive system to make it function vigorously, absorb nutrients and increase energy, and it has a strong effect on all systems of the body.

The spleen of traditional Chinese medicine is the foundation of acquired life, the source of biochemistry, and the foundation of life. Zusanli is the acupuncture point of the stomach meridian, which mainly deals with diseases of the digestive system. There is a saying that massaging Zusanli is better than eating an old hen.

Zusanli is the main acupuncture point of the stomach meridian. It has the functions of regulating the spleen and stomach, regulating qi and blood, regulating digestion, and replenishing weakness.

Diabetes patients mostly suffer from dysfunction of the spleen and stomach, unable to digest and transport food well. Massage Zusanli can strengthen the digestion and transport functions of the spleen and stomach, so that the five internal organs can get sufficient nutrition. Promote the transformation of the diabetic patient's condition in a better direction.

Zhaohai Point

It belongs to the acupoints of the Kidney Meridian of Foot Shaoyin and regulates the two meridia-ns.

Location: Inside the foot, in the depression below the tip of the medial malleolus.

Zhaohai acupoint is one of the eight channels at the intersection, which is connected to the Yinqiao channel. Therefore, Zhaohai point can not only nourish yin, clear heat and nourish the kidney, but also participate in the treatment of diseases controlled by the Yin Qiao Vessel.

Target diseases: insomnia, eyesight and nerves, fatigue of limbs, sore throat, hoarseness. Taichong Point

Taichong is one of the important acupoints on the liver meridian of the foot Jueyin.

Location: Taichong point is located on the dorsal side of the foot, in the junction of the first and second toe metatarsals. Move your fingers upward along the gap between the big toe and the second toe until you can feel the arteries reflecting your hand. This is the point.

Massage the Taichong acupoint is good for soothing the liver and regulating qi, and relieves the troubles of easy anger, poor sleep, and high pressure.

Yongquan Point

Yongquan acupoint is one of the most effective acupuncture points in the human body.

Location: The front 1/3 of the line between the head of the bottom of the foot and the heel.

Yongquan point has the effect of lowering blood sugar.

Opening up the Yongquan point can draw blood to the feet, so that aging can be relieved.

Rubbing the soles of the feet is actually massaging the Yongquan point, which can speed up blood circulation and promote the body's metabolism.

It does not take long to do these acupoint massages. I use them before getting up in the morning and before going to bed at night, each time for 15 minutes. Massage each point 100 times. Two acupoints on the legs can be massaged together at the same time, such as Fuliu and Diji, Sanyinjiao and Taixi. Massage with both hands at the same time can save time. When I massage the Yongquan acupoint, I also massage the ground tendons together. (Massage ground tendon is beneficial to the liver)

Since the acupoint massage, many of the discomforts and hidden dangers in the body in the past have disappeared. In particular, the dry mouth is basically gone, and the hands and feet have become warmer. I used to rush to the bathroom at 6 o'clock in the morning, and the stool is not forming, which is a little better than diarrhea. I can't wait to say that I'm going to pull it, and it's all right after I pull it. According to Chinese medicine, it belongs to Wugengxie, which is believed to be caused by yang deficiency of the spleen and kidney. Now I am all right, I am full of anger, my stool is formed, and my stomach is no longer gurgling. My head is no longer dizzy, and there are few blisters on my hands. In the past, Sanjiao often had tantrums, earaches and nose swelling, and was easy to be irritable. Now it is much milder and hardly loses temper. All these changes should be the result of re-balancing the yin and yang in the body.

Qigong Therapy

Qi and blood maintain a person's vitality. Qi and blood complement each other, and no one can do without. Qi is the commander of the body, and blood is the mother of the body. Qi drives the flow of blood, and blood nourishes the strength of Qi.

In the past, I have practiced the Guangming Kung fu according to books in China. Guangming Gong is a kind of Gong that is simple and easy to learn without any restrictions or requirements. Guangming Gong does not require to be done every day. Of course, it is best to do it every day. Even if it is interrupted for a few days or more, it will not have a big impact. It is still useful to pick it up and practice again. Guangming Gong can be practiced standing or lying in bed, which is very convenient. Some colleagues around me practice static exercises. Although it is very good to do static gong, it must be practiced every day. If you don't practice it will affect your gong power. After thinking about it, I picked up the Guangming Gong again. Without restraint, it is equivalent to relaxing the mind. Doing qigong in a relaxed and happy mood will yield good results.

I do Guangming Gong every night after taking a bath before going to bed, lying on the bed, first doing acupoint massage, then merging both hands to make mudra, the thumb of the left hand is held in the palm of the right hand, and the remaining four fingers of the left hand are held. Cover it on the back of the right hand, and then place this mudra on the Shenjue acupoint, which is the part of the Dantian, close your eyes, relax your whole body, and it will work inside your body after a while. At this time, I could feel as if a rotating gas was driving my body, my head was shaking gently and rhythmically, and my body was also rotating and shaking rhythmically. After more than ten minutes, as the air in the chest was exhaled from the nose, the body became relaxed. Sometimes, I feel that there is air coming out of the ear, and the air in the ear is coming out from the roots of the back teeth. After the moisture in the body is exhausted, I feel comfortable. After a day of work, my back, arms, and legs are very tired, so I am especially willing to do Guangming Gong to relieve the fatigue. After finishing the Guangming Gong, the pain in the back disappeared, and I fell asleep comfortably. In short, wherever there is a problem, Guangming Gong will clear it.

The healing method of Guangming Gong is very simple. It uses the movement of qi in the body to open up the channels of various meridians and make the blood flow smoothly. There is a saying in Chinese medicine that pain means nothing, and general means nothing. The qi and blood in the whole body are unblocked, and the muscles are not sore.

I usually do light work for 20 to 30 minutes. If I have enough time, I will do it for 30 minutes. If I don't have enough time, I will do it for 20 minutes. The biggest benefit of doing this kind of bright work is to be able to receive good results immediately. Of course, if I have enough time in the morning, or if I feel tired when I wake up, I will also do 20 to 30 minutes of Guangming Gong to smooth the whole body meridian and get up and get out of bed easily.

Cupping and Gua Sha to Clear Meridian

One winter, I was lying on the carpet one night and stretched my arms out, with my arms flat on the ground and along the carpet towards the top of my head, the left arm was very stiff, and the tendons inside were pulled, and it was painful.

Later, the left shoulder was strained again, and this time the left shoulder and arm became rigid. The doctor said it was the problem of the cervical vertebrae, so I did physiotherapy, acupuncture, and a set of massage Chinese medicine, but the effect was not very good. The whole arm is swollen and painful, and the pain is beyond descript-ion. During that time, I was in pain every day.

Later, I thought that I had brought back a set of simple cupping tools when I returned to China, so why not try it out? As a result, this test is really good. As long as it hurts, cupping will be done. After cupping, it will be relieved immediately. There are red marks, sometimes purple marks, and sometimes black and purple marks on the place where the cup was pulled. These reactions are all normal. Slowly, the blood marks on the place where it was pulled out became lighter and lighter, the congestion in the body was slowly pulled out, and the pain in the arm gradually disappeared.

Since cupping, the dark blue veins at the base of the tongue have also become thinner, no longer flying around so arrogantly, the blood supply to the heart muscle is improved. Cupping unclogs blood vessels, disperses congestion, and relieves symptoms.

The painful part from the shoulder to the arm is the route of the small intestine meridian. Chinese medicine says that the heart and the small intestine are the inner and outer parts of each other. In other words, the heart fire is transferred to the small intestine meridian, making the small intestine meridian on the shoulders and arms stiff and painful. The heart meridian and the small intestine meridian are on the arm, and the small intestine meridian runs from the head through the back shoulder to the outside of the arm. Originally, the heart fire was vented through the Sanjiao meridian, and the heart fire was transferred to the small intestine meridian when the Sanjiao meridian was not open, so it was painful.

Our human body is very smart and wise. If there is a problem with the heart, it hasn't stopped working. How can we let the outside world know about the heart disease? So its spokesperson, the small intestine, will come out to uphold justice without hesitation. If we have some knowledge of meridian, we will realize the problem and adjust the treatment in time. Also, when the heart is in the correction recovery period, its symptoms will also appear in the small intestine meridian, telling us "Hey! I am in the repair stage, please help me adjust in time if there is a problem, don't panic. "

Cupping is impossible for the finger segment, so I had to scrape Gua Sha. Scrape the small intestine meridian on the side of the hand with a scraping board, which is very comfortable. There are two acupuncture points on the sides of the fingers, Houxi and Qiangu. Qiangu is the Xing point on the small intestine meridian, and Houxi is the point on the small intestine meridian. The Xing point adjusts the heart-fire excessively, and the speciality of the acupoint lies in activating the meridians and collaterals, and is good at curing diseases of the internal organs. It can reduce the fire, adjust the heart function while dredging the meridians, transfer the excess heart fire to the small intestine, and then eliminate the body through urination. It is a good way to treat both the symptoms and root.

The small intestine meridian and the heart meridian are both on the outside and inside. Scraping the small intestine meridian can regulate the heart function, dredge the meridians and clear the collaterals and induce the fire to descend, achieving the effect of removing the heart fire. At that time, Gua Sha was only used to remove the pain, but I did not expect that the Gua Sha scraped out such an important health care route. Let me have more confidence in the cure of my thoracic aortic atherosclerosis in the early stage.

Traditional Chinese medicine believes that Gua Sha can regulate muscle contraction and relaxation, promote blood circulation around tissues, improve and adjust the functions of the internal organs, and balance the yin and yang of the internal organs. The blood vessels and nerves in the area touched by Gua Sha are stimulated to expand the blood vessels, increase the circulation of blood and lymph fluid, strengthen the phagocytosis and transport ability, and accelerate the excretion of waste and toxins in the body. After the scraped part passes through Sha, the local metabolism is enhanced, and the anti-inflammatory effect is produced.

Through this episode，I learned a Chinese medicine technique, cupping and scraping. These two traditional Chinese medicine techniques are simple and easy to learn, and they are very practical.

Stretch Body to Lower Blood Sugar and Improve Islet Function

The contraction of tendons is caused by liver problems. The liver controls the tendons, and the liver belongs to the wood. If the liver is not good, the spleen and stomach will not be good. The spleen belongs to the earth, and the wood restrains the earth. Seeing this, I suddenly realized that tendons contraction is also a symptom of insufficient blood supply to the liver.

For diabetic patients to improve the spleen and stomach, they must first make the liver healthy. Only when the liver is healthy will the spleen and stomach become healthy and produce insulin.

All kinds of books say that diabetes needs to take medicine for life, and it is irreplaceable and repairable for one's own pancreatic islets to be injured. It seems that it is not absolute. The main reason is that the key point to treat diabetes has not been found. Everything has a corresponding point, and when there is a problem, there is a solution.

The tendons belong to the category of blood vessels, and the liver controls the tendons. Stretching the tendons can nourish the liver, shrink the tendons when the liver is weak, and strengthen the tendons when the liver is strong. The tendons are strengthened and the liver is nourished, which in turn strengthens the ability to clean up blood vessels, thereby improving the secretion function of pancreatic islets, directly stabilizing blood sugar levels and improving the body's glucose tolerance.

According to ancient Chinese medicine, a person whose tendons are one inch longer increases his lifespan by ten years. It can be seen that tendons have a great role in the human body. When people get old, they shrink their tendons first, and their height when they are young becomes shorter when they get old. The reason is that the tendons in the body are shortened, and the human body is relatively short. Old people, inconvenient hands and feet, and slow movements are the reasons for muscle contractions. Regular stretching can help relax the tendons in various parts of the body. When a person feels young, people really become young. If you don't believe me, try it. After stretching, you will feel an unprecedented comfort in your whole body.

Chapter 3

Supply Qi and Blood Adjusting Pancreas and Stomach Improve Physical Function

Nutrition and Immunity

Our human beings have this or that kind of disease is related to the decline of the immune capacity in the body, and there are various reasons for the decline of human immunity, mainly because the human body lacks necessary nutrients and is weak in external combat. Therefore, foreign bacteria and viruses have the opportunity to take advantage of it. Secondly, a lot of garbage and toxins and dead cells accumulated in the body are not cleaned up in time. These are the direct reasons for the decline of immune function.

Overeating is not good for the body, a vegetarian diet is also not good for the body. The former is excessive nutrition, which consumes resources in the body excessively, and the latter is malnutrition and cell hypothalami, both of which cause more or less harm to the body's health and immunity. The best way to eat is to have a balanced nutrition, so that all parts of the body can obtain the substances they need to maintain their functions, and the accumulation and transformation of excess nutrients in the body will not cause the burden of internal organs to become garbage and toxins.

When it comes to nutrition, the human body does not get more nutrients from the more food we eat, but depends on what we eat, and the quality of our food has a great relationship with the absorption of the human body. I often meet some fat girls, who always complain that they haven't eaten anything good, even if they drink water, they will grow meat. In fact, drinking water can really make you gain weight, because there are many minerals in the water that our body needs, and the nutrients in the water are absorbed into the body. Moreover, human fatness and thinness have a great relationship with water, because most of the components in muscles are water.

To get the ideal nutrition, absorption capacity is the key. The example of those girls gaining weight when they drink water is because they are young, have sufficient energy and blood, and have very strong digestion and absorption capabilities. The food they eat and the nutrients in the water they drink have been absorbed. Therefore, the qi and blood are enough to ensure the absorption of nutrients, the body has the necessary nutrients, and the immune function can be strong. This is the way of fitness one after another. Sufficient qi and blood are the foundation of health and a necessary guarantee for the restoration of damaged bodies and organs.

Nutrition and immunity complement each other. The human body has enough nutrition and a healthy body will naturally establish a strong immune system. If the immunity is good, it can resist the invasion of foreign bacteria and viruses, and clean up the internal toxins in time. Protect us from getting sick or getting sick less often. Even if we are sick, we will get well soon.

Insufficient Qi and Blood Lead to Diseases.

Almost all diabetic doctors say to control diet, to strengthen exercise, and to insist on taking medicine. But no doctor emphasizes the need to replenish qi and blood, detoxify and remove dampness. It seems that there are only these three basic treatments for diabetes, and in the opinion of doctors, the best result for diabetic patients is to control their blood sugar. The treatment effect of some diabetic patients I know is not ideal. They often go back and forth. The more you eat, the larger the dose of hypoglycemic drugs, the weaker the body's overall resistance, and it is easy to cause diabetes complications.

Even if the blood sugar level of some diabetic patients can be kept stable, the immune function in the body is still weak, the people's spirit is not good, and they are prone to illness and fatigue. I was like this before. I controlled my blood sugar, lost weight, and my body's immune system decreased. The quality of the treatment is only judged by the level of blood sugar. The result is that the symptoms are not the root cause, and the hidden dangers of diabetes are always affecting the overall health.

Diabetes is a degenerative disease of the whole body. The treatment of diabetes requires comprehensive treatment and comprehensive adjustment to fundamentally achieve the goal of curing the root cause and improve the body's immune ability and self-healing ability. Diabetes patients not only need to control blood sugar levels, but also eliminate hidden dangers that cause diabetes. Just like the poor circulation of sewers, the flow of water is often blocked on rainy days. The problem is not to control the amount of rain, but to clean up the sludge in the sewers, so that the sewers are unobstructed and not afraid of strong winds and heavy rain.

Insufficient qi and blood cause all diseases. The disease of modern people is largely due to the lack of qi and blood. Many people may disagree with me. Nowadays, material life is extremely rich. Basically, people can eat whatever they want. As long as their stomach can handle it, they can eat a mountain. It is precisely because eating too much of the good things can backfire and cause harm to the human body. Most of the modern people are deficient in qi and blood.

Sufficient qi and blood must meet three main basic conditions: first, the absorption function of the spleen and stomach is good; second, the hematopoietic function of the liver is good; third, the food eaten is conducive to hematopoiesis. In the process of diabetes treatment, what kind of help does adjusting the spleen and stomach to supplement qi and blood play on the five zang-organs and six fu-organs, the relationship between these viscera, and what role does the rise and fall of qi and blood in the body play in the course of diabetes?. To understand these, diabetic patients can be aware of every step of the treatment, no longer blindly taking medicine, injections, and dieting.

Diabetes is a general term for diseases caused by insulin deficiency. However, the reasons for the onset of diabetes are different for each diabetic patient, so it is very important for us diabetics to understand the cause of diabetes and the relationship between the internal organs. To understand the origin of diabetes, at least we should know what adjustments we should make, so that we can prescribe the right medicine and achieve a multiplier effect.

The Role of Qi and Blood in the Human Body

Blood is a tangible thing, and Qi is an intangible thing. The movement of blood depends on qi, and blood is the best carrier for transferring the energy of qi to the organs of the body, and sufficient blood flow can carry more oxygen. Blood is born from qi, and qi must be attached to blood in order to play its role in biochemistry and movement. The two rely on each other and promote each other to maintain a relative balance. If the blood and qi lose balance, it will cause illness.

The most important function of blood for the human body is nourishment, and the nutrients and oxygen it carries are the material basis for the life activities of various tissues and organs of the human body. If the blood is sufficient, the complexion will be ruddy, the skin will be plump and plump, the hair will be smooth and shiny, the spirit will be full, the senses will be sensitive, and the activities will be flexible.

Qi propels blood and fluids in the body and is the only driving force for blood circulation. Qi transports nutrients to the parts of the body needed by the body to maintain the operation of life, and also sends various metabolites to the large intestine and bladder, which are excreted through urine and feces to remove garbage and toxins in the body. Therefore, Qi in the body is not only the main force that promotes blood flow, but also the pioneer of vitality throughout the body. Qi foot blood is abundant, Qi deficiency and blood stasis. Blood deficiency and qi weakness, lack of blood and qi deficiency.

I think the human body's qi should be divided into two categories. One is the commander's qi, which is the vitality in the body, which is inherent in the human body. It belongs to the main air flow in the body, because only the air flow can have a strong driving effect and control ability. Anyone who has done qigong has experienced that when the human body is in a static state, the whole body is relaxed, and the hands are folded together to form a handprint on the dantian, the eyes are slightly closed, and even and deep breathing, you will soon feel a surge in the body. Qi is rotating, spirally rotating in the body, dredging every part of the body. This qi is the true qi that lives in the body.

Another type of qi is oxygen, which is very important to human cells. Every living cell in our body contains oxygen, and oxygen is involved in the metabolic process of human cells. Aerobic cells are active cells, hypoxic cells are diseased cells, and anaerobic cells are dead cells. Oxygen is transmitted into our body through the respiratory tract, so the strength of lung function is directly related to the amount of oxygen stored in the body.

Chinese medicine believes that "Chi" refers to the innate qi, and "Qi" refers to the acquired qi, which is what it means. "Chi" is the vitality in the body, and qi is the oxygen coming in through the respiratory tract. In other words, the innate "Chi" is like the zymogen protein, which requires acquired oxygen to activate. The oxygen from nature is the activator of the "Chi" in the human body.

When we feel dizzy, exhausted, tinnitus, fatigued, and short of breath, the cells in the body are deprived of oxygen. In the absence of oxygen in the body, the innate "Chi" cannot be fully activated, so that the internal organs cannot be normally pushed to transmit the essence of food and excrete waste.

When cells are deprived of oxygen, it is easy to produce insulin antibodies, making insulin unable to enter the cells. It is like that when human brain cells are hypoxic, they will be slow in thinking, slow in reaction, sleepy, and feel tired and exhausted without much physical exertion. Human cells will also be slow to respond to hypoxia, not sensitive to insulin, and produce insulin antibodies.

Hypoxia is also ischemia, because blood is the carrier of oxygen, and without enough blood flow, there is not enough carrier to transport oxygen. Therefore, nourishing blood, nourishing qi, nourishing oxygen are interactive and inseparable, and this is also an effective way to treat diabetes.

Repair the Intestines and Stomach to Increase the Rate of Blood Production

Since qi and blood are so important to human life, how can we ensure that the blood in the body is sufficient?

Usually when we talk about poor digestion, we immediately think of the stomach. We all think that the stomach is not good for digestion and absorption. In fact, the stomach can only be considered as the rough processing of the digestive system. The first process, the small intestine is the main battlefield for fine processing. The small intestine has a total length of 5-7m and is the longest part of the digestive tract. Its function is to absorb nutrients and transport them. food. Of course, the absorption of nutrients in the intestine is inseparable from the cooperation of the digestive glands, liver, gallbladder, and pancreas.

Food goes down from the stomach and first enters the duodenum. It is a part of the small intestine, with a total length of about 30 cm. It is the core for the body to absorb food nutrients and produce energy. More than 70% of the body's nutrients will be absorbed here. The duodenum mixes the food delivered from the stomach with the bile flowing out of the gallbladder and the pancreatic juice digestive enzymes flowing out of the pancreatic duct. When the food arrives here, it has been decomposed and melted into a chyle s tate, and the intestines begin absorption and delivery of food to the jejunum and ileum.

How does the small intestine absorb nutrients?

The structure of the small intestine is composed of many cells with villi. There are capillary networks, lymphatic capillaries, smooth muscle fibers and neural networks in the villi. The relaxation and contraction of smooth muscle fibers can make the villi expand and oscillate. The movement of the villi accelerates the flow of blood and lymph, which helps absorb nutrients.

The mucosa of the jejunum and ileum has many ring-shaped fold villi. When these folds expand, the surface area of the mucosa is greatly enlarged, so that the surface area of the small intestine can be increased by 600 times to about 200 square meters, which greatly improves the efficiency of the small intestine to absorb nutrients. The small intestine also does self-regulatory exercise. We often hear the gurgling sound of the intestines in the abdominal cavity, that is, the small intestine is doing self-regulation to help food move and enter the large intestine. A large number of capillaries are connected to the small intestine, glucose, amino acids, cholesterol and glycerin. Triesters, various minerals and vitamins are easily absorbed into the blood by the mucosal epithelium of the small intestine, and then enter the liver to be used.

When the fat in the food continues to exceed the standard, the triglycerides and cholesterol in the nutrients severely block the mucosa of the small intestine, the villi on the intestinal cells are greasy and can not stretch, and the body is sitting for a long time, causing slow intestinal peristalsis. Resulting in a greatly reduced contact area between the small intestine and food, severely reducing the efficiency of the small intestine to absorb nutrients. Many nutrients are sent into the cecum, enter the large intestine and are excreted.

If the small intestine does not function properly to receive food, the movement of qi is obstructed, which manifests as abdominal pain. If the small intestine does not function properly in digestion, it can lead to digestive and inspir-atory dysfunction, manifested as abdominal distension, diarrhea, and loose stools. The small intestine of diabetic patients basically has problems with digestion and absorption, because there is no normal insulin infiltration in the duodenum to dissolve sugar, and the sugar in food is directly absorbed into the blood vessels, resulting in high blood sugar in the blood.

The small intestine occupies such an important position in the digestive system, it is no wonder that the small intestine and heart are both external and internal, and its status is simply the second heart of a person.

According to Chinese medicine, the spleen (intestine, pancreas) and stomach are the foundation of the acquired nature and the source of qi and blood biochemistry. To improve the nutrient absorption rate of the stomach and intestines, it is necessary to choose the preferences of the stomach and intestines, and nourish the stomach and intestines. When the function of the stomach and intestines is normal, blood production will be guaranteed. Therefore, in order to be full of qi and blood, a healthy stomach is the premise.

Stomach likes warm, irregular eating time, overeating, overeating, or overeating raw and cold foods can affect the function of the stomach and cause pain. After stomach problems, the digestive function is weakened. Therefore, the diet must be rationed on time. Digested food, the stomach likes moistening and hates dryness, while alcohol, spicy greasy and thick-flavored food can generate heat and dissolve dryness, which is not good for the stomach.

Do regular stomach and abdomen massages to strengthen gastrointestinal motility and improve the absorption capacity of the small intestine.

Abdominal Breathing Strengthens Qi in the Body

There are two types of qi, one is to eat some qi foods, such as astragalus, American ginseng, etc, and the other is to practice deep breathing. Food replenishes the vitality that the human body brings innately, while practicing deep breathing obtains the oxygen produced in the natural world.

Taoist meditation, Taijiquan's internal power, and Jinggong practice are all deep breathing, meditation is in the dantian, and abdominal breathing is also the focus on the dantian. This method of breathing pays attention to quiet, long and thin breathing. By practicing the deep breathing method of Dantian, many hidden potentials of the human body can be tapped and stimulated. Practicing abdominal breathing in diabetic patients can stimulate islet function through internal thoughts and achieve the effect of lowering blood sugar.

Most people only use shallow breathing (thoracic breathing), so only one-third of the lung function is used, and the other two-thirds of the lungs are in a resting state, depositing old air. If you use the abdominal breathing method (breathing awareness) to breathe, the lung function can be fully utilized. Abdominal breathing allows the body to fully exert its qi function, and at the same time it can take in more oxygen.

Abdominal breathing can not only purify the blood，make the blood weakly alkaline, but also promote the activation of body cells. Abdominal breathing can increase the range of movement of the diaphragm, and the movement of the diaphragm directly affects the ventilation of the lungs.

Abdominal breathing expands lung capacity and improves cardiopulmonary function. It can maximize the expansion of the thorax, allow the alveoli in the lower lungs to stretch, let more oxygen enter the lungs, improve cardiopulmonary function, and reduce lung infections, especially pneumonia.

Studies have shown that in abdominal breathing, for every centimeter of diaphragmatic lowering, pulmonary ventilation can increase by 250 to 300 ml. Adhering to abdominal breathing for half a year can increase the range of motion of the diaphragm by four centimeters. The improvement of lung function can increase the inspiratory capacity of diabetic patients, and one of the important rehabilitation methods to change the lack of air and lethargy.

Abdominal breathing can improve the function of abdominal organs. It can improve the function of the spleen and stomach, soothe the liver and promote choleretics, and promote the secretion of bile.

Abdominal breathing can lower blood pressure by lowering abdominal pressure, which is very beneficial to patients with hypertension.

Abdominal breathing has an effective effect on eliminating abdominal fat, removing waste from the abdomen, improving blood circulation in the abdomen, and promoting the life activities of the abdomen and pelvic organs.

When I first practiced abdominal breathing, I made a noise from top to bottom, that is, from the stomach, a grunt, and then the lower abdomen would respond with a grunt. This kind of grunting sound is like listening to the sound of a frog quietly when I am in the empty valley. My brain does not show the creeping animation of the large intestine and stomach at all, but it feels like empty valley or orchid. After the exercise, the fresh air enters the brain, the whole person is very energetic, and I am not sleepy at all.

If you feel that the abdominal breathing is troublesome and it is difficult to grasp the essentials, you can also simply take a deep breath, which can also play a role in calming the mind.

Splenetic of Western Medicine

In the treatment of diabetes, traditional Chinese medicine and Western medicine have different views. According to Chinese medicine, diabetes is a disorder of the spleen and stomach, and internal heat that affects the yin. In western medicine, diabetes is simply impaired islet function, which cannot secrete or insufficiently secrete the insulin needed by the body. It belongs to endocrine disorders and is a disease of metabolic disorders. In traditional Chinese medicine, the spleen and stomach disorders actually refer to the disorders of the stomach and pancreas. In western medicine, diabetes endocrine disorder refers to the dysfunction of pancreatic islets..

The spleen in Chinese medicine and the spleen in western medicine are not the same thing at all. According to Western medicine, the spleen is located at the upper left of the abdominal cavity. It is flat oval, dark red, soft and brittle. It can be said that the spleen is like a blood-filled sponge. When the spleen is hit by violence, it is easy to rupture and bleed.

Western medicine's spleen has nothing to do with digestion. It's just that no matter how much it eats, it won't hurt the spleen, because Western medicine's spleen cannot accept food at all. It is not a hollow body, nor does it belong to the digestive system. It belongs to the human immune system, a member of the team.

The spleen is an important lymphatic organ that stores blood, provides blood, participates in hematopoiesis, filters blood, clears senescent blood cells, and participates in some metabolic processes and immune responses. When the human body is resting and quiet, the spleen stores blood, and when it is under stress conditions such as exercise, blood loss, or hypoxia, it pumps blood into the blood circulation to increase blood volume. Because of its rich blood content, it can urgently replenish blood to other organs, so it is called "human blood bank".

The body's immune system has three lines of defense, tonsils, lymph nodes and spleen. The responsibility of the spleen is to deal with bacteria and viruses in the blood. If there is a problem with the spleen, the blood quality in the human body cannot be guaranteed.

Although the spleen is not part of the digestive system, the spleen governs blood. Diabetes patients' blood is not clean, which is bad for the spleen. Therefore, diabetes is related to the spleen.

The Spleen of Traditional Chinese Medicine Is the Pancreas of Western Medicine

The pancreas is a very important secretory organ in the body. It is located behind the stomach, close to the back wall of the abdomen. The head of the pancreas is just inside the small bend formed by the duodenum. The tail of the pancreas is composed of an exocrine gland and an endocrine islet, so it is a mixed gland. There is a duct in the pancreas, called the pancreatic duct, which starts from the tail of the pancreas and ends at the head of the pancreas. Most of it forms a "common channel" with the common bile duct, which opens in the duodenum. Insulin secreted by the pancreas enters the duodenum through this common channel. The tail of the pancreas is close to the back and above the kidneys, and it likes the sun and is afraid of humidity.

Regardless of the small area occupied by the pancreas, it plays a large role in the body. The pancreatic juice secreted by the pancreas is indispensable for the digestion and absorption of food. According to relevant scientific research, the normal human pancreas secretes about 1, 000 milliliters of pancreatic juice every day, which is almost equal to 10 to 14 times the weight of its own pancreas. It can be seen that its function is extremely active and its workload is extraordinary. In addition to water, the main components of the pancreas are electrolytes and zymogen protein, electrolytes can neutralize gastric acid. That is to say, the electrolyte is alkaline, which makes the food entering the small intestine from the stomach rapidly change from acid to alkaline, and provides the necessary conditions for the conversion of zymogen protein into pancreatic enzymes.

This conversion process of zymogen is called "activation", and activation is an important link in the conversion of zymogen into pancreatic enzyme to exert physiological functions. A normal adult excretes about 2-8 grams of enzymes and proteins into the small intestine every day. Like catalysts used in industry, they participate in the digestion of polysaccharides (starch), proteins and fats in food. Make them into substances that the body can absorb. If the function of the pancreas decreases due to a certain disease and the secretion of pancreatic juice decreases, the person will suffer from severe indigestion. Therefore, the pancreas is the most important endocrine organ in the human body.

In addition, the pancreas has a very important function, which is to secrete insulin. Why is it called insulin? It turns out that there are many large and small cell clusters scattered in the pancreas, especially the tail and body of the pancreas, and the head is the least. From the perspective of the pancreas, these cell clusters look like many islands distributed on the surface of the water, so they are named pancreatic islets. Insulin is secreted by islet cells.

There are about 1 to 2 million pancreatic islets. Each pancreatic islet contains at least 4 types of cells: A cells secrete glucagon, B cells secrete insulin, D cells secrete growth hormone, inhibitory hormone, and PP cells secrete pancreatic polypeptide. Various cells secrete different hormones. These hormones regulate each other to maintain the stability of blood sugar. The pancreatic islets contain the largest amount of B cells and secrete hormones. Therefore, the secretion of insulin is the most important function of the pancreatic islets.

As the most important digestive and secretory organ of the human body, the pancreas has two heavyweight offici-als under its hands, namely exocrine and endocrine function executives. The exocrine executive is responsible for the digestion of starch, protein and fat in the food, while the endocrine executive is responsible for the metabolism of sugar. Diabetes is caused by these two executives' own illnesses and slow work. Modern medical judgments let the executives of endocrine function take the main responsibility. Therefore, Western medicine puts diabetes under the treatment of endocrinology.

Diabetes patients are not only high blood sugar, but also high fat, high blood pressure, and cardiovascular and cerebrovascular diseases. These are all related to blood. At least they are potential patients in this area. I have experienced high blood pressure and high fat. When my blood sugar level was the most unstable, my blood pressure reached a high pressure of 160. Before I was diagnosed with diabetes, my triglyceride reached a severe level of 20. Later, the blood sugar was controlled within the normal value, the high blood pressure disappeared, and the triglyceride reached the normal value.

Based on the theories of Chinese and Western medicine, diabetes is a disease in which the metabolism of pancreas fat and sugar is out of balance, and it is also a blood disease in which metabolism is imbalanced.

To solve the problem of pancreatic islets in diabetic patients, it is necessary to solve the problem of pancreatic juice, which is a special function of two interdependence and support in the pancreas. When the pancreatic juice secretion is normal, the pancreatic islets will secrete more insulin.

To control blood sugar, it is necessary to control high fat in the body and reduce triglycerides in the body to reach the normal value required by the human body. After removing the oily coat covering the pancreas, the pancreas can breathe normally, and then it can regain its vitality. Restore the normal function of exocrine and endocrine.

Electrolytes Are one of the Main Components of the Pancreas

The main components of the pancreas are water, electrolytes, and zymogen protein. There is no water in the human body, and the pancreas is no exception. What is electrolyte? Since electrolytes are the main components of the pancreas, it is necessary to find out that it is quite beneficial to restore the function of the pancreas.

Electrolyte is a medical name. Electrolytes refer to trace minerals such as sodium, potassium, chlorine and bicarbonate, calcium, phosphorus, and magnesium in human serum, which participate in many important functions and metabolic activities in the body, and play a very important role in the maintenance of normal life activities. The dynamic balance of water and electrolytes in the body is achieved through the regulation of nerves and body fluids.

In other words, if there is a problem with the body's nerves and fluids, the balance of water and electrolytes in the body will be broken. Therefore, it is easy to cause metabolic disorders. Similarly, the lack of trace minerals in the human body and the inability to replenish it can easily cause cell defects to cause metabolic disorders.

The zymogen protein is an activator. In normal organisms, plasmin exists in the state of zymogen, which is a natural variety that has not been modified in the original ecology. Only through the action of plasminogen activator, plasmin has activity. Different tissues in the body have corresponding activators. These complex chemical reactions are directly secreted or produced by the pancreas, the headquarters of the chemical factory in the body.

Anyone who has made steamed buns knows that making steamed buns requires flour, water and baking powder. Our pancreas is like a recipe for making steamed buns. For example, f lour is an unaltered original ecology containing inactive zymogen protein. Baking powder is like an electrolyte. After adding water, the electrolyte dissolves in the water and becomes an activator. It is mixed into the flour to activate the zymogen protein in the flour, make it expand and ferment, and make steamed bread. The proportion of water, flour and baking powder for making steamed buns should be just right. Of course, the five elements of sufficient hot steam and time are needed to make soft and delicious steamed buns. Hot steam is the qi and blood in our body, and time is the smoothness of the meridians of the human body.

Therefore, the water, electrolytes, and zymogen protein in the pancreas must be kept in a balanced state, with nourishment of qi and blood, and the smoothness of the meridians, in order to play a good role. Disorders of water and electrolyte metabolism can cause corresponding obstacles to the physiological functions of the body's organs, especially the cardiovascular system, the nervous system, and the body's material metabolism, which can often lead to death in severe cases. We should drink plenty of water daily to avoid dehydration. In addition, maintaining a balanced diet is also very helpful in preventing electrolyte imbalances.

Understand this knowledge, We can understand why the human body needs to supplement minerals and trace elements. Why should we have balanced nutrition, not picky eaters, and eat a variety of foods?

We human beings are actually the miniatures of nature. Trace elements are indispensable substances for maintaining life and regulating metabolism. Even brain thinking cannot be achieved without the regulation of the nervous system by trace elements.

Human Digestive System

The human digestive system is composed of two parts, the digestive tract and the digestive glands. The gastrointestinal tract as we know it belongs to the digestive tract. It is a long muscular duct from the mouth, throat, esophagus, stomach, small intestine (duodenum, jejunum, ileum) and large intestine (cecum, colon, rectum) to the anus.

Another component of the digestive system is the digestive glands. There are two types of digestive glands, small digestive glands and large digestive glands. The small digestive glands are scattered in the walls of each part of the digestive tract. The large digestive glands have three pairs of salivary glands (parotid, submandibular, and sublingual), liver and pancreas. They all use ducts to discharge secretions into the digestive tract.

There are 5 digestive glands in the human body, namely: salivary glands, (secreting saliva, salivary amylase decomposes starch into maltose,) gastric glands, (secreting gastric juice, decomposing proteins into polypeptides) and liver, (secreting bile, which is stored in the gallbladder to convert macromolecules. The initial breakdown of fat into small molecules of fat is called physical digestion, also called "emulsification",) pancreas , (secretion of pancreatic juice, which is the digestive juice that digests sugars, fats, and proteins) intestinal glands (secretion of intestinal juice, It breaks down maltose into glucose, breaks down polypeptides into amino acids, and breaks down small molecules of fat into glycerol and fatty acids. It is also a digestive juice that digests sugars, fats, and proteins).

These digestive glands are extremely important. Without their participation, the human body would not get the slightest nourishment no matter how much food, no matter how good it is. It can be said that the body's absorption depends on the participation of the digestive juice secreted by the digestive glands. These digestion processes are chemical decomposition processes, which require the participation of various enzymes to complete.

The digestion process of the digestive tract and the digestive glands is as follows:

Food is eaten in the mouth, and the food is mixed with s aliva, and the enzymes in the saliva quickly decompose starch. The teeth chew the food, and then the food is sent to the stomach from the esophagus.

The food continues to be dispersed in the stomach, and the food is mixed with the gastric acid secreted by the stomach wall. At this time, the decomposition of protein begins, and the food becomes viscous and gradually enters the duodenum.

As soon as food enters the duodenum, it is immediately immersed in bile and digestive enzymes. Bile is made by the liver and stored in the gallbladder. It helps digest fat. The enzymes secreted by the pancreas play an important role in the breakdown of fat, protein and starch. The duodenum is connected to the small intestin

The final stage of digestion is in the small intestine. Enzymes, bile and pancreatic juice are further mixed to break down the food into smaller molecules, allowing it to pass through the inner wall of the small intestine smoothly. Here, nutrients are sent to the liver through blood vessels for storage and distribution, and undigested food residues enter the large intestine.

The remaining water and undigested food residues are sent to the large intestine. Here, most of the water and salt are absorbed when passing through the colon, and the rest goes directly to the rectum and is discharged from the anus. Fiber is indigestible and is the main component of feces.

Understanding the accurate components and operating procedures of the human digestive system can enable diabetic patients to better control their own body, understand the development of the disease, and facilitate treatment. After understanding the entire digestive system, diabetic patients will have a better understanding of the disease. Make accurate judgments and know where the cause of the disease occurs in the digestive system, because the best doctor is the patient himself or herself.

Kidney and Diabetes

Chinese medicine believes that the kidney is the foundation of the innate.

The kidneys are located on both sides of the spine, close to the back wall of the abdomen, on the left and right sides of the lower back. In the past, people often referred to kidney disease as waist disease, which was caused by the location of the kidney.

The human body is metabolizing all the time. In this process, some unwanted or even harmful wastes are inevitably be produced by the human body. A small part of them are excreted by the gastrointestinal tract, and most of them are excreted by the kidneys, so as to maintain the normal physiological activities of the human body. The kidneys act like a filter, retaining useful nutrients and expelling useless waste and toxins through urine. If kidney disease or kidney function weakens, the excretion of substances harmful to the human body will be hindered, and the accumulation of toxic substances in the body will cause various problems.

The kidneys have glomeruli and tubules responsible for their work. When blood flows into the kidneys, the body produces a variety of waste products in the process of metabolism. Most of the waste products are filtered through the glomerulus and secreted by the renal tubules and excreted in the urine. The urine excreted every day accounts for only 1% of the blood filtered by the kidneys. The daily urine output of a normal person is 1000-2000 milliliters. Too much or too little urine may be caused by kidney disease.

Polydipsia and polyuria in diabetic patients is an abnormal pathological phenomenon in itself. Due to excessive blood sugar, a large amount of sugar is excreted in the urine, and the human body increases the amount of water to dilute the blood for metabolism. Polyuria makes the kidney water insufficient, so it cannot reach the heart, which makes the heart fire spread and involve other organs.

When the kidney function is weak, its endocrine function will cause metabolic disorders. If the kidneys cannot normally degrade protein, the human body will lack protein support. Protein is one of the important human nutrients. Long-term malnutrition will reduce the immune capacity of the entire body, degenerate systemic functions, and cause various diseases. It can be seen that the kidney plays an important function in maintaining the stability of the body's environment.

If the blood sugar control of diabetic patients is not good, the course of diabetes will lead to hardening of the blood vessels for too long. The kidney is composed of millions of microvascular globules. Poor blood sugar control can damage the kidneys quickly and lead to diabetic nephropathy. Severe cases will lead to uremia, and they will rely on dialysis blood to maintain their lives for the rest of their lives.

Kidneys are the foundation of the innate, the place where the energy is stored, and the place where the vitality of a person resides. Whether a person's energy is strong depends on whether the person's kidney function is strong. Therefore, we should pay attention to maintaining our kidneys in daily life, especially our diabetic patients, try not to make the kidneys overworked, and control the daily protein intake. Excessive protein degradation will cause additional burdens to the kidneys. Protect our waist, don't lift heavy objects, and don't catch cold on the waist and back. In terms of diet, choose the right amount of high-protein, high-vitamin, low-fat, low-cholesterol, and low-salt foods.

High-fat and high-cholesterol diets are prone to renal arteriosclerosis, which shrinks the kidneys, and high-salt diets affect water and fluid metabolism.

Heart and Stomach

After eating something that is difficult to digest, people feel a fire in their stomach, we would say, heartburn. Rather than say, it's a stomachache. There are still many people who are confused about the feeling of heartache and stomachache. Looking at the human body picture, we know that the heart is on the upper left side of the human body, and the stomach is below. The esophagus can be divided into three parts: neck, chest, and abdomen from the pharynx. The neck and thoracic sections are close to the spine, descend behind the trachea and heart, pass through the diaphragm and enter the abdominal cavity, which is connected to the stomach. The esophagus is a flat cylindrical muscular long tube with a total length of about 25-30 cm.

The esophagus is close to the heart, and the heat and cold of food that a person eats directly affects the thermal expansion and contraction of the heart arteries. It is reported that after get off work, a guy in Beijing drank several draughts of cold beer in a cold drink shop on the side of the road due to the hot summer weather, causing a sudden myocardial infarction. There is also an example. In order to honor his mother, someone bought a few hot glutinous rice balls and took them home. It turned out that the glutinous rice balls themselves were not easy to digest, hot and sticky. The old mother swallowed them anxiously. The hot glutinous rice ball that entered the stomach couldnot dissipate the heat, and a large area of sudden myocardial infarction appeared in the heart next to the stomach. The son's filial piety harmed his mother.

Because the heart and stomach are very close to each other in the body, maintaining a good stomach means maintaining the heart. Stomach likes warmth, heart blood vessels also like warmth. The stomach does not like cold, hot and irritating food, and the heart does not like it either.

The stomach is the first granary that provides human nutrients. In the rough processing workshop, the health of the stomach is directly related to whether it can provide more valuable nutrients. A healthy stomach processes the food that is eaten int o nutritious mud, which is convenient for the small intestine to absorb. Unhealthy stomach functions are not strong, and the food that is eaten cannot be well processed, and can only be sent away hastily, which is not conducive to the fine processing and absorption of the small intestine, and most of it is discharged.

The human body needs a stomach to provide good nutrients, build fresh blood to meet the needs of the human body, and make the heart pump run with full horsepower, so as to transport sufficient blood to all parts of the body. Such a virtuous cycle makes the body function well.

Therefore, the heart and stomach are inseparable. With a good stomach and strong absorption capacity, the heart's blood supply capacity is strong. To protect the stomach is to protect the heart.

Lungs and Diabetes (1)

The lungs dominate the whole body Qi.

In the process of metabolism, the human body needs to continuously take in oxygen from the natural world and expel the turbid gas, that is, carbon dioxide. This kind of gas exchange between the body and nature is called respiration.

Both the inhaled oxygen and the exhaled exhaust gas pass through the nasal cavity and are controlled by the lungs. Chinese medicine says that the lung governs Qi. The lungs not only inhale and exhaust, but also control the Qi in the whole body. The lungs have an important regulating function on the body's Qi. The lungs are strong, and the body's Qi is sufficient, and the lungs have a strong role in regulating the distribution, operation and excretion of body fluid in the body.

Lung Chaobaimai means that the blood of the whole body continuously converges in the lungs, exchanges breathing through the lungs, and is transported to the whole body through the arteries through the heart, thereby assisting the heart to promote and regulate the movement of blood.

The main function of the lung is that the lung controls the upward promotion of lung qi and its dispersal and descending to the periphery. There is a complementary relationship between the two. The normal function of the lungs to disperse and descend, and keep the airway clean can make the airway normal and respiration harmonious, and then maintain the gas exchange inside and outside the human body, so that each visceral tissue can obtain enough qi, blood, and body fluid to nourish the body. Prevent water dampness and phlegm stagnation in the body.

If the lung function is abnormal, it will cause a series of discomfort. Common symptoms are: shortness of breath or insufficient ventilation of air bubbles on the surface of the lungs, chest tightness, cough, hemoptysis, etc.

The lungs control the water channels, which are the bladder meridians, and urine is the human waste water stored in the bladder.

The lungs are not good, and a lot of turbid gas is discharged which affects the large intestine. Therefore, the theory of traditional Chinese medicine says: "The lungs and the large intestine are on the outside and inside. " In fact, they influence each other. The meridians of the lungs run through the upper, middle and lower triple joules.

The lungs are located in the thoracic cavity, covering the heart, the highest position, the upper nasal orifice, and the outer fur. It is in close communication with the natural world and is easily attacked by external evils.

"The lungs hide the soul", the soul is semen. Chinese medicine says that the kidney meridian raises the pulse to drive semen up to the lungs. The kidneys and lungs are closely related and belong to the mother-child relationship. The lungs are the mother of the kidneys. If we want our kidneys to be good, we must nourish our lungs. The lungs have the function of purifying the blood, and maintaining the lungs is extremely beneficial to the treatment of diabetes.

The lung has two sets of vascular systems. One is the pulmonary arteries and pulmonary veins that circulate between the heart and lungs, which are the functional blood vessels of the lungs. The pulmonary artery sends out from the right ventricle and enters the lung with the bronchi. It branches repeatedly with the bronchi, and finally forms a network of capillaries around the alveoli, then gradually merges into the pulmonary veins and flows back to the left. The other set of nutritional blood vessels are called bronchial arterial veins, which originate from the thoracic aorta, cling the wall, and are distributed along the branches of the bronchus to nourish the bronchial wall, pulmonary vessel wall and visceral pleura in the lung.

From the above information, it is known that the bronchial arterial veins from the thoracic aorta cling to the bronchial wall, and bronchial inflammation directly affects the thoracic aorta, the source of the arteries and veins on the bronchial wall. The atherosclerosis of the aorta slows down the blood flow and affects the blood supply to the lungs. The blood in the lungs is insufficient and its function is weakened. On the contrary, the lack of blood in the lungs will affect the high-fat toxins in the aortic blood vessels that are difficult to clean up. If we want to improve our cardiopulmonary function, the main method is to replenish qi and blood and increase the blood flow in the body.

Lungs and Diabetes (2)

Since I was a child, I often had a cough in autumn and winter. I had a cold, and the respiratory tract was easily infected. As an adult, the symptoms gradually eased, but cough and cold still often occurred. After I came to Canada, I started coughing when the wind was blowing. With the treatment of diabetes and the improvement of my own immunity, my cough and cold symptoms have gradually improved, and now I rarely have coughs and colds.

Fresh air is a necessary condition fo r lung health care. Not only healthy people should go to places with noisy voices and air pollution as little as possible, but people with diabetes should avoid going to places with air pollution and lack of oxygen.

The lungs are responsible for the production and operation of the Qi of the whole body. Heart qi is the basic power of blood circulation. The movement of blood depends on the promotion and regulation of lung qi, that is, lung qi has the effect of helping the heart to move blood. When the qi breathed in by the body is not pure, it will affect the blood flow of the heart.

The lungs are involved in the regulation of water metabolism throughout the body. Control and regulate the infusion and excretion of body water, as well as the excretion of sweat and urine. Diabetic patients' thirst, polydipsia, and polyuria are related to the involvement of the lungs in mediating the metabolism of water throughout the body.

The heart governs the blood of the whole body, and the lung governs the qi of the whole body. The two coordinate with each other to ensure the normal operation of qi and blood and maintain the metabolism of the organs and tissues of the body. If the lung qi is weak, the blood will become weak, and the lung qi will be blocked, which will affect the new blood circulation function and lead to blood stasis in the heart. If the heart qi is insufficient, the heart yang is weak, and the blood flow is not smooth, it will also affect the respiratory function of the lungs, resul-ting in chest tightness, coughing and wheezing. Therefore, in order to restore the normal function of the heart, it is necessary to improve the function of the lungs. The heart and the lungs are a pair of complementary partners.

Why People Living in Poverty also Suffer from Diabetes

Speaking of diabetes, people always say, oh, sickness of wealth. In fact, diabetic patients have to control their diet and eat a lot less delicious food than ordinary people. It is simply a disease of poverty, hunger and thirst.

This disease of wealth does not refer to diabetes itself, but refers to the more affluent places, the more people get diabetes, so it is named. Since most of the people in wealthy regions and countries suffer from diabetes, why do many rural people in poor areas also suffer from diabetes? Some people say that this is due to diabetes caused by malnutrition. Both overnutrition and malnutrition can cause diabetes, so what do the two have in common?

People with overnutrition overeating for a long time have caused spleen and stomach disorders. The nutritious foods eaten are not well absorbed and stay in the body, and they cannot be excreted in time and become toxic substances. These harmful substances prevent the production of blood, so on the surface it looks like an overnutrition, but in fact, useful substances cannot be absorbed well, blood cannot be biochemically enough, and severe malnutrition is caused.

And those poor people suffering from diabetes suffer from long-term severe malnutrition. The carbon compounds they eat do not have enough energy and blood to break down and synthesize glucose into the cells. This is a vicious circle, which eventually leads to pancreatic islet dysfunction.

The common point that overnutrition and malnutrition cause diabetes is: both are serious insufficiency of blood in the body, causing pancreatic endocrine dysfunction.

Therefore, whether people with diabetes are overnutrition or malnutrition, they all suffer from insufficient qi and blood, and their overall function declines.

Atherosclerosis

Atherosclerosis is the most common and most important one of the vascular diseases of arteriosclerosis. It is characterized by thickening and hardening of the arterial wall, loss of elasticity, and shrinking of the lumen. The appearance of lipids accumulated on the arterial intima is yellow atherosclerosis, so it is called atherosclerosis.

Simply put, atherosclerosis is a disease in which a layer of lipids like millet atheroma is deposited on the arterial wall, which reduces the elasticity of the artery and narrows the lumen.

The cause of blood vessel problems is nothing more than excessive toxins. Toxins in blood vessels include excessive saturated fats, excessive monosaccharides, excessive chemical substances, etc. The deposition of these substances on the blood vessel wall is the hardening of the blood vessels. In the beginning, the body lacked sufficient ability to remove these toxins, the blood vessels were constantly invaded, and they were not able to get enough protective materials for repairs, and hardening was formed over time. Just as the scale in the water pipe has accumulated to a certain degree and oxidized, it is a reason that the iron pipe is rusted and blocked.

Atherosclerotic plaques are like"time bombs"that exist in human blood vessels, and their surface is a thin envelope. The envelope contains lipids, aggregated platelets, etc, like dumplings with a thin skin and a large filling, which are very easy to rupture. Without rupture, atherosclerotic plaques mainly block blood vessels, resulting in unsmooth blood flow, resulting in cardiac and cerebral ischemia and hypoxia. In emotional agitation, strenuous exercise, alcoholism, cold, etc, or when blood pressure suddenly rises, blood flow hits the plaque or vasospasm, the capsule will rupture, causing the atherosclerotic plaque, a time bomb, to be detonated. The thrombus fragments will completely block the blood vessels in an instant. If the coronary arteries are blocked, myocardial infarction or sudden death will occur. If the cerebral blood vessels are blocked, cerebral infarction will occur.

The consequences of atherosclerosis are very serious. Most diabetic patients die from cardiovascular and cerebro vascular diseases caused by atherosclerosis or arteriosclerosis. Therefore, the solution to this diabetic complication must start from the root cause.

Eat red meat in moderation, eat more fish, drink a little red wine every day to increase high-density lipoprotein levels, reduce the amount of bad cholesterol that causes plaque formation, and avoid or eat less foods with high cholesterol. Eat some oatmeal every day, because oatmeal is a killer to clean up high cholesterol. Black fungus is also a master at cleaning blood vessels.

Hypertension is the number one enemy that promotes atherosclerosis. Lower blood pressure, maintain peace of mind, don't get angry, and exercise more.

Eat food that removes dampness and detoxification, cleans up blood vessels, minimizes the toxins in the body, and reduces the dirt on the blood vessel walls. The patency of blood vessels and maintaining a certain degree of elasticity will greatly reduce the chance of suffering from atherosclerosis.

Supplement Qi and Blood to Adjust the Spleen and Stomach

Insufficient insulin in diabetic patients, doctors first want patients to control diet. Only by controlling your diet and eating small amounts of food can you keep your blood sugar within the normal range. As a result, the blood sugar level is normal, because the body does not get enough nutrients, the blood is even more insufficient, the person has no spirit, the muscles are not elastic, lose their luster, and the person becomes thin.

Although the blood sugar level remains within the normal range, I should not overeat a little bit of food. To be honest, as long as I eat an extra bite of rice, your blood sugar level will be different. In order to keep the blood sugar level within the normal range, my daily diet is rationed. I only eat a little rice at noon, which is about 50 to 100 grams rice. In the morning it is milk, oats, flaxseed meal, an egg, and potatoes in the evening. The daily diet is mainly vegetables, supplemented by meat, and one fruit a day. There is no limit to the type of fruit. Most of the time, I eat apples. Western proverb says, eat an apple a day and stay away from the doctor.

Seeing colleagues eating all kinds of delicious food without restraint, I don't feel too greedy. Seeing the plump posture of the female compatriots, it is not to mention envious. At the beginning of the year, after my blood sugar level remained stable for a few years, I decided to gain weight.

To gain weight, one needs to be able to eat, the spleen and stomach can absorb well, and the second is to be able to sleep. A diabetic can't just let go of eating and drinking. Moreover, the spleen and stomach function is poor, and the absorption rate is not high, so if I want to eat, I must eat scientifically and intelligently.

In order to nourish my stomach, first of all, I quit the habit of drinking milk in the morning for many years. Milk is cold and difficult to digest. Although calcium supplementation has a lot of nutritional value, it is not good for the digestion and operation of the spleen and stomach. I made all kinds of beans I eat in the morning into a paste, in order to allow the spleen and stomach to better absorb. Doesn't it mean that the spleen and stomach likes finely minced, soft and warm food the most?

Since the beginning of last year, I have eaten barley, yam, tash, red dates, mung bean, lily, red bean, red dates from Xinjiang Hotan every morning, and porridge cooked together. When resting at home, except for the same morning as usual, I eat a large bowl of noodle soup with broth at noon, an apple in the afternoon, and black glutinous rice, millet, red dates, red beans, sweet potatoes, etc. to boil porridge in the evening. The whole bowl is full and the whole body is warm. Take half a tablet of hypoglycemics at night. After such an experiment of replenishing qi and blood, I found that not only did the blood sugar level not rise, When I increased the amount of food, there was no immediate increase in the blood sugar level. Sleep has also been good.

After a few months, I gained weight, the digestive capacity of my spleen and stomach was strengthened, and my sugar tolerance was also enhanced.

By supplementing qi and blood, I feel that supplementing qi and blood and regulating the spleen and stomach are complementary. With sufficient qi and blood, good sleep, the function of the spleen and stomach is good, the digestive function is enhanced, and the ability of pancreatic islet self-regulation is improved.

Nourishing the Liver is the Key to Ensuring Sufficient Qi

and Blood

In Canada, apart from going to work, shopping, and returning from work, there are no leisure activities. There are also countless gatherings of friends, which is simply incomparable with the previous domestic life. People who can't resist loneliness should never emigrate, only those who like quietness can endure loneliness.

I rarely go out in my spare time. Basically, I watch news online, chat, watch TV, and connect with society and the world from the Internet. We all know that people who use the Internet a lot are very harmful to their eyesight. Chinese medicine says that looking at things for a long time hurts blood. When the blood is sufficient, the eyes are clear and bright. The color of the whites of the eyes is cloudy and yellow, indicating that the liver is insufficient. People who have been in front of the computer for a long time are mostly dull-eyed and lethargic.

The liver is an organ in the body whose main function is metabolism. Its function is to deoxidize, store glycogen, and synthesize secreted proteins. The liver also produces bile in the digestive system.

The liver is the largest digestive gland in the human digestive system and an important organ for metabolism in the human body. The liver is also the largest detoxification organ in the human body. Toxins, wastes, poisons eaten in the body, drugs that damage the liver, etc, must also be detoxified by the liver. The liver breaks down toxic substances absorbed by the intestine or manufactured by other parts of the body, and then secreted in the form of harmless substances into the bile or blood and then excreted from the body.

The fat content of the normal liver is very low, and the liver itself has the function of transferring and synthesizing fat. However, if the fat in the liver increases and cannot be resolved and transferred, the liver will harden and become cirrhosis. When I checked before going abroad, the doctor told me that I had a mild fatty liver. Although there was no major problem at the time, I should not take it lightly. Most diabetic patients have more or less fatty liver problems, which are liver diseases caused by metabolic disorders, and belong to metabolic diseases like insufficient insulin secretion.

To protect the liver and nourish the liver, we must first pay attention to food hygiene. Do not drink cold water, do not eat cold seafood. Because clams, oysters and shellfish are susceptible to hepatitis A virus infection. I used to eat raw seafood occasionally in China. After I lived in Canada, I never drank cold water or eaten cold seafood.

Excessive consumption of cooked seafood can also cause problems for the liver. Once, I ate seafood, which was dried clams with their shells removed. The clams have a high protein content. I scrambled eggs with clams, it was very fragrant, and I ate a lot at once. In the afternoon, my stomach began to feel uncomfortable and pained. I started to have a fever at night, and then my urine was red and bloodshot. I was horrified, I don't know why this happened. I just ate scrambled eggs with clams, but I ate twice as much as usual. I checked the information online and said that eating too much seafood would increase the burden on the kidneys and cause the kidney capillaries to rupture. Now I am relieved, it is not a kidney disease.

That night, I kept drinking water, and the color of my urine gradually changed from red to yellow. By the next morning, the color of my urine became normal, light yellow and transparent. Why does this happen. The liver is an organ for detoxification. Eating too much clams at once causes an extra burden on the liver. The liver has no time to detoxify, so it delegates the task of breaking down high protein to the kidneys. Excessive protein is beyond the ability of the kidneys to decompose, so the kidneys can't stand it, causing the rupture of the kidney capillaries, causing mild hematuria. From this point of view, the five internal organs of the body are all the same and affect each other, and the disconnection of one link directly affects the next link. Therefore, it is more certain that the treatment of diabetes is a systematic project.

My biggest worry is that eating too many health supplements will affect the liver. I have to eat essential vitamins and mineral health products every day, which brings a lot of burden to the liver. Necessary health products must be eaten, so you should eat propolis and lecithin that protect the liver at the same time, and eat some bloodenriching foods, increase fresh blood, ensure sufficient blood, and make the liver work effortlessly, detoxify and detoxify easily.

Ensuring sleep is also the key to nourishing and protecting liver. 1 to 3 o'clock in the morning is to enter a deep sleep state, this time is the best time to nourish liver and blood, on the contrary, there will be insufficient blood nourishment. I go to bed at 11 and a half every day, no more than 12 o'clock at the latest, and I am guaranteed to enter a deep sleep state between 1 am and 3 am. Get 7 to 8 hours of sleep a day. As the saying goes: " The liver hides blood. " It means that the blood flows to the limbs during daytime activities, and the blood is hidden in the liver at night when sleeping. If you stay up late for a long time, the blood cannot be cleaned and replenished, the liver will be overdrawn, the internal organs of the human body will not be able to get normal blood supply, and people's health will be in trouble.

Conditioning Tendons and Repairing the Liver

Chinese medicine believes that the length of the tendons is one inch, and the longevity is ten years.

The main function of the tendons is to restrain the bones, connect the muscles of the limbs, and maintain various tissues and organs. The most basic function of the tendons is to stretch and pull the joints to make various movements. The tendons need to be moved frequently, that is, stretched, to maintain stretch and elasticity.

We generally focus on physical health care on the internal organs or qi and blood. Few people are interested in the maintenance of tendons, except for some special occupations, such as athletes and dancers who need to stretch, protect tendons, and strengthen tendons..

The poor coordination and flexibility of the body are not only the result of long-term inactivity, but also contraction, which is one of the characteristics of accelerating body aging. People with contractions are almost less agile than before, walking not vigorously, lower back tends to bend, limbs stiff, and legs and feet do not fall well. The muscles in the body shrink, forming uneven lumps, which can also compress nerves and cause pain, pressure blood vessels and cause insufficient blood supply, dystrophy of muscles and veins, numbness, and numbness. We saw some old people bending over, walking very hard, moving step by step, this is the obvious back contraction phenomenon.

Many diseases are caused by contractions, such as dizziness, headache, and neck and shoulder pain can be caused by contractions in the neck and shoulders. Chest tightness, back pain, and fatigue can be caused by contractions in the chest and back. Sore waist, soft knees, pain and numbness in the buttocks and lower extremities can be caused by the contraction of the waist, buttocks, and hamstrings.

A few years ago, I did an experiment. Lying on the carpet, I lifted my hands up against the ground. I stretched my left arm to the number 2 of the clock, and I couldn't lift it up anymore. The tendons inside were tensed and painful. Carefully touched on the arm, found many small bumps, uneven. I sat cross-legged on my feet, and the pain in my feet was unbearable, the tendons inside were pulling and hurting. I pulled my legs, the tendons on my legs shrunk severely, and my thighs had no elasticity at all, and they protested to me stiffly. It turns out that most of the muscles in my body started to contract.

The theory of traditional Chinese medicine, the liver governs the tendons. If we want to nourish our liver, we must nourish our muscles. Nourishing good tendons is an effective way to restore the normal function of the liver. People with weak liver function also have stiffness in their tendons. Chinese medicine believes that blood vessels belong to the category of tendons, and nourishing tendons is equivalent to assisting in strengthening the function of blood vessels.

Chinese medicine believes that the tendons benefit from blood and can walk and work. Once the blood cannot supply nutrients in a timely manner, the tendons will be starved, lose their original elasticity, and will shrink, resulting in "blood does not nourish the tendons, and the tendons do not solid bones". Staying up late, working in front of the computer for too long, or long-term use of the eyes by the copywriters can hurt the liver the most. the liver stores blood, blood nourishes the muscles, and nourishes the liver, and the muscles are strong.

Strengthening tendons can open up the governor channel and bladder meridian on the back. The governor channel is the meeting of all yangs, the channel of vitality, this channel will strengthen the kidney, and if the kidney is strong, the energy of the person will become stronger. The bladder meridian is the body's largest detoxification system and an important barrier against wind and cold. If the bladder meridian is unobstructed, it is difficult for wind and cold to invade, and internal toxins are discharged at any time. Strengthening tendons is extremely beneficial to assist in curing diabetes.

The knee is the home of tendons, and kneeling is a good way to nourish tendons. After get off work, sometimes I kneel in front of the computer and watch the news. There are also some ways to strengthen the tendons, such as raising both arms, and stretching the whole body as much as possible, which is a bit like a yoga exercise, and then stretch left and right, and rotate the left and right waist. Tired of typing, I knelt on the carpet with my hips sitting on my feet, my whole body lay down, stretched my hands forward as far as possible, and pulled the whole arms and back muscles. Or stretch your arms and waist as much as possible on the ground like a dog crawl. There is also sitting on a yoga mat with alternate legs sitting cross-legged, or straight legs and two hands to hold the feet, stretch hard, the tendons of the legs and back will be pulled very comfortably, and the legs will be easy to walk.

In short, there are many ways to stretch the tendons. We can do it as convenient and comfortable as we can. We don't have to practice the soft skills of a dancer, as long as it can relieve fatigue, invigorate the spirit, and make people feel good and full of vitality. The legs and feet are strong, the limbs are flexible, and the coordination of the whole body is good to achieve the goal.

The tendons of the body become softer, the side effects of the liver are less, and the blood can be concentrated to provide fresh blood.

Gallbladder and LiverBile is a special fluid that flows in the bile ducts, is secreted by the liver, and is stored in the gallbladder. Studies have shown that high-protein and high-fat foods can cause a large amount of bile secretion and excretion, while carbohydrate foods have less effect. The human body controls the secretion and excretion of bile through both nerve and humoral pathways.

The role of bile is mainly the role of bile salts or bile acids. Bile salts or bile acids can be used as emulsifiers to emulsify fat, reduce the surface tension of fat, emulsify fat into microdroplets, and disperse in aqueous solution, thus increasing the area of action of pancrelipase. Bile acids can also be combined with fatty acids to form water-soluble complexes and promote the absorption of fatty acids.

Liver cells continuously secrete bile, but during the non-digesting period, the bile secreted by liver cells is stored in the gallbladder. During digestion, bile is directly discharged from the liver and from the gallbladder into the duodenum to neutralize part of the gastric acid. When the biliary tract is blocked and bile cannot enter the duodenum, the digestion and absorption of fat will be hindered, which can cause steatorrhea. Bile salts can inhibit the absorption of sodium and water by the colon. If the small intestine absorbs bile salts obstructively, a large amount of bile salts enter the colon, often causing watery diarrhea. Bile can stimulate the movement of the bowel, so the lack of bile will cause the weakening of the bowel movement and the accumulation of food in the intestine.

Bile is a digestive juice that emulsifies fats, but does not contain digestive enzymes. Bile plays an important role in the digestion and absorption of fat.

The functions of various parts of the human body can neither be overused, causing fatigue and exhaustion, nor can they not cause local function atrophy if they are not used for a long time. The enzymes secreted by the pancreas include proteins, fats, and various enzymes that decompose other substances. Insulin secreted by the pancreas is a special enzyme that decomposes sugar. The bile secreted by the liver is mainly used to break down fat.

If a vegetarian is determined not to eat animal fats and stays vegetarian for a long time, then what are these enzymes and bile that break down fats for? If the bile secreted by the liver does not have the opportunity to digest and decompose fat, the information fed back to the liver is that the bile is useless. After a long time, the liver will refuse to secrete bile. This is why people who have been vegetarians for a long time suddenly can't stand the stomach after eating meat, and it is difficult to digest.

Bile is used to digest fat, and if fat and moisture enter the liver, the gallbladder will also be eroded by fatty fluid and moisture. The bile biochemically produced by fatty liver can only be fatty bile, or the bile duct is blocked resulting in poor bile excretion, which affects the need for bile to be sent to the small intestine for digestion, causing indigestion diseases.

If the liver and gallbladder function is weak, bile cannot work normally, and fat cannot be well decomposed, absorbed and excreted. Some people have to have their gallbladder removed due to gallstones or other gallbladder diseases. Without the gallbladder, bile cannot be stored, which will cause bile reflux, and the food eaten is easily excreted. Usually, they have to go to the toilet soon after eating.

The bile secretion is normal, the digestion ability is good, and the gastrointestinal absorption ability is good. The absorption capacity is good, the hematopoietic material in the body is sufficient, the blood is abundant, the internal organs are full, and the body has the strength to work. On the contrary, insufficient bile secretion affects normal digestion and poor gastrointestinal absorption.

If the liver is healthy, the gallbladder is healthy, the liver secretes enough bile, and the ability to digest fat is normal. If there is a problem with the liver, the secretion of bile will be affected, and the fat cannot be broken down and digested if there is not enough bile.

Red Dates

There is a folk saying that "eat three jujubes a day, and you will not be old at a hundred years old". Jujube is a cheap and beautiful tonic in ordinary people's homes. Almost every Chinese family can't live without jujube in their diet. Red dates have been the best blood-supplementary ingredients since ancient times, especially women who have just given birth to children need more nourishment from red dates.

However, there are many medical and health care books that say that people with diabetes are not suitable for eating red dates. They believe that red dates are high in sugar and are not suitable for supplementing for diabetics, so as to avoid the increase of blood sugar and the deterioration of the disease. Therefore, since I got diabetes, I followed the doctor's instructions to control my diet and control foods with high sugar content, so I said goodbye to red dates.

Due to the comprehensive treatment of diabetes, my blood sugar level has been controlled within the normal range in recent years, and my blood sugar level has also been normal. However, due to the instability of blood glucose levels during the initial period of diabetes, the problem of weight loss, coupled with diet control, has never gained weight.

Therefore, I decided to increase my qi and blood to increase the body's self-healing ability and at the same time increase my weight. I started to eat beef, red dates, red beans, black glutinous rice, these fast-acting blood-enriching foods. At the beginning, I ate 8 red dates a day, and then increased to 20 a day. I just take half a hypoglycemic medicine after dinner, and I also eat some fruits. My blood sugar level can still be kept within the normal value. I have eaten red dates every day for six months. Obviously, the sugar tolerance in my body has increased. Sweet food is no longer a ban on me. Once, after eating dinner, I bought a medium-sized pizza. I couldn't help but ate two more pizzas and took half a hypoglycemic drug. The blood sugar level was normal the next day.

By eating red dates, I feel that my body is full of qi and blood, the saliva in my mouth increases, and the sticky feeling in my mouth is much less. The veins at the bottom of my tongue were thick and big, like two earthworms lying there, black and blue. Now the two large earthworms at the bottom of the tongue are gone, the veins have become gentle, and the tongue has changed from purple to pink. This shows that the fat congestion in the blood vessels has been gradually cleared.

According to the research of relevant experts, red jujube is rich in cyclic adenosine monophosphate, which is an essential substance for human energy metabolism. It can enhance muscle strength, eliminate fatigue, dilate blood vessels, increase myocardial contractility, improve myocardial nutrition, and have good effects on the prevention and treatment of cardiovascular diseases.

Jujube has the functions of nourishing deficiency and replenishing qi, nourishing blood and calming the nerves, strengthening the spleen and stomach, etc. It is a good health care nutritional product for patients with weak spleen and stomach, insufficient qi and blood, fatigue and insomnia. Jujube has good curative effect on acute and chronic liver inflammation, liver cirrhosis, anemia, allergic purpura and other diseases.

Red dates protect the liver. The carbohydrates, fat and protein contained in red dates are nutrients that protect the liver. It can promote the synthesis of protein in the liver, increase the content of serum globin and albumin, and adjust the ratio of albumin to globulin.

Autumn is dry and easy to get angry. Cooking Tremella can nourish yin, nourish body fluid, put some red dates to nourish blood, and put some lilies to moisturize dryness.

Autumn is dry and easy to get angry. Cooking white fungus can nourish yin and body fluid, put some red dates to nourish blood, and put some lily to moisten dryness.

We have to try everything before we know if it is appropriate. Through my experience in eating red dates, I personally think that red dates are suitable for us diabetic people. However, it should be noted that eating red dates should be done after the blood sugar level has stabilized for a period of time. And we have to be aware of our physical condition in order to treat the symptoms, otherwise blindly eating red dates will increase our blood sugar level. At the same time, when the blood sugar level is stable, we should not be greedy to eat more red dates. After all, the sugar tolerance of diabetic patients is limited.

Chapter 4

REMOVE DAMPNESS AND DETOX, CLEAR BLOOD VESSELS AND INTESTINES, AND CLEAR OBSTACLES FOR ISLET RECOVERY

The theory of traditional Chinese medicine believes that all diseases are caused by blood stasis, and blood stasis is the cause of disease. The blood vessels and internal organs in the human body are like rivers, lakes and seas. Once the stasis is blocked, it will flood into a disaster. If it is dredged in time, the waterway will be smooth, the river will be safe, and the disease of the human body will be solved.

People all know the importance of Qi and blood for life maintenance, and they pay more attention to nourishing blood and nourishing Qi. But few people put dampness and detoxification in the key position of treatment. In today's diseases, due to the environment, diet, and living habits, there are more and more opportunities for cold and dampness to invade. As the saying goes, most diseases are caused by cold and dampness.

In fact, our human health has been harmed and we have suffered various diseases, which are largely related to the cold and dampness in the body, the toxic substances in the blood and the cells that have died of old age and disease have not been cleaned up in time. These residues do no harm to the body and accumulate in various parts of the body. Wherever the weak part is, it is easy to cause disease, and the occurrence of diabetes is no exception. If we want to make our body really relaxed, we need to clean up, thoroughly remove dust, garbage, all kinds of toxic substances, dead cells and free radicals.

Metabolic Disease

There is life, there is death, this is the irresistible natural law of mankind. The continuation of human beings evolved from the combination of eggs and sperm, then from infant growth to maturity, becoming a vigorous adult, and gradually aging and toward death. All of this is a process that follows the laws of nature and also shows the process of human evolutionary history.

Cells in all parts of the body have the law of growth and shrinkage. The metabolism of the human body is to excrete the dead cells and toxins to make room for the production of new cells.

There are a lot of toxins in the blood, which is the main cause of cardiovascular and cerebrovascular diseases. The blood is metabolized, and the old blood is constantly being rewashed to keep the blood clean. The liver needs to generate fresh blood every day to replace the consumed blood.

The intestine is a place where nutrients from food are absorbed and waste is eliminated. It is a pollution source of toxic substances in the body. Therefore, cleaning the intestine is as important as cleaning the blood vessels.

However, the metabolism in the body is carried out regularly, too much or insufficient metabolism can cause metabolic diseases. Diabetes is a metabolic disease caused by endocrine disorders in which insulin is relatively or absolutely lacking in the body.

There are many causes of metabolic dysregulation, but most are due to insufficient raw materials to generate these fresh cells, and certain obstacles that affect the ability of intrinsic tissue generation. We all know that the raw materials for generating these cells come from the food we eat every day, and the quality provided to the hematopoietic organs depends on the absorption capacity of the spleen, stomach, pancreas, and small intestine. If the spleen, stomach, pancreas, and small intestine suffer from cold and moisture, they cannot absorb the essence needed by the body normally. Therefore, the liver cannot produce the blood needed by the human body with high quality and quantity. If the liver cannot provide the fresh blood that the human body needs, it cannot detoxify normally, resulting in insufficient food for the various organs, malnutrition, and weakening of the immune system, leading to diseases.

The blood vessels and intestines of the human body are the most easily contaminated places. Cleaning the blood vessels and intestines is like removing dust at home, wiping the table and sucking the floor every day to keep it clean and tidy. If the floor of the house is not cleaned, the table is not cleaned after eating, and the dishes and leftovers that have been eaten are piled in the cleaning pool, the air in the house will definitely be filled with sour smell after a long time, and it will b e dirty everywhere. Our intestines and blood are the same. Contaminated intestines and blood are prone to problems and cause various diseases. Therefore, blood vessels and intestines should be cleaned every day.

Ten Diseases and Nine Cold Dampness

Most of our diseases are caused by cold. As the saying goes, there are ten diseases and nine cold. Here I add a wet after the cold, because the humidity in the body is more harmful to our health than the cold.

A person is born with a physique with sufficient yang energy. Many people still remembers that there were no diaper stickers in the past, and two- and three-year-old children still wore open-crotch pants, because children in this age group have poor self-control and can't take care of themselves, so it is convenient to wear open-crotch pants. A child who has just learned to run, running in the snow with bare buttocks, dancing and playing, is not afraid of the cold at all. As the saying goes, a child's buttocks have three fires. It means that children are physically active and are not afraid of cold, but they are more afraid of cold as they get older.

In daily life, most of us know how to avoid cold, but do not know how to avoid moisture, so the harm of moisture to the human body is often ignored and not easy to be detected. It has been lurking in the human body for many years, slowly hurting our body until it appears. People become alert only when they have the symptoms of harm. However, the disease has already appeared at this time, causing harm to the health of the body.

Humans come out of their mother's womb with yang energy, and their bodies are soft and soft. From the moment we start eating food, the body begins to change. In daily life, people inevitably eat a lot of cold food, and when people come into contact with nature, they inevitably encounter a lot of cold weather. These chills enter our healthy body little by little, and slowly stiffen our warm internal organs and bodies. There are many personal behaviors contaminated with cold and humidity that can be avoided, such as, try to avoid eating cold food, do not walk in the rain on rainy days, do not swim in cold water, do not camp in the wild, do not wear wet clothes, wet shoes, etc. But people's nature is to choose what they like, even if it goes against their health, especially when we are young, relying on our own health, we don't care about anything.

I remember that when I was young, I liked to walk in the rain. I didn't care about getting wet from the rain. On the contrary, I liked the feeling of being wet by drizzle. The surrounding is rainy and foggy, very poetic. I also like to go barefoot in the rain, and I don't even think of any sequelae caused by getting wet in the rain.

After washing my hair often, I like to have wet hair floating in the wind or wash my hair before going to bed and fall asleep with wet hair. The result of these inadvertent bad habits is that the cold and dampness camps in our body, step by step, devouring our healthy body, until we get sick.

What is Poison

A toxin is a substance that can interfere with normal physiological activities and disrupt body functions. Intrinsic toxins such as: free radicals, stool, cholesterol, fat, uric acid, lactic acid, water poisoning and congestion.

Exotic toxins such as: air pollution, pesticide residues in vegetables, automobile exhaust, industrial exhaust gas, chemicals, radiation, preservatives in food, excessive heavy metals in cosmetics, junk food and other toxic side effects brought about by modern civilization, pathogenic microorganisms.

Endogenous toxin: Metabolic waste produced in metabolism. When angry, the human body will produce a kind of acid poison, intestinal stool and toxins produced by disorders of sugar and fat and protein metabolism.

What is Dampness

The water in the human body is like rivers and springs in nature, as well as fog and humidity in various forms. The blood in the blood vessels is like a river, the lymph in the lymph glands is like spring water, and the moisture in the human body is like the dampness and mist in nature. The water is flowing and clear, and the dampness is foggy and wet. Anyone who lives in the Yangtze River Delta in China knows that during the plum rain season at the turn of spring and summer, it rains non-stop, the air smells of dampness everywhere, and the house is no exception. The quilt at home was stained with moisture and felt damp on the body. So when the sun is out, every family pulls up the rope in the yard, and takes out the quilt and clothes to dry in the sun to remove dampness.

Although dampness is also water, it does not belong to the scope of water metabolism, which means that the water metabolism system in the body cannot control dampness. Therefore, dampness is unscrupulously destroyed in the body. Among the pathogenic wind, cold, summer heat, dampness, dryness, and fire, the "six evil qi", Chinese medicine is most afraid of dampness. Dampness is the easiest to penetrate, and the dampness evil never fights alone, but always combines with other evil spirits. With dampness in the human body, it is easy to become lazy, sleepy, and tired, and lack energy.

The dampness is divided into internal dampness and external moisture. Internal dampness is moisture generated through food, and external dampness is moisture introduced through the skin.

Endogenous moisture: some moisture comes from food, sugar generates moisture, sticky food also generates moisture, excess meat also generates moisture, and long-term consumption of rice made by rice cooker will also generate a lot of moisture in the body. I have done a comparison, the rice made by the rice cooker is sticky, and the rice grains are not easy to separate from the rice grains, and they are mainly lumps. In the traditional way of making rice in the past, rice and water are put into the pot together, put more water in the rice cooker, wait for the water and rice to boil, boil for a while, and pour out the excess water in the pot. Rice soup is called rice soup oil. The rice made by this method is very fluffy, the rice grains are scattered one by one, and it is not sticky in the mouth at all. Some comments on the Internet said that the moisture of the rice was boiled in the rice soup and poured out. I feel that the rice may be sticky because of the moisture. The method of removing the rice soup to remove the moisture is a traditional folk diet. Now it is rare in the cities, including the rural areas, because it is very easy to cook with an electric rice cooker, pour the water and rice into the pot, press the switch, and you are ready to eat. Although modern innovation has brought us a lot of convenience, it has also impacted our fine traditional way of life.

Exogenous dampness: Some moisture penetrates from the skin when dealing with water, such as walking barefoot in the rain on a rainy day, and sleeping after washing your head. When a person sleeps, the pores of the hair are open. The skin temperature is also high, so the water from the hair slips into the body through the hair hole that opens the door. If the shoes are wet, they should be changed in time, and wearing wet shoes is also easy to enter the dampness. People living in North America like to travel, often as a family, or as a group of relatives and friends, camping in a tent near the water or in the mountains at night. At night, the damp mist from the waterside and the forest penetrates into the human body through the pores of the human body unconsciously. When sleeping on the ground, the moisture of the land will also erode into the body. Many rheumatic diseases are caused inadvertently in this way.

There is also moisture that remains in the body from infection and destruction of tissue fluid. Once dampness enters the human body, it does not appear in the form of water, but mainly adheres to various parts of the body with moisture, which is the same scourge as high blood sugar. The Five Elements Theory of Traditional Chinese Medicine believes that the pancreas has the characteristics of "earth", and earth can easily absorb water, so the spleen (pancreas) is most likely to be damaged by moisture entering the body. The ancients said that "when the spleen is deficient, the lung qi first disappears, "indicating that the functions of the spleen and the lungs are interrelated and affect each other. When the spleen is deficient to a certain extent, and the lungs are not nourished, it is easy to have shortness of breath, lack of qi and lazy words, and shortness of breath when moving.

Dampness becomes cold and damp when it encounters cold. This is like in winter, if the climate is dry, no matter how cold it is, people can still accept it, but if the humidity is heavy, people will be uncomfortable. The winter in the south is more uncomfortable than the winter in the north, because the humidity in the south is heavier, and the cold and humidity are overwhelming. The cold and dampness in the human body can damage the blood circulation system of the human body more than the cold air, making the blood flow not only slow and astringent.

Dampness becomes hot and humid when it encounters heat. This is like the hot and humid summer in Lingnan, China, which makes people breathless, while the summer in Northeast China is scorching, the climate is dry, and it feels good to sweat.

When dampness encounters wind, it becomes rheumatism. It is easy to drive the wind, but once it becomes rheumatism, it is often a chronic disease, and rheumatoid arthritis is difficult to cure. When moisture is under the skin, obesity is formed, and puffiness is also a health problem that is difficult to deal with.

When moisture encounters high blood sugar in the blood vessels, it becomes sugar dampness. This is the patent of our diabetic patients. Originally, high blood sugar in the blood vessels is troublesome. When mixed with moisture, it becomes sticky and astringent, which is more harmful to blood vessels, causing various complications.

When moisture meets fat in the blood vessels, it becomes phlegm. For patients with type 2 diabetes, phlegm dampness is one of the main causes of pancreatic disease and insulin deficiency.

There is an old saying: "Thousands of colds are easy to get rid of, but wetness is hard to get rid of. The wetness is sticky and turbid, like oil into the noodles. " If the dampness does not go away, no matter how many supplements and medicines are taken, it will not work at all. In life, many people suffer from fatty liver, asthma, hypertension, diabetes, cardiovascular and cerebrovascular diseases, and even malignant tumors. In fact, these diseases are related to dampness and phlegm.

Dampness and Pancreas

Here in Chinese medicine, the spleen is the pancreas. Traditional Chinese medicine has always believed that the pancreas likes dryness and hates dampness, so the pancreas is most afraid of excessive moisture and causes diseases. The pancreas belongs to the soil, and the soil needs water to be irrigated. Therefore, the pancreas controls the transportation and transformation of water and is the biochemical source of body fluids.

Chinese medicine believes that the pancreas has the function of transporting water and dampness. The so-called transport and transformation of water and dampness means that the pancreas plays an important role in regulating and maintaining the metabolism of water and fluid in the body.

The pancreas transports the excess water from various tissues and organs of the body to the corresponding organs (such as lungs, kidneys, bladder, fur, etc.) in time, and turns it into sweat and urine to be excreted from the body. Therefore, in the whole process of water metabolism, the pancreas plays an important pivotal role, promoting the circulation and excretion of water. The transportation and transformation functions of the pancreas are normal, and the digestion and absorption of food, as well as the transportation and distribution of subtle nutrients are all functioning well, so as to ensure the distribution, transportation and excretion of water in the body and maintain a normal and relatively balanced state.

Conversely, if the pancreas does not function normally and the spleen is weak, not only will abdominal distention, unformed stools, fatigue and other digestive disorders occur, It will also cause abnormal water metabolism, resulting in a variety of pathological changes of water stagnation. In life, some people have edema, some people usually have a lot of phlegm, some people like diarrhea, and some people have thick and greasy tongue coating. These conditions seem to be unrelated, but Chinese medicine believes that they are related to pancreas deficiency and excessive moisture in the body. The pancreas is easily troubled by dampness, so it is easy to generate internal dampness.

The pancreas neither likes wetness nor dislikes dryness. It likes to take the middle way, to balance dryness and dampness, to maintain the balance of yin and yang of the pancreas, and to operate normally.

When the land is flooded, the soil contains too much water and the crops under it will rot. If the water content in the land is too low, drought will occur. If the crops are not moisturized by water, good food will not grow, and even the grains will not be harvested. The same is true for the pancreas in the human body. The growth laws of nature are the same for all living organisms.

Whether the pancreas is excessive or lacking, it will cause the pancreas the source of body fluid biochemistry, to become unbalanced, resulting in a shortage of pancreatic islets in the pancreatic endocrine system in the body, leading to diabetes.

Dampness and Lymph Nodes (1)

The blood circulatory system of our human body is the most harmful to dampness, and the blood circulatory system is composed of the cardiovascular and lymphatic systems.

Invasion of cold and dampness in the blood and lymphatic system is just like the ice layer on a river in winter causes qi stagnation and blood stasis in the blood vessels of the human body, and lymphatic swelling. Wherever the cold and dampness is, blood stasis and lymphatic inflammation are prone to occur.

We are all familiar with blood stasis and know how to clear it, but we are seldom clear about diseases of the lymphatic system. The lymphatic system not only secretes lymph fluid to participate in the circulation in the blood, but is also an important immune system of the human body. It can be said that the lymphatic system is the bodyguard of vascular circulation. The consequences of lymphatic disease are very serious. It can easily lead to the imbalance of body fluids in the body, resulting in systemic edema and heart failure.

Once the human body enters the moisture, and a large amount of moisture accumulates in the body, no matter what kind of evil it encounters, it will form a greater lethality. When a person suffers from cold and dampness, it is also possible to suffer from dampness and heat. Both cold and heat are linked to dampness. The interweaving of cold, heat and dampness increases the negative energy of dampness.

The vascular system is most afraid of cold and lack of oxygen. Cold is like natural ice, freezing the water on the river, making it unable to flow and stagnating blood. The lymphatic system is most afraid of dampness and hypoxia. The dampness makes the lymphatic system cover a layer of damp cloth, swelling, and lymphatic fluid cannot be secreted and diffused well. I used to live in the basement for two years. During that period, I often caught a cold, my throat was often inflamed, and the lymph on both sides of my jaw always bulged up with two large lumps. A colleague of mine also lives in the basement. She also had a small cold and her lymphatic inflammation has not been well for several months. Later, I moved out of the basement and lived in a sunny room, and the inflammation of the lymph gradually disappeared.

Lymphopathy, in addition to bacterial infection and other factors, are mostly related to the invasion of dampness. Luo Jing, a famous CCTV announcer, suffered from lymphoma and died young. I noticed in the photo that he has big eye bags. When he first joined CCTV as a news network host, he had eye bags. It is not normal for a person of his age. By the last time he hosted a news network, the bags under the eyes were already slack. The bag on the left side of his eye is obviously larger than the bag on the right side, which confirms the Chinese medicine says that the symptoms are manifested by men on the left and women on the right. Large bags under the eyes indicate that there is a lot of moisture in the body. There is moisture in the body for a long time, and the destruction of the endocrine system can be imagined.

After Luo Jing's stem cell transplant operation, the cancer cells in the lymph nodes in his body have disappeared. It can be said that the operation was a success. But after 9 times of chemotherapy, it not only killed cancer cells, but also killed normal cells, doubled the destruction of body fluids in the body, and made the body's water metabolism dysfunctional. His oral ulcers have been unable to heal and the pain is unbearable. It can be said that the immune system in the body has been completely destroyed.

After the operation, the leaders of CCTV went to the hospital to visit Luo Jing on the Dragon Boat Festival, and several people including the attending physician. Luo Jing went home for dinner in the evening, but he didn't feel well the next day and he immediately returned to the hospital and never went home again. Then, May 29th was his birthday. CCTV came to a group of colleagues to celebrate his birthday. On June 1st, his condition suddenly deteriorated. He suffered from heart failure on the 4th and passed away in the early morning of the 5th.

Why in a short period of time, the lymph nodes that have no cancer cells have relapsed, and there is no power to recover.

According to the treatment of Western medicine, Luo Jing's stem cell transplantation was successful, but the nursing work after transplantation was unsuccessful. Although the stem cell transplantation is successful, it is only a temporary cure. He should also follow the treatment of traditional Chinese medicine to remove dampness and detox, increase qi and blood, and support the reconstruction of the immune system. This is the cure. The treatment of lymphoma can be successful only when the symptoms and root causes are combined. For a long period of time after the operation, the patient must absolutely rest and avoid any public places and people that carry bacteria. Any factors such as excitement, exhaustion, and labor may cause the disease to worsen. In a real sense, Luo Jing's death was not due to lymphoma, but the sequelae of uncontrolled body fluid disorders and high-dose chemotherapy in the body.

Any disease of the lymphatic system needs to repair the pancreas, the biochemical source of body fluid, and fully repair the waterways. Restoring the normal function of the lymphatic system is a long-term task. Until the system is truly consolidated, it must not be taken lightly.

Dampness and Lymph Nodes (2)

Another example is former US First Lady Jacqueline. Kennedy, who also died from lymphoma. From many photos of her life, we can see that she likes to wear skirts, especially in the cold winter with her calves exposed and wearing stockings. In some books, it is described that she likes to party near the fireplace when she is young, which is obviously due to insufficient heat in her body to keep warm.

Jacqueline's voice was soft, a little hoarse, and not too loud, like an underdeveloped child with a lack of breath. The volume of a person's voice reflects Yuanyin (also known as True Yin, True Water, which is interdependent with Yuanyang, and is the essence of life), body fluid, blood, and the size of the air flow exhaled during pronunciation, the strength of the sound can also reflect the sufficiency of Yuanyin and Yuanyang in the human body. The volume is also closely related to the qi in the human body. A person's volume is related to the lungs, because the lungs are equivalent to the human body's music resonance box. With it, the sound volume can be effectively amplified. Therefore, when the resonance effect of the lungs is weakened, it will also lead to changes in the sound wall, resulting in hoarseness or even aphonia. Obviously, Jacqueline suffers from respiratory disease and qi stagnation and blood stasis.

Jacqueline found an induration on the back of her neck and was diagnosed with lymphoma after examination. The illness came suddenly, and she was completely unprepared psychologically. In fact, it was the dampness in her body and the result of years of living habits. Not only does Jacqueline not pay attention to keeping warm in the cold weather, she likes to eat ice cream, she likes to sit in the wetlands near the water and read a book.

Jacqueline has smoked since she was young. She is a cultural worker, works as an editor in a publishing house, and reads a large number of authors' manuscripts. She often works until she goes to bed at 2 o'clock at night and wakes up at 12 o'clock the next day. She has guaranteed sleep time. But the liver has no time for blood purification and hematopoiesis (human blood purification and hematopoiesis time from 12:00 to 3:00 in the night), although she rides, swims, and runs, she cannot replace the precious time and opportunity for the liver to purify blood and make hematopoiesis at night. Therefore, the blood in Jacqueline's blood vessels is basically old blood, which is easily damaged by bacteria and toxic substances in cigarettes. The role of the lymphatic system is to filter bacteria and help the body fight disease. If the blood is not purified for a long time and lacks the supplement and support of fresh blood, a large number of bacteria will make the lymphatic system too busy and overworked, until it becomes paralyzed, thus losing the normal function of the immune system.

Tobacco and alcohol are extremely acidic substances. People who smoke and drink for a long time can easily lead to an acidic constitution. Jacqueline. Kennedy has been smoking for many years, and her bad habits and smoking have acidified her constitution. She works as an editor of a publishing house. Long-term reading with her head down not only consumes a lot of her blood, but also the ischemia of her body is unable to clear the congestion on the cervical spine. Congestion of the cervical spine leads to poor lymphatic circulation, and the operation of the body is linked to each other and affects each other.

In our lifetime, the lymphatic system will almost inevitably experience more or less and inflammation, resulting in lymph node enlargement of varying degrees. In most cases, the swollen lymph nodes will return to their normal size after the inflammatory response is resolved. However, if it is a long-term, chronic inflammatory stimulation, hyperplasia, and enlarged lymph nodes, it is difficult to completely recover. Lymphoma is the result of lymphatic injury in prolonged fighting against the enemy.

In fact, lymphoma is the induration that Chinese medicine calls it, but this induration is not the induration of the blood vessels, but the induration on the lymph nodes. Chinese medicine explains that lymphoma is caused by wind, fire and blood dryness externally (the cause of hypofunction of metaplasia and blood, deficiency of blood, lack of body fluid), or stagnation of cold phlegm (the phlegm cannot be removed by freezing cold), the internal cause is worry, moodiness and anger, liver Stagnation of qi, phlegm and fire, qi stagnation and blood stasis, the internal deficiency of the internal organs due to insufficient nutrition, the loss of liver and kidney, and the loss of both qi and blood, it has become an induration. Lymphoma and what Chinese medicine calls shirong (neck tumor lump), Diseases such as malignant nucleus (cancer of a lump in a limb) and gangrene (a poisonous sore lump as hard as a stone) are similar.

Lymphoma and lymphatic inflammation are the same thing, but the length of the disease is different. Lymph has evolved from inflammation to a lethal lump, so it takes more time to resolve it in treatment.

Kennedy Jacqueline died less than half a year after fighting the disease. Her final death was not because of lymphoma, but because of the same high-dose chemotherapy as Luo Jing, her immune system was severely damaged. The treatment method of chemotherapy, for cancer patients, is to kill one thousand enemies and lose eight hundred for themselves. It should have taken a resting therapy to maintain physical strength and gradually restore the function of the immune system. But in a state of extreme frailty, she was eager to exercise to help her recover. In the cold wind of early spring, Jacqueline wore a thin silk scarf and went for a walk in New York's Central Park near her home. This rush to recover is undoubtedly equivalent to pulling the seedlings to encourage growth. Once the roots are separated from the soil, they cannot survive. Cancer patients after chemotherapy must absolutely rest and wait patiently for the gradual blooming of their vitaliy.

Dispelling dampness and detoxification are necessary measures to clean up various diseases. Only by removing the culprit of moisture, removing the toxic substances in the body, and eliminating the reserve army of the sick, can there be hope of recovery. Diabetes and lymphadenopathy are disorders of the endocrine system, both of which are blood problems. One is red blood and the other is white blood. They are two branches of the blood circulatory system. Most patients with diabetes have experienced lymphatic inflammation. In the first few years when I suffered from diabetes, my lymph nodes were often swollen and I took a lot of laxatives. (I said before)

Diabetes is a problem with the pancreas, the pancreas is the biochemical source of water in the body, and the lymph fluid is a component of the body fluid. The two are closely related. Protecting the lymphatic system is equivalent to keeping viruses and bacteria out of the door. Adds positive energy to the repair of the pancreas.

Dampness and Diabetic Foot (1)

Why is it that diabetic foot is not easy to heal, and antibiotics are not effective, and inflammation cannot be eliminated. Instead, the inflammation continues to worsen, and the limb is amputated as a last resort?

There are two main reasons for this. One of the main reasons is that the patient did not follow the doctor's instructions to strictly lower blood sugar. They eat what they want, drink what they want. Continue to maintain high blood sugar levels in the blood. The second is that the moisture in the body of diabetic patients is large, and the water transport and transformation function is poor. Water itself is a sinking substance. As the saying goes, water flows down. Humans are like plants. Too much water accumulates in the roots, and the roots will rot. If the feet of the human body accumulate too much moisture, they are easily infected and spread by bacteria, and slowly corrode and deteriorate to the surrounding area.

Diabetes patients are more likely to develop diabetic feet if they have heavy moisture in their bodies. Moist places are prone to mold and bacteria, and humidity generally occupies low-lying places. We often see swelling of legs and feet. We rarely hear of swelling of hands and arms. Because feet are the roots of people, moisture tends to stay in the feet. Once the water metabolism in the body is imbalanced, the legs and feet are prone to swelling. Similarly, it is not easy to heal after an external wound.

We store white sugar at home generally in jars and put them in a dry place. The small particles of white sugar are dispersed, just like sand. If the white sugar enters water or is heated, it will become sticky, and it will form a hard block after a long time. The high sugar in the blood can be easily lowered with hypoglycemic drugs, but if the high sugar in the blood seeps into the moisture, the blood will become sticky and thick, and the effect of taking the same hypoglycemic drugs will not be so good.

Dampness generally likes to go down in the body. People's lower limbs are most vulnerable to moisture damage. High blood sugar causes nerve lesions in our diabetic patients. The feeling is not sensitive, and it is easy to cause lesions in the large blood vessels and microvessels, and the blood flowing to the lower limbs is insufficient. Once the skin is traumatized, the nerves feel insensitive and the blood supply is insufficient to purify and nourish the wound, so the moisture starts to play a negative role. The first thing affected by moisture is the liquid. The lymph in the blood begins to swell and spread. Due to the effect of moisture and high sugar in the blood, the pancreatic drainage and absorption functions are blocked. There isn't enough positive energy to resist the damage of moisture.

I read on the Internet the experience of a diabetic friend before and after he became ill. This patient used to be a chef. He was born with a love for food, and his life and work were irregular. He became a fat and strong man at a young age. He once ate a food stall with his friends, threw the cigarette butt on his feet, and the meat was burning with oily smoke. He didn't feel it, others reminded him after seeing it, At the time, a large blister was burned on his toe by a cigarette butt.

A young man with a big blister on his foot is not a serious illness. He applied some burn medicine to the wound himself. After a week, there is no sign of improvement, and the toes are still inflamed and pus. Moreover, the color of the toes near the wound began to darken, first dark red, then purple, and then the toes turned black. He went to the doctor and the hospital diagnosed him with diabetes. The doctor instructed him to take hypoglycemic drugs, adjust his diet and so on. However, this little brother was born fond of food. He ate and drank a lot while taking medicine, which caused the wound on the right foot to never heal, continued to be infected, and had a fever that did not go away. He took all antibiotics, the infection kept getting worse, and finally, the entire right foot turned the color of charcoal. To save his life, the doctor had to amputate his right leg.

There is also a case of diabetic feet, which a colleague of mine told me happened to her good friend. This friend of hers loves rice and eats rice three times a day. Unfortunately, she has diabetes. The doctor said that her blood sugar level was very high, and she couldn't go down even after taking medicine. It had something to do with her love of eating rice. In order to lower her blood sugar level, the doctor asked her to give up rice. If she insists on eating, try to eat as little as possible, just eat one meal of rice a day. But she didn't listen to the doctor and continued to eat rice, and insisted on three meals a day. Soon, she suffered from diabetic foot, one leg began to swell, slowly turn black and necrotic. The doctor said, you must stop eating rice and lower your blood sugar, otherwise it will be life-threatening. However, the diabetic patient loved rice more than her own life, so she did not change her habit of eating rice. Before long, the inflammation of the diabetic foot spread to her upper body and took her life. For this sugar friend, life is precious, and the price of living is higher. If it is rice, both can be thrown away.

Since the infection caused by sugar dampness in the body is very rapid and serious, when a diabetic patient has a foot infection, the first thing to do is to lower the blood sugar level as soon as possible. Not only need to take hypoglycemic drugs, but more importantly, adjust the diet, mainly light vegetables, avoid all foods that may cause blood sugar to rise, and aquatic products, seafood, dairy products and other foods that are easy to cause wound infections and attacks. Excluding the destruction of the main enemy's high blood sugar, leaving the moisture to fight alone, it is relatively easy to deal with. To deal with the diseases of our human body, we must also learn to grasp the main contradictions, solve them separately, and overcome them individually.

The second is to remove dampness and detoxification. Anyone with a bit of common sense knows that an inflamed wound is the result of an invasion of bacteria that usually prefer to live, multiply, and expand in damp and dirty places. Thus, cleansed blood and lymph, free of moisture and toxins, helps to heal wounds.

If the moisture and toxins are left alone, the wound will continue to deteriorate and the cell tissue will die. The water metabolism of the necrotic site is imbalanced, the good body fluid in the body cannot enter and moisturize other good cell tissues, and the contaminated fluid cannot be absorbed and dissolved. The harmful substances in the water fluid quickly kill a large number of cells and tissues that are still good. Eventually leading to necrosis of the entire leg.

Dispelling dampness and detoxification can prevent the infected water from deteriorating in time, prevent it from flowing to the surrounding area, try to restore the body's ability to absorb the water, let the body absorb it naturally, and slowly heal the wound.

Dampness and Diabetic Foot (2)

I have had such an experience. One year I wore a pair of new leather shoes to work and walked back and forth for more than an hour. Fortunately, my feet didn't feel uncomfortable when I went there. When I got off work, my feet were not right when I walked halfway, and my big toe felt painful. I forcibly walked home, took off my shoes and checked, the big toenails on both feet were congested and a little purple. Changing into old shoes and walking were not affected, so I didn't take it seriously. I took a shower as usual, with my toes soaked in the shower. After a few days, I got up in the morning and felt something wrong. My right toe felt a little itchy. I thought it was a good symptom. It didn't hurt even if I touched it with my hands. Because the toenails were a bit long, I used nail scissors to repair them. Unexpectedly, as soon as I cut it off, the place where the toenails and the flesh were connected opened, and a puddle of water rushed out.

I looked down and shocked me. It turned out that all the toenails were inflamed inside. It's all liquid and bulging. I immediately became nervous at the time, because I knew the consequences of a diabetic foot inflammation.

My heart tightened suddenly, and my brain started to work at a high level. What should I do? The gill of the big toenail is already inflamed, but it must not spread any more, and the inflammation must be controlled in a local area. After a few seconds, I immediately wiped off the dripping water with cotton wool. The water in the nails was constantly flowing, and I kept using cotton wool to wipe it off, because the affected area did not feel any pain under the water soaking. So I started to squeeze gently on the nail cap, trying to squeeze out all the water inside until the water stopped flowing out. My blood sugar level was very stable. It has been a long time since I took hypoglycemic drugs, but I was afraid that the inflammation of my toes would affect the stability of blood sugar level, so I started taking hypoglycemic drugs on the same day.

In order to prevent the disturbance of high blood sugar and prevent all possible deterioration, in the days when the wound is inflamed, I absolutely do not eat seafood, foods and vegetables that are easy to cause severe wounds, and eat some light food. Eat barley soup every morning to remove dampness, and wrap injured feet with plastic bags when taking a bath to avoid water. In this way, because of the good self-protection measures, the inflamed toenails did not worsen, and there was no pain, and there was no inconvenience in walking as usual. After a few days, the inflammation on my right toe was completely gone, the swollen big toe was as thin as normal, and then the injured toenail fell off with a new cap. Strangely, my left toe was also squeezed black and purple by the new shoes, but it was not inflamed, nor did the nails fall off, but the new long nails came up little by little to replace the black and purple nail cover.

A colleague of mine went out to play once, accidentally kicked her big toe on the threshold, and the toenail kicked purple, just like my toenail cover was purple. It has been several weeks. Not only has the inflammation of her toenails not been good, but it has become more serious. The inflammation of the toes is slow to walk and turn. After seeing Chinese and Western medicine, the doctor prescribes anti-inflammatory drugs and takes the every three hours. The Chinese doctor says to be patient and it will take a while to be effective. This colleague of mine does not hav e diabetes, but he likes to eat all kinds of sweet foods. Eating too much sweets is prone to moisture in the body. Her calf is thicker, which is the result of moisture accumulating under the skin. She and I are in the same situation. I am still a diabetic, and the probability of wound deterioration should be greater than hers, but the situation is just the opposite. After my wound became inflamed, it quickly healed, and her wound worsened after inflammation, although In the end, no major harm was caused, but the inflammation lasted for almost two months, which brought a lot of inconvenience to her life.

From the comparison of these two examples, my colleague was caused by the moisture in the body, which caused the inflammation of the wound to worsen. At the same time, during the period of inflammation, she didn't stop eating and continue to eat sweets, without removing dampness and detoxification, and my own immune system will not be able to play its role under the dampness. Therefore, when people have inflammation and edema in their lower limbs, they must pay attention to removing dampness and detoxification, and pay attention to the diet.

In the case of good blood sugar control, removing dampness and detoxification is very important for diabetic foot patients. It is also very important for non-diabetic patients with foot infections and inflammations to remove dampness and toxins.

Although the glucose metabolism and water metabolism of our diabetic patients are dysfunctional, if we can deal with problems scientifically following the law of development of things and practice self-help, we can still reverse the adversity. Instinctively speaking, the cells of the human body do not want to die abnormally. It is because we humans do not understand how to help ourselves, which leads to negative results that can be restored.

Rigid Fingers in the Morning

When immigrating to Canada, the easiest job to find is manual work, as long as you are willing to do it and you are not afraid of hardships.

I had just arrived in the city at that time, I was not familiar with the city, and I didn't dare to go far, so I went to the nearest supermarket to inquire about it. I didn't expect that the supermarket really wanted to recruit employees, so I went to work the next day.

There are only a few types of jobs in the supermarket, such as delivery, cabbage, and cashiers. I'm a new employee, and the old employees are just behind the storefront, making me go to the seafood department at the front to sell fish and wrap fish. I used to work in an office, and it feels very new and exciting to switch to another labor force. As soon as I go to work every day, I pull out a truckload of frozen fish from the freezer, pack them into boxes, measure the weight on an electronic scale, and type out the price, and then stick the price label on the packaged box, and then, delivered to the freezer in front of the shelf for sale.

There is also a male employee in the fishery department. He only sells live fish, kills fish for customers, and changes the water in the fish tank. He never touches frozen fish. Later, the male employee moved to Vancouver, and the task of selling live fish was handed over to me. In the days of working in the supermarket, I listen to music every day and work non-stop. If there are no customers to buy live fish, I will pack all kinds of frozen fish. The frozen fish that guests buy from the freezer is packaged by my hand. When a customer comes to buy live seafood, the fish is picked up from the big fish tank according to the customer's request, weighed, cleaned and placed in a clean and transparent plastic bag, and a price tag is attached to it and handed to the customer. When customers buy sea crabs and lobsters, they don't need to dissect them, just weigh them and put a price tag on it.

Gradually, when I woke up in the morning, I suddenly found that my hands became stiff. The symptoms were very obvious. I have never had this problem before. I don't know how this happened. Is it the result of my daily hands with frozen fish. Frozen fish is very cold, but as soon as my fingers feel the pain of being frozen, I turn on the hot water faucet to warm my hands.

During that time, the fingers of both hands were always stiff when I woke up in the morning, and I couldn't bend them freely.

The blood sugar level began to be unstable. Before taking this job, the blood sugar level of taking the Chinese patent medicine Xiaoke Pill was very stable, below 6 mol. Since the morning stiffness of the fingers, the blood sugar level of taking the same dose of medicine has reached more than 7 mol. I quit my first job after a few months and got a job that doesn't stick to frozen objects or food. The stiffness of the fingers is also relieved a lot.

The Meniscus on the Nail Is Sparse, and the Stool Cannot Be Flushed Cleanly

I have never paid attention to my nails. Many health care books say that you can know whether your body is cold and damp by looking at the meniscus on your nails, and you can judge the severity of cold and dampness in your body according to the proportion of the meniscus to your nails. Most of my nails can barely see the meniscus, which is a symptom of severe cold and humidity in my body. This is also a symptom of ischemia in the body

The human body is cold and humid, which is also reflected in the hair. Usually people with a lot of humidity have little or no hair on their arms and legs, light and sparse. The growth of hair is controlled by the lungs. When cold and damp air enters the lungs, the water and fluid cannot be distributed effectively, so it is not good for the growth of hair.

I have never paid attention to stool before, but since I got diabetes, I have also started to pay attention to it. Sometimes the stool is not flushed cleanly, leaving some residue on the water surface, and it is mistaken for a problem with the toilet. After reading the knowledge of health care, I realized that if the human body has moisture, the stool will not be flushed cleanly, and there will always be some floating objects on the water surface. I have observed it several times. Whenever the floating objects are stuck in the water and do not want to be flushed away, no matter how many times I flush it, it will not help. I have to take a bucket of water and slam it down the toilet，only then did the floating objects get forced away.

Dampness and Obese

Moisture in the skin, it forms obesity. Wherever the moisture goes, it will foam and gain weight. When the moisture stays on the lower eyelid, bags under the eyes will appear, swelling and bulging. Some people have very serious moisture, and the bags under the eyes look like goldfish eyes. Moisture generally likes to go down the lower body, and the wet weight will naturally fall, which will cause the lower body to appear fatter than the upper body. If the moisture stays under the skin of the whole body, obesity will be formed. Many fat people have excessive moisture in the body. Moisture is water, and the fatness and thinness of a person is the amount of water.

The human body is dominated by water, and the body's water accounts for about 60% of the total, and it runs along normal waterways. Once the water enters through other paths and exceeds this specific gravity, it is excess water, that is, moisture, which not only cannot help the human body, but has the opposite effect.

In order to maintain a moderate body shape, it is necessary to control the content of water in the body and eliminate the dampness in the body in time, that is, to eliminate excess water. Therefore, people do everything possible to lose weight and take various diet pills, but they forget to remove dampness and detoxify to maintain the water balance in the body.

Dampness Lead to Knee-Joint Pain

One morning in June 2004, I went to the sports center to exercise, I wore a skirt, and soon after I went out, it started to rain lightly. I didn't go back to add clothes because I walked halfway. At night, the knee of one leg hurts faintly, and the joints of going up and down the stairs will not bend.

In 2005, when I went back to China to visit relatives, the climate in China was very hot in the early summer, and it suddenly rained for several days in a week. It is very comfortable to wear a skirt in the rain, but the moisture in the rain sneaks in through the gap in the knee, and then stays in the knee to set up camp. After returning to Canada, the damp knee started to hurt, and the symptoms could not be relieved for a long time. The knee was stiff and could not bend freely.

These two knee joint pain because of wear skirts in the rain on the occasion of the spring and summer, the knee is exposed to the outside are attacked by moisture caused. Rainy, cold easily invade the joints muscle, making the muscle and joint pain, severe acid, adverse events involving the stomach is not comfortable, diarrhea is a common practice. This is for people with diabetes, worse, worse.

In Canada, the hands of some elderly people are often seen deformed in public places, especially the thick, bent and twisted finger joints, which are caused by the long-term cold and dampness in the body. Canada is close to the North Pole and has a high latitude. The summer is very short. There are more than half a year in winter, except for Vancouver, which has the rainy season for half a year. However, the rain and humidity in Vancouver brings more moisture to people's bodies. On the one hand, the joint deformation of middle-aged and elderly people in Canada is caused by the cold and humid climate in Canada, and on the other hand, the water quality in Canada is very hard, which damages human cartilage.

During my years in Canada, I rarely or hardly wear skirts, especially after my knee hurts. I pay special attention to protecting my legs. Even in summer, I wrap my legs tightly and wear knee pads.

Dampness Lead to Sleepy

Before diabetes, I started to suffer from sleepiness, because of the high blood lipids in the body, it is even more so when I have diabetes. Every morning at ten o'clock, I came up with sleepiness, breathing hard, and wanted to sleep. The whole body is lack of strength, short of breath, lack of energy, and people look tired, as if they always don't get enough sleep.

There is dampness in the blood of the human body, which is like wearing a wet coat, which affects the normal operation of the blood, and becomes slow and heavy. The combination of dampness and high blood lipids makes the blood of the human body astringent, so people become easily sleepy and have no energy.

Diabetic Patients Are mostly Yin Deficiency and Fire

As the saying goes, illness comes from the mouth. To sum up, the main reason for my own diabetes is gluttony and bad habits. I used to like to eat braised pork, especially the pork knuckle nest. It is fat and lean, soft and delicious, and not greasy. I also like to eat chili. Every time I cook, I always need some chili as a supplement. When I was young, I knew how to exercise every morning when I got up, and I ran around the campus. Since I got married, I gradually slack off and I no longer have the habit of morning exercises.

Excessive consumption of fatty food, and no way to consume fat, so the body's phlegm and dampness accumulate more and more, the yin qi is getting insufficient, the body's serious yin and yang imbalance, the thick phlegm and dampness accumulation of heat seriously hinder the pancreas normal operation, finally went on strike.

Yin deficiency should eat some supplements, but for a long time I couldn't eat warm and nourishing food, and I would get angry when I eat it, so I dare not eat these ingredients that are beneficial to the body's qi and blood. Later, after learning some health care knowledge, I realized that people with yin deficiency are not really hot, but false fire, which is an appearance. Only by removing the virtual fire, we can supplement some ingredients with curative effect and nutrition.

Yin in the human body represents water, blood, and body fluid. Yin deficiency means blood deficiency in the body. Water and body fluid are insufficient. The pancreas is in charge of the water, which is the spleen in Chinese medicine. The spleen is soil in the five elements, and the earth is lacking. The water will dry and crack, so the yin deficiency and the fire are prosperous. This fire is not the yang qi in the body, but the symptoms of disease caused by yin deficiency. Only by replenishing the yin fluid and rebalancing the yin and yang in the body can we truly get rid of the symptoms of yin deficiency and fire.

What Is Phlegm Dampness

People with a little bit of common sense in life know that greasy substances flow more slowly than water-based substances. The presence of moisture in the blood increases the resistance to blood circulation in the blood vessels, and the greasy liquid in the blood combines with moisture. , The circulatory system in the human body is like being forcibly installed with a reducer, and the blood flow becomes astringent and weak. This combination of greasy liquid and moisture should be what Chinese medicine experts call phlegm.

This viscous and greasy liquid is phlegm-dampness, which adheres to the internal organs as the blood flows. Wherever the weak part of the body is, it adheres there. If it adheres to the liver, it is fatty liver. If it adheres to the blood vessels, it is arteriosclerosis. leading to various cardiovascular and cerebrovascular diseases. Adhesion to the microvessels will cause fundus lesions, hand and foot lesions, and neurological lesions. Adhesion to the pancreas, the islets of the pancreas are blocked by phlegm and dampness and lose their normal secretory function, and the endocrine and exocrine secretions of the pancreas are damaged to varying degrees, causing diabetes. Gout is also a type of phlegm-damp vascular occlusion. It can be said. Where the phlegm-damp blocks the blood vessel, pathological changes will occur.

These greasy liquids-phlegm and dampness are the accumulation of human body toxic substances and countless free radicals plus moisture. Phlegm and dampness not only blocks the normal functioning channels of the internal organs, but also hinders the normal hematopoietic and detoxification function of the liver, and has great lethality and destructive power to the body.

Diabetes patients not only have phlegm and dampness in the blood vessels, but also have high blood sugar, which has a double destructive effect, which seriously damages our blood vessels and the body.

In 1996, the hospital found that the triglycerides in my body were several times higher than the standard, and my hands were often numb. After taking the lipid-lowering drugs prescribed by the doctor, the symptoms were relieved, but little was known about the serious consequences of hyperlipidemia, and there was no awareness of health care at all. After controlling my mouth for a few days, I started to eat and drink without restrictions. It seems that health issues are all the concerns of the elderly, not my own.

In 1999, before I went abroad, it was found that I had a mild fatty liver. The symptoms of hyperglycemia were already obvious in my body. I felt tired, weak, thirsty and hungry all day long. If I had a little bit of health awareness at the time, I would have controlled my eating, controlled the consumption of high-fat and high-protein foods, overcome bad eating habits, and strengthened physical exercise, and my body would slowly return to good operation. My body was delayed by my own ignorance of health care, and diseases that could have been avoided occurred, and gradually deteriorated from high blood lipids to mild fatty liver, to diabetes.

Phlegm Dampness is Acidic Feature

The human body not only balances yin and yang, but also balances acid and alkali in the body.

The blood of the human body is weakly alkaline, and the PH value is about 7. 35-7. 45. When we were first born, we had a weakly alkaline physique, and the appearance of an acidic physique was the result of acquired bad eating habits.

Our human body faithfully reflects what we eat every day, and what kind of physique we eat will be given to us by what we eat. Excessive consumption of big fish and meat not only makes the body produce phlegm dampness, but also makes the physique become acidic. Think about it, there is a layer of oil and fat flowing in the blood vessels of the body, how terrible, there is such a time bomb hidden in the body, it may block a certain place at any time and cause disease.

Acidic physique is the source of all diseases.

According to Japanese medical research, when the PH of the human body drops by 0. 1, the insulin activity of the human body drops by 30%. The decline of insulin activity aggravates the disorder of human metabolism. The disorder of human metabolism increases the acidic substances in the body and increases the acid-base imbalance in the body. In such a vicious circle, the utilization rate of blood sugar in the body is getting lower and lower, which aggravates diabetes. It can be seen that patients with type 2 diabetes have a typical acidic constitution.

If we want to change our acidic physique, we must first clean up the blood in the blood vessels and remove toxins from the blood.

The Composition and Function of the Large Intestine

The large intestine is the last part of the digestive system. The diameter of the thickest part of the large intestine is about 5 to 8 cm, which is about twice that of the small intestine, and the length is about 1. 5 meters. The large intestine does not digest food. Its main function is to absorb water and electrolytes, make stool and excrete it. After the food is absorbed, the remaining pasty residues enter the large intestine from the small intestine to absorb water and electrolytes and turn the pasty residues into solids to form stool.

The large intestine can be divided into cecum, ascending colon, transverse colon, descending colon, sigmoid colon and rectum. The cecum is located in the lower right abdomen and is connected to the small intestine. Although the appendix extending from the cecum has nothing to do with digestion and absorption, recent studies have found that it is also a part of the body's immune system and has the effect of preventing infection cecum inflammation is actually appendicitis.

The large intestine starts from the cecum, first as the ascending colon, extending above the right abdomen， under the liver, it changes to the transverse direction, passing through the abdomen as the transverse colon， then under the spleen, it changes direction to become the descending colon， it extends down to the pelvis, Forms the sigmoid colon， it curves toward the center of the abdomen, and finally forms the rectum, which connects to the anus.

The cecum is the thickest, shortest, and most accessible section of the large intestine. The cecum is bounded by the ileocecal valve, the ascending colon and the ileum. The ileocecal valve is the two half-moon-shaped valves at the end of the ileum. Its function is to prevent the contents of the small intestine from flowing into the large intestine too quickly, so that food can be fully digested and absorbed in the small intestine, and prevent the reflux of cecal contents into the ileum.

The main function of the colon is to absorb water and electrolytes, and to store and excrete feces. The absorption of water and sodium is mainly in the right colon, while the descending colon and sigmoid colon also absorb some water, but the main function is to store and excrete feces. Therefore, if we do not defecate in time, the stool will stay in the colon for too long, and the water in the stool will be absorbed by the colon, making the stool dry and hard, making it difficult to defecate.

The rectum and anus are located at the end of the digestive system and control the excretion of feces. The size of the upper end of the rectum is the same as that of the colon, and the lower end is enlarged into the ampulla of the rectum, which is the temporary storage site for feces. Food residues form feces in the large intestine. After the feces reach the rectum, they will stimulate the rectal wall, and the signal will be sensed by the brain through the spinal cord to promote rectal peristalsis and defecation.

The sphincter used for defecation is divided into the internal sphincter and the external sphincter. The internal sphincter is not controlled by consciousness and mainly plays the function of closing the anus. The reason why we can endure the urge to defecate to a certain extent is the credit of the external anal sphincter that can be consciously controlled.

After food is digested and absorbed, it takes about 5 to 10 hours to reach the end of the small intestine, and 9 to 16 hours to reach the large intestine to absorb water. Bacteria in the gut ferment and spoil food scraps to make stool. After the stool is formed, it usually accumulates in the sigmoid colon. Soon, as the stool moves to the rectum due to its own weight, the receptors in the rectum are stimulated, resulting in the urge to defecate.

Intestinal is Largest Place of Hiding Toxin

The small intestine absorbs nutrients, and the large intestine excretes stool. Although their division of labor is different, they are all places where a lot of toxic substances are hidden. Speaking of it, intestinal cleansing is more important than blood cleansing, because the small intestine is related to the body's absorption, and the uncleanness of the small intestine will directly affect the quality of nutrients that penetrate into the blood. The small intestine is like the kitchen of a restaurant. The kitchen violates the sanitation regulations and allows sewage and pollution sources to enter the food, which is the main reason for customers to get sick after eating. Therefore, if we want to eat healthy, not only food is healthy, but hygiene is also very important. Cleaning the small intestine is the key to prohibiting toxic substances from entering the blood.

Large intestine excretion is also very important. Stool on time can excrete toxic substances in time. If the large intestine can not defecate on time and the stool accumulates in the venue, toxic substances will be reabsorbed into the bloodstream. This is the reason why many people with long-term constipation have various bowel diseases, and some people also get various bowel cancers for this.

Diabetic blood problems are also associated with unclean guts. Cleaning up the intestines is helping to clean up the blood, because cleaning up the blood and cleaning up the intestines are a unity, and they are linked together. Only when the upstream water is clean can the downstream water be kept clean.

We all know that Soong Meiling, the widow of President Chiang Kai-shek of the Republic of China, is a legendary figure who occupies a place in modern Chinese history. She has spent 106 long years and tenaciously spanning 3 centuries in her life. She is a politician, she is very busy, she was not in good health when she was young and middle-aged, she suffered from severe pneumonia and almost died, and suffered from severe stomach problems. When she was forty, she suffered a back injury in a car accident, a broken rib, hives and sinusitis. She had gallstone surgery in her sixties and breast cancer in her seventies. Then a car accident also damaged her sciatic nerve, severely sprained and dislocated her spine, and severely traumatized her central nervous system. Benign ovarian tumors were detected at the age of 90.

Soong Meiling was once addicted to cigarettes, staying up late, it can be said that not only is in bad health, butalso in bad habits. She had so many diseases in her life, why did she live so long? However, what is the secret of Soong Meiling's lifelong life? In addition to Song Meiling's emphasis on diet, painting, and nourishment, she also maintains a very important traditional health maintenance measure, which is to use water enema to detox. Since she was young, Song Meiling has been used to regularly enema every day, using enema utensils and water, not only to complete the daily laxative, but also to clean the intestines.

Everywhere in the world has its own custom of enema detoxification. In the non-fiction "Sahara Desert" by the late Taiwanese female writer San Mao, there is a description of the experience of a local woman detoxifying with seawater enema under the cliff by the sea. In the Bay of Bojardo in the Atlantic Ocean, a naked Saharawi woman poured sea water into a large jar, inserted the water tube connected to the jar into the woman's body, and poured three jars of water in a row, begins to expel dirt and feces from the intestines. This detoxification process needs to be cleaned 3 times a day for 7 consecutive days, and the intestines have been cleaned up.

For others, perhaps this ancient traditional enema method is to solve the problem of constipation, but for Soong Meiling, the importance of enema is actually the detoxification of the body. Song Meiling is not constipated, but every day she insists on having an enema before going to bed to defecate early. Because the longer the stool is in the human body, the greater the chance of contamination and the greater the toxin. Use water enema to defecate in advance, excrete the stool in advance, reduce pollution sources, and keep the lower part of the intestines such as rectum, sigmoid colon, descending colon and other parts clean. After doing this, she took a bath and went to bed, and she was clean inside and out.

Because Song Meiling knows that human stool contains the most toxins, if a person wants to keep the body clean and the skin flawless, she should start with the excretion of stools that contain more toxins. Soong Meiling's experience after years of practice is that it is indeed an important health care method to let the food waste of these poisonous bacteria be excreted as soon as possible. This not only keeps her skin clean and prevents harmful substances overnight, but also prevents or greatly reduces the entry of foreign toxic substances into the bloodstream. Enema is indeed a good way to detoxify the intestines.

Judging from the large and small diseases that Song Meiling has suffered in her life, cancer, lung disease, gallstones, and stomach disease, that is, there is no cardiovascular disease, no lymphatic system disease, that is, no blood circulation system. This is all due to the detoxification effect of enema, which has been used for decades. The detoxification of the intestinal tract effectively prevents foreign toxins from entering the blood and avoids blood and blood vessel diseases.

Song Meiling's longevity has a lot to do with her insistence on enema for several years. It removes toxins from the intestines and prevents the chance of internal and external toxins entering the bloodstream. A body without toxins, even if she encounters accidental injury or suffers from disease , and can recover quickly.

There is a saying that the large intestine is the "source of all poisons" in the human body. For example, when people experience diseases such as difficulty in excretion, various toxins in the feces stay in the body for a long time, which will cause acne, reduce antibodies, intestinal flora imbalance, stomach problems, bad breath etc. Severe cases can lead to fatty liver, coronary heart disease, arteriosclerosis and other diseases. The longer the stool is in the body, the greater the chance of contamination and the greater the toxins.

How important is detoxification. Although we will not use the old-fashioned detoxification method of enema, we can use the food on the table to achieve the effect of detoxification.

To clean the intestines, eat more fiber to make stool normal and keep the intestines functioning normally. Foods rich in fiber include:

Sweet potato: The fiber contained in sweet potato is soft and easy to digest, which can promote gastrointestinal motility and help defecation.

Bamboo shoots: It is a good helper to clean up blood trash. Traditional Chinese medicine believes that bamboo shoots have the effects of clearing heat and resolving phlegm, moisturizing the intestines and laxatives, and digesting food. Bamboo shoots are rich in dietary fiber, which can help break down food residues, reduce blood cholesterol, and long-term consumption can also prevent bowel cancer.

Oat bran: rich in cellulose, mixed with vegetables and fruit juice has the effect of removing cholesterol and regulating blood sugar.

Wheat bran: rich in cellulose b family members, help the large intestine to distend and excrete feces in time.

Baking Soda: Cleans the intestines, blood, and blood vessels.

Cardiovascula and Arteriosclerosis

Ten years ago, I went to the hospital for a physical examination, and the film showed that I had visible atherosclerosis in my thoracic aorta. Cardiovascular disease is a major concern for people with diabetes, and it is the most feared and most likely complication. Atherosclerosis is the most common and most harmful disease, which shows that corrosive high fatty acids penetrate into the inner layer of blood vessels and damage the blood vessels. It is difficult to clear them.

When I got the inspection report, my brain was confused. In order to control my blood sugar level, I have been strictly controlling my diet. The daily diet is definitely more than half of vegetables, and the other half of meat, fish and staple food. How can there still be atherosclerosis, and it is still the thoracic aorta. I used to have the phenomenon of rapid heartbeat and chest tightness, but I haven't had it in the past few years, and the triglyceride in the blood test is also normal. How can there still be atherosclerosis in the thoracic aorta?

Before, I thought that since the blood sugar level was normal and the heart no longer had chest tightness and tachycardia, there should be no cardiovascular problems. After calming down, I thought carefully that the atherosclerosis of the aorta was not entirely caused by the course of diabetes, and most likely it was the residual poison of the previous high fat in the body, which has not been cleared up so far.

As a result, a hospital inspection report gave me a new understanding of curing diabetes. With a new direction in the treatment of diabetes, I started a new round of comprehensive body conditioning methods.

Human life coexists with its own arteries. In other words, the life span of arteries is the life span of a person. If people want to live long, they must keep their arteries healthy. To care for arteries is to care for life, and to prevent arteriosclerosis is to prolong life.

Arterial blood vessels are the widest blood vessels in the body. When a person is born, the arterial blood vessels are elastic, the walls are smooth, soft, and the ability to transport blood is also the strongest. In fact, the reason is very simple. The blood vessels of the human body are like water pipes. There is no problem with using new ones, but after a long time of use, if they are not cleaned, the inner walls of the pipes will be scaled and rusted, which will gradually lead to the obstruction of the pipes, and the water supply is small or not available.

The scale produced in the blood refers to cholesterol, triglycerides, etc. The blood of diabetic patients also contains sugar, which accumulates more and more in the blood vessels, making the blood thicker and slower. When the toxic substances in the blood accumulate more and more, the elasticity of the blood vessel wall will decrease and the blood flow will be blocked. Eventually, the heart and cerebrovascular diseases will be caused by ischemia. Diabetes cardiovascular complications are the main cause of death in type 2 diabetes, and the consequences are really terrible.

Why does atherosclerosis not cover the entire area of the inner layer of the blood vessel, but attach to the blood vessel wall like atherosclerosis. The blood vessels in the human body have a complete endothelium. Under the influence of hyperlipidemia, high blood pressure, diabetes and other factors, the human vascular endothelium will be corroded and damaged, and the endothelium is no longer complete and smooth. Dead cells and other toxic substances make their home in the damaged areas, gradually forming atherosclerotic plaques, affecting blood flow to the heart, brain and the entire circulatory system. Atherosclerosis is a dispersion one by one, scattered on the walls of blood vessels.

The heart is the hub of the whole body's blood circulation system. It is like a pump. The main function of the heart in the circulatory system is to pump blood to meet the needs of the body's metabolism. When the heart expands, it receives blood returning from different parts of the body, and when it contracts, it pumps out blood and sends it to various organs in the body, and it starts over and over again. This is the most important duty of the heart. The pump has enough energy to pump and drain. The same is true for the heart, which needs enough blood to do its job.

The heart pumps 3 to 5 liters of blood to the whole body every minute. Human blood accounts for about 1/13 of body weight. A healthy heart beats in a stable and regular rhythm every minute, which is called normal sinus rhythm. The heart beats about 100, 000 times a day. The heart cannot directly use the blood in the heart cavity, but relies on special blood vessels for its blood supply. This task is completed by the coronary arteries. Coronary arteries are arteries that supply blood to the heart. If the coronary arteries are blocked, the ability to supply blood to the heart is greatly reduced, and myocardial ischemia can easily cause heart disease.

The contraction and relaxation of the heart keeps blood circulating in the body. Blood circulation is divided into systemic circulation and pulmonary circulation. The systemic circulation, also called the macro circulation, is the main way of nourishing the human body. Pulmonary circulation is the way to purify human blood. The blood releases carbon dioxide in the lungs, exhales from the lungs, receives the oxygen inhaled by the lungs, becomes arterial blood, and then returns to the heart. Functionally, the heart and lungs are interdependent and closely related.

When diabetic patients suffer from atherosclerosis, blood vessel channels become narrow, which seriously affects the blood transfusion function of the heart, causing systemic blood supply shortage, causing systemic functional deterioration and various diseases.

Diabetes can cause systemic arteriosclerosis, and most diabetic patients die of cardiovascular disease.

Without sufficient fresh blood in the body, there is no certain energy to clean the heavy oil stains on the blood vessel walls and repair the damaged parts of the blood vessels. It's like the sewers are blocked, there is not enough water and pressure, and the silt and dirt cannot be washed away. The hidden dangers in the blood vessels still exist, lurking like a time bomb.

The heart is an unsung hero, working silently, never complaining, unless it is a last resort. The blood vessels are blocked by 50% and continue to work, until the blood vessels are blocked until more than 80% before they start to call for help. Shouldn't we take the initiative to rescue our unsung heroes to keep our lives going?

3. Inspiration of Hot Water Boiler for Blood Vessel

The hot water boiler in the house I used to live in has been used for more than ten years. Later, the hot water always flowed very slowly, and the leather pipe also leaked water. Every time I took a shower, the water flow of the hot water was always twisted to the maximum point, and the faucet flowed. The water is weak and the water temperature is not high. I always thought that there was a problem with the water supply pipe. When the technician who repaired the water pipe came to check and said that the main problem was the aging of the hot water boiler, the inner tank and outlet of the hot water boiler were blocked by scale, and the hot water boiler should be replaced.

After replacing the new hot water boiler, as soon as the faucet is turned on, the hot water rushes out, and when the faucet is screwed to the highest point, the hot water is like a blowout. The hot water flow is several times what it was before the repair! This is shocking! At the same time, the faucet and leather tube will not leak water.

The great enthusiasm of the new hot water boiler, the rushing hot water flowing happily all the way, not only deeply impacted my heart, but also touched me a lot. This is life force! Powerful vitality!

This example reminds me of the blood vessels of the human body. The blood vessels that have been used for half a lifetime are blocked by blood stains before various diseases appear. After the blood vessels are blocked by blood stains, the blood flow is slow, the blood flow is severely insufficient, the blood circulation is not good, the hands and feet are always cold, the whole body is rarely warm, and the sticky blood does not come out after a needle squeezed on the fingertips for a long time. This is the same reason that the hot water boiler is blocked by scale. Replacing the hot water boiler with a new one solves the problem. If the blood vessels of the human body are cleaned of blood stains, they can be rejuvenated with new vitality.

The comparison between the accumulation of blood scale in the blood vessels of the human body and the accumulation of scale in the hot water boiler is surprisingly similar:

The Accumulation of Blood Scale in the Blood Vessels of the Human Body.

1. Slow blood circulation.

2. The blood flow is small and small.

3. Cold hands and feet.

4. High blood pressure, high fat, high blood sugar, hardening of blood vessels.

Scale Build up on Hot Water Boiler

1. Hot water flows slowly.

2. The flow of hot water is very small, and the maintenance time is very short and there is no hot water.

3. The hot water boiler is covered with scale, the pointer is turned to the maximum heat, the thermal efficiency is still not enough.

4. The faucet and the water pipe are leaking, and the water inlet and outlet of the hot water boiler are filled with scale.

Diabetes patients are not only a blood disease, and long-term lack of qi and blood in the body of diabetic patients, and various functions of the body are impaired. Diabetes is also a degenerative disease of systemic functions.

In conclusion, according to my own problems, I think that in order to completely cure diabetes, we must clean the blood vessels, replenish qi, blood and oxygen, so that the internal organs can get enough blood supply, In this way, various organs can not only function normally, but also have the ability to clean up the dirt in the blood vessels in the body, repair themselves, and restore the elasticity of blood vessels. Allows the heart to circulate well.

Dampness in Stomach Causes Indigestion

Saliva, gastric juice, and pancreatic juice all contain a variety of biological enzymes, among which amylase can help digest food, and lipase in pancreatic juice can break down fat.

The human stomach is the foundation of the acquired nature, and the stomach is an important supplier of life support. Injury to the stomach is tantamount to having trouble with oneself and plundering one's own nourishment for survival.

People with diabetes basically have weak digestion in the spleen and stomach. I have a good appetite, and everything tastes good. Why do I always eat a lot and people don't gain weight? I have a colleague who is fatter than me, but I eat almost twice as much as hers. At work, every time we take a break, she just drinks some water, and I drink and eat, no matter how much I eat, I don't grow meat.

Although I eat a lot and eat deliciously, my mouth is often sticky and my saliva is not refreshing. Also, I can't eat cold food, I want to keep warm because my stomach can't get cold and can't eat hard food, otherwise my stomach will be very uncomfortable.

In the past, I used to get up and drink water every morning. After drinking some water, my stomach felt full and I didn't want to drink any more.

I don't have acid reflux, it's not that I have too much stomach acid. I usually eat food without a stomachache, not a stomach ulcer. I eat a lot and don't grow meat because of poor absorption. Why can't it be absorbed. I checked the information about the digestive system and learned that the food people eat is digested by an enzyme, and diabetes is a disease of the endocrine system in Western medicine. There is a problem with the endocrine of the human body, and the enzymes secreted by the body are not enough to maintain the needs of the body's absorption. Only human saliva, gastric juice and pancreatic juice contain this digestive enzyme.

The cause of my diabetes is high blood lipids. The phlegm and dampness produced by long-term greasy and fat food has long disrupted the function of the stomach, making it impossible to secrete a certain amount of digestive enzymes in the gastric juice. As the pancreatic islets of diabetic patients have problems, the pancreatic juice also has troubles, and will not secrete the necessary digestive enzymes. Saliva is produced in the mouth, and the source of acceptance is the liquid delivered from the stomach. If the ground fluid is insufficient, the mouth will become dry and sticky. Therefore, there is not enough digestive enzymes.

The digestive system does not secrete enough enzymes, and my stomach is like a big funnel. It leaks as much as I eat. No wonder I am not fat and not energetic.

To eliminate the symptoms of indigestion, it is necessary to increase saliva, gastric juice and pancreatic juice to secrete enough digestive enzymes to digest food. Lack of body fluid is the main problem of diabetic patients, so the digestive enzymes in body fluid are also lacking. To increase body fluid, the saliva in our mouth must first become moisturized. (For massage points to increase saliva in the mouth, please see the relevant chapter) The saliva in the mouth is continuously fed into the body from the mouth, solving the problem of diabetic dry mouth will gradually solve the problem of lack of digestive enzymes.

The pancreas and stomach have four fears, namely: the spleen and stomach are afraid of cold, catch cold, sweet, and too full. We should eat hot food, keep warm, avoid sweets, and not eat too much. Follow these four points to eat and regulate, the pancreas and stomach will be happy, and it will gradually restore its elasticity and increase its digestive ability.

Excessive Sweets Can easily Produce Dampness

When I was young I loved chocolate, cream cakes, cookies, summer watermelon, all kinds of ice cream. In winter, before going to bed, drink a glass of hot milk and add a few spoonfuls of sugar to get a good night's sleep. Because the company distributes a lot of white sugar every year, in addition to giving it away, I also eat a lot of it myself. Every time I go shopping, I always like to visit the dessert shop and taste sweets such as glutinous rice wine in sugar water, red bean cake, chocolate cake and so on.

Anyone who loves desserts knows that after eating sweet food, the mouth will be sweet and sticky, and the throat will be a little congested, so we have to drink some water.

In the past, it was always believed that diabetes was caused by too much sugar, but later I realized that it was not. Although diabetes is not caused by eating too much sugar, excessive consumption of desserts will produce dampness in the body. According to the theory of traditional Chinese medicine, sweet and greasy can reduce dampness. Usually, we store white sugar in glass bottles in a cool place. If we put it in a sunny, hot place, the sugar will melt. Excessive sugar cannot be properly transported and absorbed in the body, and the sticky moisture produced is the same as the moisture produced by fat, which is a harmful substance that poisons our body.

Clearing Dampness First Yin-nourishing Second

Yin-tonifying foods are beneficial to the production of yin fluid in the human body, and have the effect of nourishing body fluid and promoting body fluid and moisturizing dryness.

Body fluid is the water in the human body, used to nourish the internal organs of the human body and our body, skin, hair, etc. The production, operation, and excretion of body fluid are necessary conditions for maintaining the metabolism in the body.

The balance of Yin and Yang in the body of diabetic patients is lost, and the Yin fluid in the body is insufficient, which can not normally nourish our body and internal organs, and cannot restrict Yang Qi.

Just as the land is exposed to the sun, dry and cracked, and no rain is irrigated for a long time, even some artificial water irrigates the land with little water and thirsty, which cannot solve practical problems. As a result, people with diabetes will feel thirsty, upset, and swollen and painful facial features.

Due to the imbalance of body fluid in diabetic patients, if we want to balance the yin and yang in the body, it is necessary to replenish yin.

Eating yin-tonifying herbs and ingredients is the fastest way to supplement yin. However, most of the foods that nourish yin are sweet, cold and greasy, which are not good for people with weak gastrointestinal functions such as stomach cold, gastrointestinal indigestion, abdominal distension, etc. It can be seen in traditional Chinese medicine shops that many Yin-tonifying ingredients are marked with advice that people with weak spleen and stomach, and those with indigestion should not eat. Why is there such a situation. Is it because those of us who are weak in the stomach in urgent need of yin supplementation have no way to enjoy these yin supplementing ingredients?

Later, it was found that the reason was dampness in our stomach and intestines, and it was the dampness that refused all external help, and also used these Yin-tonifying foods to create new conflicts and worsen the original ones. To avoid problems, herbal stores generally offer well-intention advice. At first, I ate ingredients for nourishing yin, and my stomach became more afraid of cold, and the problem of dry mouth was not solved. The nourishing ingredients are even more afraid to eat. After eating, they will definitely catch fire, and this fire is virtual fire. Later, through my own yin replenishing process, I figured out that if I want to replenish yin, I must first remove dampness and drive the dampness out of the body, and then yin replenishment can really be effective.

The Ways for Clearing Dampness

I have tried several methods to solve the problem of removing dampness, removing dampness through food, removing dampness through massaging the meridians, soaking feet to remove dampness and detoxification, and cupping to remove dampness and detoxification. These are all simple and easy to do. They can be done in daily life. Food costs less, and we don't need to spend money to massage yourself. Soaking your feet in hot water every night can relieve fatigue. It can be said to serve multiple purposes. There is no need to see a doctor to formulate any medicine.

Food to remove dampness:

Barley is the most effective in removing dampness. Once it arrives, the moisture will be scared away. Barley can cure dampness, benefit the stomach, reduce edema, invigorate the spleen and stomach, and take a long time to lighten the body and replenish qi. Regular boiled barley soup can continuously remove the moisture in the body and keep the body light.

Chixiaodou- has obvious effects of diuresis, swelling, invigorating the spleen and stomach, and can nourish the heart and blood.

Mugwort - is also a master at dispelling dampness, and has special knack for cold dampness and evil.

Winter melon- clears away heat and relieves phlegm, relieves irritability and quenches thirst. It has the effect of eliminating phlegm, clearing away heat and detoxifying water. If people with damp-heat constitution have edema, fullness, excessive phlegm, heat boredom, diminished thirst, eczema, boils, etc, they can eat it.

Massage Acupoints to Remove Dampness

Yinlingquan Acupoint- Foot Taiyin Spleen Meridian Point. On the inner side of the lower leg, when the medial condyle of the tibia is posterior and inferior to the depression. The combined points of the spleen meridian of the foot Taiyin..

The functions of its acupoints: clearing away damp-heat, strengthening the spleen and regulating qi, tonifying the kidney and regulating menstruation, and activating the meridians and collaterals.

Yinlingquan literally explains that body fluid is yin fluid, yinling spring has yin, spring is water, and it is also the place where the water is produced. Therefore, the main way to grasp the yin fluid is to massage and we can get the desired effect. Yinlingquan points can also assist in the treatment of diabetes.

Chengshan Point-In the middle of the lower calf, where the muscles are divided into a "person" shape, Chengshan Point is in the middle of the word.

Chengshan acupoint is a large acupoint for removing moisture from the human body. Chengshan is on the bladder meridian of the foot sun, and the bladder meridian hosts the yang energy of the human body. On the one hand, Chengshan acupoint is the gathering place of the tendons, bones and flesh that are under the most pressure in the whole body, and on the other hand, it is the hub of the meridian with the most yang qi in the human body, expel body moisture.

Normally, as long as we lightly press the Chengshan point, there will be obvious soreness and pain. This is all because of the wetness in the body. But after pressing and rubbing Chengshan for a period of time, we will feel our legs relax and our body will feel slightly warm. This is the yang energy on the bladder meridian is working, and the dampness on the body is radiating outward with the slightly elevated body temperature.

Soak Our Feet to Detoxify the Cold and Dampness

Soak our feet with a bucket of hot water before going to bed every night, which can remove dampness and detoxification, make the meridians of the whole body smooth, and also help we fall asleep better.

There is an important acupoint on the sole of the foot called Yongquan acupoint, which is the most important detoxification point on the kidney meridian. Yongquan acupoint can also eliminate fatigue, edema, muscle soreness, and improve kidney function. Yongquan acupoint can help improve sleep, improve dizziness, cold hands and feet and other problems.

There is a view that if we can stick to soaking our feet every day, we can prolong our life by ten years.

Cupping Therapy

Cupping therapy is a commonly used method of traditional Chinese medicine to treat diseases. This therapy can remove cold and dampness, dredge the meridians, remove stagnation, promote qi and blood circulation, reduce swelling and pain, remove toxins and diarrhea, and can adjust the balance of yin and yang of the human body. Relieve fatigue, enhance physical function, so as to achieve the purpose of strengthening the body and eliminating evil and curing diseases. Moreover, cupping is relatively easy to operate, which is very suitable for self-maintenance and moisture removal at home.

It is best to reduce exposure to humid environments in daily life, especially for people who are sensitive to moisture, and do not directly sleep on the floor. The moisture in the air will drop and the floor will be heavy, which can easily invade the body and cause sore limbs. It is best to sleep on a bed at a distance from the floor. Reduce going out on wet and rainy days. Reduce the time spent on air conditioning. Don't wear damp, wet clothes, and take proper amount of water. People in North America like to go camping and sleep by the water, which can attract moisture.

It is best not to live in a humid environment in daily life, especially those who are sensitive to moisture, do not sleep directly on the floor. The moisture in the air will drop and the floor moisture will be heavy, which can easily invade the body and cause pain in the limbs. It is best to sleep in a bed that is some distance from the floor. Go out less on rainy days. Reduce the time of blowing the air conditioner. Don't wear wet clothes, water intake should be appropriate. People in North America like to go out camping, and sleeping near the water will attract moisture.

Dampness Gets Hot it Becomes Heat Toxins

Apart from the eczema on my hands that had been exposed to the sun for the first few years, there are few other skin problems. Last year, I had some problems with my cervical spine. After seeing a Chinese medicine practitioner, the Chinese doctor used a Mitsubishi needle to tap on several acupoints on my neck and shoulders. Then cupping, some moisture and light blood flowed out.

On the same day, I bought leeks at the nearby supermarket by the way. The next day, I ate leeks at home and basked in the sun for more than ten minutes. On the third morning, I was woken up by severe itching. When I got up to check, there were dense patches of eczema on both sides of my neck, arms, and chest. Fortunately, these eczema did not continue to expand, and it disappeared automatically after a few days of itching. Since then, whenever there is heat in my body, eczema or rashes will appear on both sides of my neck, which tortures me for a few days and then withdraws. My colleague brought back a traditional Chinese medicine hot pack from Thailand and lent it to me to warm the cervical spine and shoulders. I used it once, and the next day my neck was a lot of red, it disappeared, and I used it again. After a few times, I couldn't bear the itch. It was so uncomfortable that I had to return it to my colleague.

I checked the relevant information, people with endocrine system problems will have eczema after applying heat. Diabetes is an endocrine disease. Why do people with endocrine diseases develop eczema after applying heat. This shows from one side that there is a lot of dampness on the body of diabetics. When the dampness encounters a certain amount of heat, it becomes heat poison. The vent of this heat poison is the skin. At the same time, it also proves why the eczema or rash on the skin does not develop malignantly. The damp-heat poison generated by the combination of hot air and dampness will be vented from the skin, and it will be fine after it dissipates. So, having eczema or rashes on our skin isn't necessarily a bad thing, it's also a way of detoxifying our body.

Eczema and boils on the skin of people with diabetes are the external manifestations of the detoxification of the body's heat toxins. In the past, I didn't know why the skin of diabetic patients could not be exposed to strong sunlight. Now, through my personal experience, I believe that it is the heat toxin produced by the moisture in the diabetic body when it encounters heat energy, which is excreted through the skin. Diabetes is a blood disease caused by the accumulation of a large amount of phlegm and dampness in the blood vessels, so the dampness in the blood vessels can only be diffused out through the skin.

For the past two years, I have been eating blood-enriching food, and the digestion of the spleen and stomach has improved significantly. Glucose tolerance was enhanced, and weight was gained. There is more blood in the body, and the body's ability to repair itself is strengthened. I still have a red rash on my neck that is itchy, but it's gone for a few days. The left arm will also be swollen severely, and a bluish-red lump will appear when it is tapped. These are all manifestations of the body's detoxification. At the beginning of last year, I had two hopes for my health, one is to clear the fat on the walls of blood vessels, and the other is to gain weight. Now, the detox is still going on and I've gained several pounds. This is not a small improvement and deserves congratulations.

Eczema and Lungs

The lungs participate in the purification of human blood.

Eczema on the skin is a blood problem, which means that the blood is detoxifying through the skin.

According to traditional Chinese medicine, the lungs dominate the skin. In other words, eczema on the skin is a problem of the lungs, and the moisture in the lungs can not effectively purify the blood.

On the days when my body had eczema, I woke up on time at about four in the morning every day to check the duty schedule of each meridian. That time was when the lung meridian was on duty. The excretion of heat poisoned the moisture in the body, especially in the blood, the moisture is brought out, and at the same time the moisture in the lungs is brought out.

My skin is only eczema, and there is no coughing phenomenon. There is no problem with the trachea and the lung organs. It is just that the cold and damp air flowing into the blood of the lungs becomes heat toxins and is excreted through the skin. The outlet of the skin is in a limited way, a large amount of heat toxins accumulated around the sweat pores, forming blockages, so eczema occurs.

Body Dirty Reflects the Health Condition

Speaking of the three turbidity seems very indecent, almost no one has ever met and asked, is your bowel movement normal today? Are you urinating normally today? Did you fart today? In people's minds these are unclean rubbish. In fact, farting, urinating and defecation are as important as eating, and are closely related to our physical health, and are also necessary activities that we perform every day. In particular, diabetics should pay close attention to ventilation and bowel movements, because these normal excretory functions can tell us the state of our body in time. Urine and waste gas are the waste of the human body, and they must be cleaned every day. If they are not excreted in time, they will become toxic substances in the body and corrode our body.

When people breathe, they will produce qi, and they will also enter some qi when they eat. These qi operate in the body, and when we breathe in and out, once we breathe in more than the expelled breath, the qi will be noisy in the body and will be excreted through farts and hiccups. No one doesn't fart, some fart loudly, some smelly fart, some fart. The smell of fart can tell whether the human body is exhausting or detoxifying. Usually, I like to eat some legume foods, these foods like to produce farts, but it is very comfortable to put it, the whole internal organs are empty, and it is not smelly. If one day eats too much high protein, the fart from high-fat food will smell bad, the smell of high-protein and high-fat fart is also different, farts from high-fat foods are very smelly, and farts from high-protein foods should be gentle, the smell has a characteristic sourness of protein.

Once I was so tired after taking a shower, I fell asleep in bed. My hair was half wet, and I had a thick coat over my belly, and my arms were exposed. When I woke up, I didn't feel anything bad. Waking up the next morning was not right, with heavy, sore arms, and the body seemed to be wrapped in a wet suit, tight and uncomfortable. The stomata in the body are blocked by moisture and cannot be excreted smoothly, and the body is swollen, especially the blocked part, the swelling and pain is simply a kind of torment. No matter how I rub my stomach, I don't fart, and I look forward to farting as I look forward to amnesty. If the turbid qi cannot come out, the body will be very uncomfortable, and the qi will travel in the body, and the muscles will swell to the point of cracking pain. Until one day I finally farted, my body suddenly felt relaxed, and the feeling of swelling and pain suddenly weakened. Afterwards, the turbid qi was expelled, the qi became smooth, and the swelling and pain in the body healed by itself.

Urine is the best evidence to test the condition of the kidneys and blood. Fluctuations in blood sugar levels can also be monitored. If the blood sugar level exceeds 10 moles, the urine will be cloudy, and the urine will contain protein taste and slight sweetness. When the blood sugar level is high, there will be more bubbles in the urine, and there will be a string of bubbles. When the blood sugar level is normal, the urine is clear, there are a few bubbles, and it disappears quickly, and the amount of urine is normal. Sometimes, drinking the same amount of water, but the amount of urination is small, the water cannot be excreted in the body, and it turns into moisture in the body, which becomes edema. If ou urinate less, our eyes will become swollen and water will stagnate in our body. A few times, when I encountered less urination, I would increase the amount of water I drank, until the water channel was smooth, and the urine would be excreted with a rush.

Diabetics are mostly accompanied by cardiovascular problems, large and small, and have heartburn. I always feel a fire going out in my heart. When the heart is hot, the smell of pee is a little nasty. In this case, it is necessary to replenish yin in time and eat some moisturizing and tranquil foods. The blood enters the kidneys every day for filtration, excreting toxins through urine. Therefore, when the body is detoxifying, the smell of urine is also very heavy. With strong kidney function, more toxins are filtered out, and the smell of urine is strong.

Stool has always been normal, and it will be excreted on time at a certain time every day, without constipation. Despite this, I have had diarrhea or loose stools for a long time. Sometimes the stool looks well-shaped and has a soft texture. After washing with water, there will be some residue. I began to think it was a flushing faucet problem, or that the leafy vegetables were not digested and excreted directly.

At the beginning of last year, during the process of removing dampness and detoxification, I learned a lot of online medical and health knowledge before I realized that these problems are serious symptoms of cold and dampness in the body. When this happens in the stool, my body is directly telling me that there is severe cold and dampness in my body, reminding me to pay attention. However, I didn't know anything about it, so that it was delayed for so long. Cold and dampness in the body is a big obstacle to the treatment of diabetes, and severe cold and dampness can also affect the stability of blood sugar in the body.

The normal stool is golden yellow banana shape. When the body is wet, the color of the stool is grassy blue, soft and unformed, and there is always a feeling that it is not clean. It is an important sign of spleen deficiency, and many people have it.

At first, my blood sugar level was very unstable. When the blood sugar level was high, the smell of stool was sweet and greasy, exuding a taste like rotten apples. I am very afraid of the sweet smell of stool, as long as I smell the smell of this apple-smelling stool, the blood sugar level will definitely rise. Usually, if I eat a lot of high-fat foods, my stools will smell like farts. I eat a lot of high protein, and the stool exudes the unique sour taste of protein. There are many vegetables, and the stool is tasteless, or a light stool smell. During detoxification, the stool will smell bad. If we eat too much meat, the stool will also be very smelly. If we drink soda water to detoxify, we will excrete a little sticky stool the next morning.

Since insisting on food, acupuncture points and hot foot bathing to remove dampness and detoxification, stool no longer appears floating, stool is formed, basically yellow, and the body has become relaxed, indicating that the main force of moisture in the body has been basically expelled.

Damp Evil Hurts Tendon

The tendons of our human body are like the reinforced ropes of the bridge, which play a fixed role. The strength of the reinforced ropes indicates the reliability of the bridge, and the strength of the human muscles and bones can prolong the life of people.

Injured tendons are common diseases in daily life. Almost everyone encounters them. People who like sports and those who do physical labor will often encounter the problem of tendon injuries. Injuring tendons is the concept of traditional Chinese medicine, and modern medicine is called soft tissue injury. bump bump, it is almost a small accident that is inseparable from daily life. These are secondary and will be fine in a few days. What makes people troublesome is the external evil, and the cold and damp evil is the most common cause of tendon diseases. When the human body encounters cold and dampness, the pores of the human body tend to shrink, and then the tendons also begin to shrink. If the cold and dampness does not go away, it will stay between the skin and muscles, causing the body's qi and blood to coagulate and block the blood vessels and the muscles and veins, causing injuries. The nutrient imbalance in the part of the body causes the tendons to contract easily, resulting in muscle soreness, numbness, stiffness, and inability to stretch.

Anyone who has bought analgesic plaster knows that it is obviously a soft tissue injury, but almost all plaster will indicate that its efficacy is to remove dampness, dispel wind, dredge bones and muscles, and activate qi and blood. The famous wound dampness relieving ointment is our commonly used bruises ointment. This shows that traditional Chinese medicine is very concerned about removing dampness when treating bruises, and puts dampness in the first place in the treatment. It can be seen that the influence of dampness on tendons is great.

Almost every adult has suffered more or less injuries to the soft tissues (tensions) of the limbs. Although most people do not have any sequelae, the old injuries will become swollen and sore before it rains, which is more accurate than the weather forecast. In the later years or in old age, some people have rigid and deformed hands and feet, and some can't take care of themselves in life, which seriously affects the quality of life. These are all due to the failure to remove dampness in time when the soft tissue is injured.

Therefore, cold and dampness is not only the main enemy of the blood circulation system, but also the main enemy of the human body's bridge steel cables-tendons.

Clearing Poison and Garbage of Blood

The blood seems to be very clean, but in fact, there are many toxic substances and garbage hidden in the blood, such as lipid-containing toxins such as triglycerides, cholesterol, and phospholipids. There are also toxins such as dust, harmful metals, and some chemical agents that we inhale. The garbage in the blood is the free radicals generated by the oxidation process. These garbage are generated at any time. These toxins and garbage are extremely harmful. It is the main cause of people suffering from cardiovascular and cerebrovascular diseases. Blood toxins are also the main culprits in developing high blood pressure.

The human body itself has the function of self-purification, which is under normal circumstances, the human body implements self-rescue. However, due to excessive hyperlipidemia and hyperglycemia in the body of diabetic patients, the body's self-help function is out of balance and can not purify the blood itself. As a result, a largeamount of toxic substances accumulate in the blood of diabetic patients.

The reason why diabetic patients have an acidic physique is because the body accumulates a large amount of high fat and other harmful substances, and the acid-base balance in the body is destroyed. The consequence of the body's self-purification ability not working.

If we want to change our acidic physique, we must first clean up the two large reservoirs of poison in our body, namely the blood and the intestines, and remove the toxins in the blood and intestines.

Detoxification of blood and intestines is a very important method of treatment, rehabilitation, and health care. The purpose of blood and intestinal detoxification is to remove the waste in the blood and intestines, so that the body can return to the best life state.

There are many ways to remove toxins from the blood and intestines, the easiest of which is through food. The human body itself will respond to what we eat. We can change the acidic constitution by eating some alkaline foods, and gradually achieve the acid-base balance in the body. And actively dissolve and clean up blood vessels and intestines and toxins in cells through these alkaline foods.

Food Clearing Poison

Vegetables: All kinds of fresh vegetables contain a large amount of alkaline components, which can dissolve the toxins deposited in the cells and excrete them with the urine. They are the best "purifier vitamins" for the blood.

Kelp: It is rich in kelp gum, which can promote the excretion of radioactive substances in the body.

Mung bean: It has the effect of eliminating toxins. It is very effective when adding mung bean when boiling soup or making rice porridge.

Mushrooms: have the effect of lowering blood pressure and blood lipids. It can resist viruses, protect the liver, and is a supplementary food for the treatment of hepatitis. It has strong detoxification ability and is a master at purifying blood.

Yeast is rich in chromium, which can strengthen the function of insulin and have a therapeutic effect on diabetes. Drinking a glass of fruit juice for breakfast and half a teaspoon of yeast can also remove excess fat and cholesterol.

Oat bran: rich in fiber, mixed with vegetables and fruit juice can remove cholesterol and regulate blood sugar.

Pig blood rich in plasma protein , after being decomposed by gastric acid and digestive enzymes, it produces detoxification substances, which are effective against a variety of poisons and are the best in detoxification foods.

Black fungus: can remove various toxins in the blood.

Oatmeal has the effect of lowering cholesterol and blood fat. Because oatmeal contains rich soluble dietary fiber that other grains do not have, this fiber is easily absorbed by the body and has low calories. It is not only good for weight loss, but also suitable for the dietary needs of people with heart disease, high blood pressure and diabetes.

Corn is rich in calcium, phosphorus, magnesium, iron, selenium and vitamins A, B1, B2, B6, E and carotene, etc. It is also rich in fiber. Regular consumption of corn can lower cholesterol and soften blood vessels, and has an adjuvant therapeutic effect on cholecystitis, gallstones and diabetes.

Onions and garlic: onions contain compounds such as cycloaliin and thionine, which help dissolve blood clots. Onions contain almost no fat, so they can inhibit the increase in cholesterol caused by a high-fat diet and help improve atherosclerosis. Garlic can lower serum total cholesterol, and methacrylic trisulfide, a secondary metabolite of allicin, can prevent blood clots.

Yam: Its mucin protein can prevent fat deposition in the cardiovascular system, maintain blood vessel elasticity, prevent arteriosclerosis, reduce subcutaneous fat deposition, and avoid obesity. The dopamine in yam has the function of dilating blood vessels and improving blood circulation. Yam can also improve human digestion. If we have indigestion, we can cook yam, lotus seeds, and gorgon.

Sweet potato has a strong effect of lowering blood cholesterol, maintaining blood acid-base balance, delaying aging, preventing cancer and anti-cancer. Sweet potatoes are rich in defecation substances such as dietary fiber and colloids, which can be described as "intestinal scavengers".

Red dates: eating more can improve the body's antioxidant and immune capabilities, and it is also very effective in lowering blood cholesterol and triglycerides.

Millet is gluten-free and will not irritate the intestinal wall. It is a relatively mild fiber and is easily digested, so it is suitable for eating with a detox meal. Millet porridge is very suitable for detoxification, has the effect of clearing heat and diuresis, is rich in nutrients, and also helps in whitening.

After a period of detoxification, the body will feel relaxed. Detoxification is a continuous process, just as people need to eat to maintain life, to feed, and clean up. This is a life cycle process.

Drink Water Clearing Poison

Drinking water to detox is the easiest and easiest. Water can overturn and carry a boat. We know that most of the weight of the human body is water, therefore, the water in the body must not only be sufficient, but also healthy.

Many people think that drinking water is to quench thirst, so they will drink water when they are thirsty, and they will not drink water when they are not thirsty. If you are not thirsty all day, you will not drink water all day. This was how I was when I was young. In fact, drinking water is not only to quench thirst, but to meet the needs of the body's metabolism. Nearly 80% of the water that is drunk will quickly enter the bloodstream directly, which is extremely important for maintaining life and health.

Water in the body is responsible for transporting nutrients and oxygen, regulating body temperature, excreting waste, coordinating metabolism, lubricating body joint functions, circulation, absorption, and digestion.

80% of blood is water. It is like crisscrossing rivers and streams on the earth, continuously transporting various energy and nutrients to our various organs to ensure their normal operation. Moreover, the various immune substances contained in the blood and the lymphocytes in the blood make the human body immune. At the same time, blood can maintain the acidity and alkalinity of itself and other body fluids, so that the human body always maintains a weakly alkaline healthy physique.

Water accounts for about 70% of the human body. Normally, the water in the human body is renewed every 15 days. Health care experts recommend that in order to maintain the normal renewal of body water, adults should drink no less than 2000 ml of water per day. If we drink less water, the water in our body cannot be updated in time, which will result in a decrease in the quality of body fluids and the accumulation of various "garbage" in the body, which cannot be eliminated in time, thus affecting the health of the entire human body.

The intestine is the body's largest detoxification organ, and it is responsible for most of the body's detoxification tasks. The intestine itself is full of folds, and it is the base camp where most of the body's toxins and metabolites are concentrated. However, modern people's diet is too fine, irregular diet, diet safety and other issues, as well as Asian people's intestines are longer and curved, which makes it easy to hide toxins in the intestines.

Drinking hydrolyzed toxin is not only to ensure that we have to drink eight glasses of water a day, but also to learn to drink water the right time to get double the effect. The following is the method of drinking water on duty in the Four Classics that I learned on the Internet.

Four classics on duty drinking water method:

Large intestine meridian detox method: the human large intestine meridian is most active at 5-7 in the morning. At this time, you should drink 200ml of boiled water (preferably cold water) on an empty stomach. It can relieve constipation and is beneficial to skin care.

Heart meridian detoxification method: the human heart meridian is most active from 11 am to 1 pm. At this time, we should drink water on an empty stomach to dilute the blood and help eliminate toxins in the cardiovascular.

Kidney meridian detoxification method: 5-7 pm, the human kidney meridian is the most active. At this time, we should drink water on an empty stomach to clean your kidneys and bladder.

Pericardial meridian detoxification method: the human pericardial meridian is most active at 7-9 in the evening. Drinking water on an empty stomach at this time can reduce blood viscosity and help prevent excessive blood concentration at night. But before that, we should do a proper amount of exercise (such as walking) to promote blood circulation, so as to achieve the best results.

Massage Acupoint Detoxification Method

Massage acupoints Detoxification is to start from the meridians and find out the corresponding diseases of the acupoints. The result of massage is to dredge the meridians, the meridians are smooth, the qi and blood are smooth, and the effect of detoxification is naturally achieved. When massaging acupuncture points, if you feel swelling, soreness, and hard lumps in the massaged area, it means that there is moisture congestion in the corresponding area, which blocks the normal circulation channels of Qi and blood, and needs to be dredged immediately to guide the removal of toxic substances to outside the body.

In fact, as long as we listen carefully to the language of the body, we will find that many of the problems in the body are manifested in the acupuncture points. Understand the role and efficacy of acupuncture points in the body, and know our own physical condition, so as to minimize the negative impact and easily eliminate the disease in the bud.

Each major organ has a main detoxification point that serves it. The human body is a magical medicine library. As long as we are willing to learn and listen to the language of the body, we will easily learn and master the seemingly profound but simple acupoint health knowledge. We are our own doctors, removing dampness and detoxification for ourselves.

The heart is the most important organ of the human body. It never rests at work all day long. Even when a person is sleeping, the heart is still working non-stop. It is very important to maintain the heart's safe operation. The first is to detoxify the heart, remove the toxic substances in the cardiovascular system, and let the heart work easily.

The key point for detoxification of the heart-Shaofu point, located in the palm of the hand, between the 4th and 5th metacarpal bones, between the little finger and the end of the ring finger when making a fist. Use a little bit of strength for the massage, alternating left and right hands.

The liver is a blood-forming organ of the human body, which is easy to accumulate toxins. If the toxins in the liver accumulate too much, people have a big liver fire, and they like to have a nameless fire, and they love to have spots on the skin. Toxins in the liver affect the quality and quantity of hematopoiesis.

The main point of the liver's detoxification organ-Taichong point, is located in the depression before the junction of the first and second metatarsals on the back of the foot. Press and knead with our thumb for 3 to 5 minutes to feel a slight soreness. Do not use too much force and do it alternately with our feet.

Chinese medicine believes that the lungs and large intestine are a system. When there are toxins in the upper lungs, there will be abnormal stasis in the lower intestines, resulting in constipation, and the face is dull and

The key point for detoxification of the lungs - Hegu Point, is located on the back of the hand, between the 1st and 2nd metacarpal bones. We can pinch this part with your thumb and forefinger and press it hard.

When there are pigment spots on the face, excessive leucorrhea, or abnormal breath, it indicates that the toxins in the spleen have begun to spread outward. At this time, it is time to detoxify the spleen.

The key point for detoxification of the spleen - Shangqiu point, is located in the depression in front of and below the inner ankle. Press and rub the point with our fingers to maintain a sore and heavy feeling. Each time about 3 minutes, alternate feet. Shangqiu acupoint just corresponds to the lower body lymphatic reflex area in the plantar reflex area, so it can treat various inflammations.

At the same time, it also illustrates a medical truth: inflammation is generally caused by bacterial infection. Because the spleen is a tube for blood supply, it can transport fresh blood to the lesions. After the dirty things are removed, the inflammation will naturally be eliminated.

The key point for kidney detoxification - Yongquan point, located in the third of the sole of the foot, is the lowest point of the human body. If the human body is a building, then this point is the outlet of the sewage pipe. Massage the Yongquan point every day the detoxification effect is very obvious. This acupoint is more sensitive, and it is best to combine massage and rubbing for 5 minutes each time. When there are toxins in the kidneys, symptoms such as body edema, mandibular acne, physical fatigue and mental fatigue will appear.

The cells of the human body are undergoing metabolism all the time. Once the metabolism of the human body fails, it will cause many diseases, such as diabetes.

The key point of human metabolism and detoxification - Quchi point, this point is located on the inner side of the elbow. Quchi point is closely related to the metabolism of the human body. When massaging the elbow, press the depression here with our thumb, and we can feel it. Slight soreness. Press slightly harder with our thumb, take a slight pain as the benchmark, press and hold for 5 seconds and then release, and press alternately with both hands for 3-5 minutes.

Intestinal detoxification point - Tianshu point. This point is three finger widths on both sides of the navel. Massage method: Before going to bed, rub the Tianshu acupoint 50-100 times with the forefingers of both hands at the same time, repeating counterclockwise and clockwise each time. It is closely related to the gastrointestinal tract, and has an obvious bidirectional effect on regulating the intestines. It can not only stop diarrhea, but also clear the bowels. Long-term maintenance and massage of this point can ensure the health of the intestines and clear the accumulated stools in the intestines.

Baking Soda Water Detox

Edible baking soda is usually used to make bread and soda. The canned drinks all contain baking soda. When we open it, bubbles appear, that is, the baking soda is chemically reacting. Baking soda also has a cleaning function. Adding a little baking soda to the dishwashing water will not burn our hands, but can also wash the bowls and dishes very cleanly. We can also use baking soda to scrub stainless steel pots, copper pots or iron pots, baking soda can also clean the scale in the thermos. In addition, baking soda can also remove peculiar smells, etc. Baking soda has many uses.

Since the baking soda is edible, it can also clean up the dirt, the same reason, then the toxic dirt in the blood vessels can also be cleaned up. Do people drink Coca-Cola also contain a lot of baking soda? People in European and American countries like to drink soda. Soda water is water made by baking soda, which is weakly alkaline, and the human body environment is weakly alkaline. Diabetes patients have an acidic body, long-term drinking can remove acidic metabolites in the body, adjust the body's acid-base balance, and change the acidic body. Medically, baking soda can be used to treat hyperacidity, indicating that baking soda has the effect of regulating acidity.

General food and vegetables can only remove toxins in the blood and intestines, but there is no way to deal with the stubborn toxins on the blood vessel walls. However, the baking soda water has an osmotic function, which can pass through the cell membrane to carry toxic waste out of the cell, keeping the body clean, smooth and full of vitality. Baking soda can promote insulin secretion and cholesterol decomposition, keeping the body away from high blood lipids.

Cardiovascular atherosclerotic plaque adheres to the damaged blood vessel wall. It is uneven and forms a hard protective film on the outside, so it is not easy to be cleaned off. At present, general doctors do not advocate oral thrombolytic drugs to solve atherosclerotic plaques, because thrombolytic drugs can cause large plaques on the blood vessel wall to fall off and easily form embolism, which is very risky.

While soda water is weakly alkaline, the most obvious is its osmotic dissolving function. I scrubbed the greasy kitchenware with soda water, and saw that the oil on the kitchenware was quickly dissolved by the soda water, and then I washed it with water. So, I thought that since baking soda is edible, it should also be a good scavenger for the blood vessels of the human body. Because the principle of soda cleaning is to first penetrate and then dissolve, and then take the dissolved toxic substances out of the body.

Soda water can be made by ourself, which is very convenient. For a period of time, I got up every morning, mixed a half spoon of edible baking soda in a glass of boiled water, and then drank it. In the morning, the blood in the body is relatively viscous. The plain water washed with baking soda can not only quickly dilute the blood, but also dissolve and clean up the old oily and fatty plaques hidden on the blood vessel walls. Every time I drank baking soda, the stool on the next day formed, but it must be a little sticky, and the stool came out with a slight sensation. I have observed many times, and I can conclude that the soda that I drink in the morning dissolves and excretes the fat in the blood vessels.

Using baking soda to clean up fatty plaques on blood vessel walls is effective. However, everything has two sides. Although baking soda can help human body descaling, it can also take away a lot of bone, prone to osteoporosis. Therefore, don't drink it every day, drink it every other day, or drink it at different times. Or sometimes eat too much meat and fish, and then drink a glass of baking soda to neutralize it. Everyone's physical condition and physique are different, so we should drink soda reasonably according to our actual condition.

Table Vinegar Detox

Vinegar is the most commonly used condiment in the home and has a strong antibacterial ability. In the past, every cold season, vinegar was boiled at home, and the smell of vinegar circulated in the room to achieve the purpose of sterilization. The liver likes acidic foods, and vinegar can enhance liver function and promote metabolism. Vinegar can also soften blood vessels, dilate blood vessels, help lower blood pressure and prevent the occurrence of cardiovascular diseases. Vinegar enhances kidney function, has a diuretic effect, and can reduce urine sugar levels. It can also convert excess fat in the body into physical energy consumption, and promote the metabolism of sugar and protein, which can prevent obesity. Vinegar stimulates gastric acid secretion and aids digestion. In short, there are many benefits of vinegar, which are very helpful to the human body.

Edible vinegar and fruit vinegar are made from grains and fruits and have no side effects on the human body. Because the raw materials of vinegar are different, the production method is different, and the taste and acidity of vinegar are also different. Shanxi old vinegar has a strong flavor and a strong sour taste. Zhenjiang balsamic vinegar is light in taste, moderately sour and mellow, making it the first choice for home. I like to mix cold dishes with Zhenjiang vinegar. Shanxi old aged vinegar takes time to taste, and the more delicious it is, the more fragrant it is. The taste of fruit vinegar is single, mainly sour, all sour, and the throat and eyes are sour after drinking it.

I cross-drink these vinegar and try each one. In addition to adding some vinegar to taste when cooking every day, get up in the morning, mix a spoonful of Shanxi aged vinegar or Zhenjiang balsamic vinegar in a glass of boiled water and drink it. Or put two spoons of fruit vinegar in plain water. After drinking the vinegar water, be sure to drink a few sips of pure boiled water to wash the vinegar in your mouth. Because acetic acid will corrode teeth, rinse with pure white water and it will be fine.

Although vinegar has many benefits, it cannot be overdone. Excessive drinking of vinegar will not only not help the human body, but will damage the gastric mucosa. There must be a degree in everything, not too much vinegar. As long as we eat a little vinegar every day, we can have a significant detox effect in the long run.

Chapter 5

Pancreas is fountain of body fluid

It is very interesting to accidentally see the distribution of water and land on the earth. The structure of man and nature is so similar that I can't help but marvel at the magic of the creator. According to statistics, the area of the world's oceans is about 361 million square kilometers, accounting for 71% of the earth's surface area. The land area is only 29%. The total area of the ocean is almost two and a half times that of the land. Let's take a look at the water in our human body, which accounts for about 70% of the body weight, which is the same as the water share on the earth. Is this a coincidence? No, I don't believe this is an accidental number. It is that the creator of nature has shaped human beings according to the standards of nature since the day he created man, or the origin of man is naturally generated and evolved in the environment of nature, The structure of man is entirely inherited from nature.

Nature is based on water, and the human body is based on water. Everything revolves around water to survive, develop, and continue. It can be said that without water, there is no continuation of human beings. Human embryos develop in the amniotic fluid in the mother's womb. The amniotic fluid in the womb is the ocean world of embryos, and is the nutritional base for embryo development and formation.

The occurrence of various diseases of the human body is also related to water, which is a phenomenon that we usually rarely notice.

Water is the key to our health, the root cause of all diseases, and modern civilization diseases are usually caused by water-related causes, such as immunity from fatigue, cell poisoning, cell oxidation, abnormal blood circulation, etc. These are all closely related to water. Water is the solvent for many substances in the body. During the whole life process, the stream circulates endlessly throughout the body, keeping the volume of body fluid inside and outside the cell and the concentration of the substance, pH, temperature, osmotic pressure and other conditions relatively stable.

Diabetes is caused by a lack of water in the body. To be precise, the body cannot secrete or insufficiently secrete a specific body fluid - the hypoglycemic hormone insulin. Diabetes is not only related to high blood sugar, but also has a more direct relationship with body fluid.

Chinese Medicine Says Diabetes is Damaging Yin, What Is Yin?

Body fluid is the general term for the normal water of the human body, and it is the basic substance that constitutes the human body and maintains the life activities of the human body. Water is yin in the body, and yin in the body represents water. Injury to yin is to damage the production of body fluid and affect the distribution of body fluid.

Each of us comes out of this world through a channel, and this channel is the mother's vagina. The vagina is a natural outlet that continues human life for generations, and is the door of life for new life to pass baptism. And when people come to this world and open their eyes, they see the light. Why did the ancients give this door of life the name of vagina instead of Yang Dao? It can be seen that Yin occupies a very important position in the continuation of human life.

According to the theory of traditional Chinese medicine, blood belongs to yin, and water also belongs to yin. The continuation of human beings cannot be separated from blood or water. A woman's egg is combined with a man's sperm. The man's sperm is wrapped in semen and runs to the egg. The woman's egg is also pushed by the fluid secreted in the tube to enter the uterus. Therefore, the combination of sperm and egg to create life is inseparable from the help of water. During pregnancy, a woman's uterus is filled with amniotic fluid, which is a sea of embryos. The formation and development of human embryos are carried out in amniotic fluid, human reproduction is established in water. Therefore, yin is an important birthplace of life, and hurting yin is to damage the basic living conditions of the body, resulting in the degeneration and imbalance of the body as a whole.

The goddess who dominates the water in the body is our dear pancreas. It is our ignorant lifestyle, overeating and vegetarian diets that have brought destruction to our lovely goddess. The vibrant body of the past, now weary and struggling between life and death. The process of curing the disease of our diabetic patients is to try to restore the original beauty and health of the water goddess. For this reason, understanding the water family is also a necessary part of the road to health.

Body Fluid Family

Modern medicine believes that body fluid is the general term for all normal water fluids in the human body. It is customary to also include urine, sweat, snot, and tears in the metabolites. Body fluid is mainly composed of water and contains a large amount of nutrients. Body fluid is one of the basic substances that constitute the human body and maintain life activities. If the body fluid is not produced enough or lost too much, many diseases will be caused. Diabetes and tumors are typical cases of body fluid deficiency and yin injury.

In traditional Chinese medicine, there is a saying that "the five internal organs transform into five liquids". Sweat is the product of the heart, snot is the product of the lungs, tears come from the liver, the spleen produces mouth watering, and the kidneys produce saliva. Therefore, Chinese medicine believes that body fluid is composed of five fluids: sweat, snot, tears, mouth water, and saliva. Most of the five fluids referred to by traditional Chinese medicine are metabolites of modern medicine, excluding other important fluids in the human body.

We can learn from the analysis of body fluids in traditional Chinese medicine, and intuitively learn a lot of medical knowledge from the superficial phenomena of the human body, so as to judge what obstacles are caused by the lack of body fluids, so as to avoid unnecessary water consumption.

Chinese medicine believes that body fluid is an important part of blood, and blood is dominated by the heart, so sweat is the heart fluid. Those who sweat too much will consume the heart's blood and hurt the heart and yang.

The nasal mucus can moisturize the nostrils, and the nose passes through the lungs, so the nasal mucus is lung fluid. Lung heat, dry lungs will cause less nasal discharge, dry nose, and insufficient lung qi will cause nasal congestion and runny nose.

Tears are hidden in the eyes and do not flow out, and can nourish the eyes, while the liver is related to the eyes, and tears are liver fluid. If there are few tears, the eyes will be dry, which is liver yin and liver blood deficiency. Weeping in the wind is due to a large fire in the liver meridian, or deficiency of both liver and kidney.

Saliva can moisten the throat cavity, and the spleen is related to the mouth, so saliva is spleen fluid. If the spleen and stomach body fluids cannot go up to the mouth, the saliva will be less and the mouth will be dry.

Two saliva are body fluids in the mouth, collectively called "saliva", which is what we often call "Mouth water".

The saliva, which is thicker, is raw under the tongue, spit out from the mouth, has the function of dissolving food to facilitate swallowing and protecting and moisturizing the mouth, and is transformed by the kidney essence. The liquid, which is thinner, overflows the mouth and flows out from the corners of the mouth. Salivation protects and cleans the mouth, moistens and dissolves food, making it easier to swallow and digest, and is governed by the spleen. Saliva contains a lot of enzymes, which are chemicals needed by the human body to help digest food, moisturize the mouth, and resist the invasion of foreign bacteria. If the salivation secreted by the spleen is not enough, the mouth will be dry, the digestive enzymes will not be enough, the spleen and stomach will be out of balance, and the normal secretion of insulin will be affected, which will eventually lead to diabetes.

In addition, gastric juice, intestinal juice, joint fluid, pancreatic endocrine fluid, exocrine fluid, etc are all critical to human body fluid, which contains a variety of enzymes and is the human body's chemical plant. Modern medicine calls these body fluids hormones, which regulate human functions. Indispensable chemical elements for metabolism all the time.

It can be said that the human body's internal organs, muscles, bones, etc. are human hardware, and body fluid is the human body's software. This is my definition of the division of body fluids in the body. To understand body fluid, we must first understand the endocrine system.

Endocrine System

In humans or higher animals, some glands or organs secrete hormones, which are carried to the whole body by the blood without passing through the catheter, thereby regulating the growth, development and physiological functions of the organism. This secretion is called endocrine.

The main endocrine glands of the human body are: pituitary gland, thyroid gland, parathyroid gland, adrenal gland, gonad, pancreatic islet, thymus and pineal gland, etc. These glands secrete high-efficiency organic chemicals called hormones, which pass through the blood circulation to transmit chemical information to organs or cells that can receive hormone stimulation from endocrine cells to exert excitatory or inhibitory effects. Hormones are also called endocrine as the first messenger.

Medically, the endocrine system is defined as an important regulatory system of the body, which complements the nervous system and jointly regulates the growth and development of the body and various metabolisms, maintains the stability of the internal environment, and influences behavior and controls reproduction.

Pancreatic islets are a cluster of cells scattered between the pancreatic acinar cells, accounting for only 1% to 2% of the total pancreatic volume. Pancreatic islet cells are mainly divided into five types, of which A cells account for about 25% of the total islet cells and secrete glucagon. B cells account for about 60% of the total islet cells and secrete insulin. D cells secrete somatostatin in small numbers. In addition, PP cells secrete pancreatic polypeptide.

The main role of insulin is to regulate the metabolism of sugar, fat and protein. It can promote all tissues of the body, especially can accelerate the uptake of glucose by liver cells and muscle cells, and promote their storage and utilization of glucose. After liver cells and muscle cells absorb a large amount of glucose, they convert it into glycogen and store it on the one hand, or convert glucose into fatty acids in the liver cells, which are transported to adipose tissue for storage. On the other hand, it promotes the oxidation of glucose to produce high-energy phosphoric acid compounds as an energy source.

Another function of insulin is to promote the synthesis of fatty acids by liver cells. The glucose that enters the fat cells can be used to synthesize fatty acids. Insulin can also inhibit lipolysis. Sugar cannot be stored and used when insulin is lacking, which not only causes diabetes, but also causes fat metabolism disorders, increased blood lipids, arteriosclerosis, and serious cardiovascular system disease.

Insulin also plays an important role in protein metabolism. It can promote amino acids to enter cells, and then directly act on ribosomes to promote protein synthesis. It can also inhibit protein breakdown, which is very important for the body's growth process.

Endocrine disorders are extremely harmful to the body, making the body unable to carry out normal growth, development, reproduction, and normal metabolic activities. There are many kinds of endocrine glands in the human body, and different endocrine glands have different harms to the human body when diseases occur.

If the pancreatic islets are affected, too much insulin secretion will cause hypoglycemia, and too little insulin secretion will lead to diabetes. If the thyroid gland produces too much thyroid hormone, it will cause hyperthyroidism, overeating, weight loss, fear of heat, and palpitation. Hypothyroidism occurs when thyroid hormone is produced too little, and the symptoms are just the opposite of hyperthyroidism.

If the pituitary gland produces too little growth hormone, dwarfism occurs, and the height of an adult is less than 130 cm. If the pituitary gland function is low, it can affect the thyroid, gonads, and adrenal glands, resulting in sexual underdevelopment, hindered growth and development, poor physical strength, and poor intelligence.

Insulin is the only hormone in the human body that can lower blood sugar, and it is also the only hormone that promotes glycogen, fat, and protein synthesis at the same time.

Next, we need to understand the blood circulation system, and get to know the unsung hero's lymph fluid behind the scenes, the family members of body fluid。

Blood Circulatory System

Blood is the main substance that nourishes the body, and the quality of nutrition directly affects the activities of the human body, including heart function.

The ancient Chinese medicine book "Nei Jing" says: "The heart governs the blood of the body". Therefore, people with insufficient blood and body fluids are most likely to suffer from heart disease. The blood circulation system is the channel through which blood flows in the body and is divided into two parts: the cardiovascular system and the lymphatic system. As we know, the blood circulatory system basically refers to the cardiovascular system. Few people associate the lymphatic system with the blood circulatory system.

Cardiovascular system

The cardiovascular system consists of blood, blood vessels and the heart. The heart is the power organ that drives blood flow. Blood vessels are the series of tubes through which blood flows, and blood vessels in the human body are found throughout the body. According to the structure and function of blood vessels, they are divided into three types: arteries, veins and capillaries.

Arteries are the blood vessels that carry blood out of the heart. Veins are blood vessels that carry blood back to the heart. Capillaries are very thin blood vessels connected between arteries and veins. Arteries and veins are pipes that transport blood, and capillaries are places where blood and tissues exchange substances.

The cardiovascular system is a "closed" system of pipes that consists of the heart and blood vessels, including arteries, veins, and capillaries. The heart is the muscular power organ that pumps blood, and the vascular system that transports blood. The cardiovascular system is responsible for transporting the blood pumped by the heart to various tissues and organs throughout the body to meet the various nutrients required for the body's activities, and to transport the end products (wastes) of metabolism back to the heart, excreted from the body through the lungs, kidneys and other organs. The total number of capillaries in an adult is more than 30 billion, about 110, 000 kilometers long, enough to circle the earth 2. 7 times.

Lymphatic System

The lymphatic system is another tributary of the blood circulatory system. The lymphatic system is composed of lymph, lymphatic vessels and lymph nodes. The lymphatic system is an important defense system of the human body, and it is closely related to the cardiovascular system.

The lymphatic system produces white blood cells and antibodies, filters out pathogens, participates in immune responses, and plays an important role in the distribution of fluids and nutrients in the body. Lymph fluid produced by the lymphatic system enters the bloodstream and is circulated throughout the body by the blood vessels of the heart. The lymphatic system is also known as the body's immune system.

The main functions of the lymphatic system are as follows: 1. Recover the liquid that has penetrated into the interstitial spaces from the capillaries and divert it to the blood. 2. The digested fat can be transported to the blood vessels. 3. It can produce lymphocytes and antibodies to defend and filter and reduce lymphatic pathogens.

Between the tissues and capillaries of the human body, a part of the liquid in the blood will become tissue fluid in the tissues. After the tissue fluid enters the lymphatic vessels, it is the lymph fluid, which is a substance that is as clear as water and resembles blood plasma. We have all had this experience. When a certain part of our body is accidentally bruised or burned, the tissue becomes inflamed, and the injured part swells, the lymphatic system is required to drain the accumulated fluid.

At first, there was some watery fluid in it. It keeps flowing out, until the liquid water stops flowing, the wound will begin to heal, and the human body will resume normal fluid circulation. Also, when the virus invades the human body and the infection occurs, the lymph nodes will become swollen and painful. For example, when the throat becomes inflamed, two lumps will be felt under the chin, that is, the lymph nodes. After the inflammation disappears, the lymphatic mass will naturally shrink and disappear.

The combination of the cardiovascular and lymphatic systems is our blood circulatory system. The cardiovascular system is the main circulation of our body, and the lymphatic system is the bodyguard and patron saint of the cardiovascular system. Lymph fluid is a part of body fluid and belongs to the body fluid family.

Saliva

Saliva contains a variety of enzymes, and we people feel sweet when eating. It is the result of the chemical action of the enzymes in the saliva. The quality of a person's appetite is closely related to the saliva in the mouth. People with a dry mouth will never have more appetites than those with moist saliva.

Saliva not only allows us to taste delicious food, it has a digestive effect, but also helps our oral cavity clean and hygienic, moisturize the mouth, easy to speak and swallow, and saliva can sterilize.

Once in a health program, I saw a Chinese doctor teach us to identify diseases on the tongue. He said that the root of the tongue is

Xia Jiao. If the root of the tongue is greasy and sticky, it means that the kidneys have damp heat. In the past, I always thought that the sticky tongue was a problem of the spleen and stomach. Through the advice of experts, I understood that it was caused by dampness and heat in the kidneys. The kidneys are hot and humid, and the hot kidney water cannot cool the heart fire, so the saliva under the base of the tongue is thick and sticky. Wrong judgment leads to wrong treatment, so the effect is not good. Eating food that purifies stomach fire for a long time not only does not change the symptoms of sticky mouth, but aggravates the cold in the stomach. Makes the stomach uncomfortable and indigestion.

Saliva is a part of body fluid. We usually feel dry mouth and lack of saliva moisturizing. It is because the small salivary glands in the mouth are malfunctioning due to the function of the internal organs, which can cause abnormal secretion. In the five elements, the kidney is restricted by the spleen (pancreas). The spleen is not good, the kidneys are affected, and the spleen and kidneys are hot and humid. It is inevitable that the water channels are blocked, the saliva is insufficient, the tongue is sticky, and the smell in the mouth is not pure.

For diabetic patients, the pancreas, the biochemical source of body fluid, malfunctions, causing systemic water shortage.

Pancreas Is the Biochemical Source of Body Fluid

The physiological function of the pancreas is similar to that of the spleen, but not the same. The relationship between the two is like a pair of twin brothers. The spleen controls the blood and the pancreas controls the body fluid. The spleen is the source of blood biochemistry, and the pancreas is the source of body fluid biochemistry. The pancreas is responsible for the coordination of the whole body, managing the intake of nutrients, controlling the water metabolism in the body and nourishing the human body.

From the perspective of human organ function, the problem of blood is the spleen, and the problem of body fluid is the pancreas. Is there a problem with the blood or the body fluid in a diabetic? Is this the dereliction of duty of the spleen or the pancreas?From the appearance point of view, the sugar content in the blood of diabetic patients is high, and the high blood sugar flowing in the blood vessels does bring great harm to the human body, but the cause of this harm is the endocrine disorder of the pancreas. It does not secrete the insulin that the human body needs to lower blood sugar. Therefore, to catch the thief must capture the king, and to solve the problem must grasp the main contradiction, so as to achieve the desired results with half the effort.

In the process of self-treatment of diabetes, I repeated many times, and gradually explored more feasible methods of self-care and treatment. I put qi and blood in the first place. This is because qi and blood are the most basic living material of the human body. If there is insufficient qi and blood, the body's self-healing cannot be achieved. In other words, without the aid of qi and blood, the human body cannot be I repair broken and broken bodies. When the human body's qi and blood meet the needs, the human body begins to become stronger and the immune system is enhanced, before it can automatically start the repair work.

We still haven't really understood the important role the pancreas plays in the human body. We all understand blood. The human body cannot survive without blood. So, can the human body not survive without body fluid?

The answer is yes. This is why pancreatic cancer has the highest degree of malignancy and the highest mortality rate among common tumors. If there is a problem the five internal organs of the human body, it be replaced by surgery, such as heart replacement, kidney replacement, liver replacement, etc, to save the patient's life, but if it is the endocrine system, the lymphatic system has a major problem and it is impossible to replace it. Just like the computer has a problem, the hardware can be replaced, and the entire system is paralyzed if the software is broken.

Does that mean that a problem with the body fluid command system cannot be resolved? I think it can be solved, because everything in the world has a cause and effect. Since disease has a path, it must also have a way back. It depends on whether we can find the golden key to solve the problem. At least no one can really solve this difficult medical problem. Insulin is the only hypoglycemic hormone, there is no replacement hormone in the body.

Chinese medicine believes that the pancreas belongs to the yin in the viscera, is surrounded by the viscera, is yin in the meridians, and is sandwiched among many yang meridians on the back, and is the yin meridian of the yang. Inside, the pancreas distributes body fluid to the three burners, the upper burner is like a mist to nourish the five organs of the viscera, and the lower burner is like a stream to dissolve silt and rot and clear the intestines. Outside, it emits meridian qi, replenishes skin fat, and keeps it elastic and energetic. It can be seen that the pancreas is not only the source of biochemical yin fluid, but also an important minister controlling the distribution of yin fluid.

Since the pancreas is the biochemical source of yin fluid, it controls the production and distribution of body fluid in the body. If there is a problem with this source, problems will occur in the water channels in the body, and various water supply units will have problems successively. To solve the problem of dehydration in diabetic patients, I mainly use body fluids and massage the pancreas. I think that since the body fluid is insufficient, the top priority is to replenish it from the outside, and at the same time use the theory of TCM meridians to resolve the internal blockage of the pancreas. TCM says that as long as the road is open, there will be no pain. As long as the heat and humidity in the pancreas is removed, Clean up the silt in the waterway, so that the pancreatic cells are full of oxygen and breathe freely and smoothly. Its function will slowly recover, at least it will not deteriorate.

Massage the pancreas before and after every morning and evening. In fact, massaging the pancreas and even the natural kidneys is done together. After each massage, the back of the waist is warm and the saliva in the mouth is filled. The skin has not been dry, and drinking eight glasses of water every day is a crucial guarantee.

The most effective way to invigorate body fluid is to boil white fungus and red jujube lily soup. Tremella is a yin-tonifying liquid to moisturize dryness, red dates are to replenish blood, and lily is to clear lung heat. When these three are combined, the nourishing body fluid is very effective. At least it is very effective for me.

Milk is also an excellent food for replenishing yin. Milk is biochemically formed by the blood in the cow's body, which is yin, the best nourishing yin fluid. Drinking a large bowl every day will not only help you sleep better, but you will also rarely get skin diseases.

Because I have been insisting on hydrating my body and replenishing yin. When my skin accidentally suffers external damage, it will heal quickly. The self-maintenance of the lymphatic system in the body is normal and there is no mistake, and there has been almost no swelling of the lymph nodes in recent years. Therefore, the blood sugar level is also easy to maintain within the normal range.

Regulation of Water Metabolism by Human Organs

Water-liquid metabolism is the main link to maintain the body's balance. The human body is a closely cooperating team, and the entire process of human body water metabolism is completed by the cooperation of the functions of the various organs. Any dysfunction of the viscera will affect the production, transportation and excretion of body fluids, which will hinder the metabolism of body fluids. We now look at how the liver, spleen (pancreas), lungs, triple-burner, (Based on the theory of traditional Chinese medicine the upper, middle and lower triple burners are used to divide the internal organs of the human body)and small intestine participate in the water metabolism in the body from the perspective of Chinese medicine.

The regulation of water metabolism is closely related to the liver. Liver governs dredging, regulating qi, and the operation of water also depends on the promotion of qi. The liver regulates the metabolism of water and fluids, mainly through three ways: First, adjust the qi movement of the Sanjiao, so that the waterway of the Sanjiao is fluent. The second is to promote the ascending and descending of the qi of the lungs, spleen, kidneys and other viscera, so as to play their role in hosting water and fluid metabolism. The third is that when qi travels, blood travels, blood travels, water conservancy, qi and blood run smoothly, and water and fluids run normally.

If the liver has pathological changes, it is not easy to disperse, and the movement of qi is not smooth, which will affect the movement of blood and water. Blood stasis and water resistance, qi stagnation and water stagnation, which lead to water and fluid metabolism disorders, will cause water metabolism disorders such as liver ascites.

The spleen (pancreas) plays an important role in the process of human body water metabolism. The meaning of transporting water is very broad, including the process of elevating, distributing, excreting, etc, of water in the body's various organs, tissues and organs.

The spleen (pancreas) is in the middle focal point, which is the overall regulation of the body's qi lifting and lowering, and the water and liquid metabolism. In the body, water drops from the lungs to the kidneys, or from the kidneys to vaporize and rise to the lungs, both of which rely on the transmission of the spleen (pancreas) to maintain normality. The spleen (pancreas) has sufficient qi, and the function of transporting and transforming water is strong, and the body's water metabolism can be coordinated and balanced. If the spleen (pancreas) is insufficiency, it will be difficult for the water to be transported and excreted, causing the water to stop internally and produce a variety of symptoms.

Ancient Chinese medicine believed that "all dampness and swelling belong to the spleen. " Various lumps and moisture in the body are attributed to the problem of the spleen (pancreas), which emphasizes the important role of the spleen (pancreas) in the process of water and fluid metabolism.

The lungs are in charge of lifting and lowering, and regulate the function of water channels. There are clear and turbid water, among which the clear, through the lung's propagating and dispersing effect, distributes to the body surface and viscera to nourish and moisten the viscera, skin, and fur. The turbid water in it, through the descending action of the lungs, descends into the kidneys through the Sanjiao waterway, and is converted into urine for excretion.

The regulating effect of the lungs on water and fluid metabolism is mainly achieved by regulating perspiration and the Sanjiao waterway, so "the lungs are the source above water". If the lungs are diseased, the water metabolism will be abnormal, which can lead to edema and inconvenience in urination.

Chinese medicine believes that if the kidney qi is strong, the water will return to the sea, and if the kidney qi is weak, the water will disperse in the skin. Qi can promote water, and kidney yang is the foundation of yang qi in the human body, and it plays a warming and biochemical effect on the functions of the body's various viscera.

The gasification of kidney yang plays an important role in the propagation and suppression of the lungs, the transport and transformation of the spleen, the opening and closing of the bladder, and the dredging of the water channels of the triple burner. Therefore, the kidney plays an important role in regulating the balance of water and fluid metabolism.

Sanjiao is a term unique to traditional Chinese medicine. It is one of the six fu-organs. It is a pathway for the movement of qi and water and liquid, and it is one of the important viscera that participates in the metabolism of water and liquid in the human body. The triple focus is located in the cavity between the body and the internal organs, including the thoracic cavity and abdominal cavity. The internal organs of the human body are all in it. Upper focus, including heart and lungs. The internal organs from the transverse septum to the belly button are middle focal, including the spleen, stomach, liver, and gallbladder. The lower part of the umbilicus is the lower focal point, including the kidneys, large intestine, small intestine and bladder.

Sanjiao is sick, which often affects water metabolism. The triple-burner is impassable and the water is blocked. Systemic edema such as skin and muscles can occur, as well as ascites, pleural effusion and other diseases.

The small intestine also has the physiological function of identifying turbidity. It not only absorbs nutrients, but also transports food residues to the large intestine, and also absorbs water to participate in water metabolism. When the small intestine absorbs the essence of food, it also absorbs part of the water, and descends the bladder to form urine, so it is also called"the main liquid of the small intestine". If the small intestine is diseased, the turbidity is not distinguished, and the water and residues flow into the large intestine together, and diarrhea occurs, and the urine is also short and yellow.

Cells and Insulin

Normal human tissue cells must be in a suitable acid-base environment in order to carry out normal life activities.

Insulin is a protein hormone secreted by pancreatic beta cells in the pancreas. Insulin is involved in regulating glucose metabolism and controlling blood sugar balance. Insulin is the body's only hypoglycemic hormone and the only hormone that promotes the synthesis and storage of nutrients (sugar, protein and fat) in the body. Insulin acts on liver cells, fat cells, muscle cells, blood cells, lung cells, kidney cells and testicular cells, etc, but mainly acts on liver cells, muscle and fat cells.

The secretion of insulin is divided into two parts. One part is the insulin secreted to help maintain normal fasting blood sugar, called basal insulin, and the other part is the insulin secreted to reduce postprandial blood glucose rise and maintain normal postprandial blood sugar, called prandial insulin.

In the liver, insulin mainly promotes glycogen synthesis and inhibits the production of glucose. Since the source of glycogen is glucose, the increased production of glycogen will utilize blood sugar, and the concentration of blood sugar will decrease. In addition, the liver is the factory that produces glucose, and this function will be inhibited by insulin, which will also have the same hypoglycemic results.

The liver of people with type 2 diabetes releases too much glucose, especially at night, (normally the liver only releases a small amount of glucose) resulting in higher blood sugar levels in the morning.

In adipose tissue, insulin can inhibit the breakdown of fat, because blood sugar (glucose) can be used as energy, so there is no need for fat to break down. In other words, insulin can promote energy storage in the form of fat.

Every cell in the human body has a part where insulin can act, called the insulin receptor. The combination of insulin and receptors is like inserting a key into a keyhole. Insulin is the key that opens the door of a cell, allowing glucose to enter the cell and providing energy to the cell. The important job of insulin is to help glucose enter cells.

Diabetes patients are because there is a problem between the key to open the cell and the cell. Glucose cannot enter the cell, which causes the sugar content in the blood to increase, and the human cells cannot get the nutrition of glucose. When the concentration of sugar in the blood reaches a certain level, the kidneys will try to excrete it into the urine, so frequent urination, thirsty, or hunger will cause the body to lose weight.

Therefore, human cells need the participation and help of insulin to be adequately nourished. Human cells that lack insulin participation die off rapidly, which is why diabetes causes systemic degeneration.

Insulin resistance

Insulin resistance refers to the failure of normal amount of insulin to lower blood sugar, that is, antibodies are produced in the body for the lowering blood sugar effect of insulin, and fat cells, muscle cells and liver cells are not sensitive to the effects of normal concentration of insulin. For example, just like a normal person, one unit of insulin can lower 10 units of blood sugar, while in type 2 diabetic patients, the same unit of insulin can only lower 5 units of blood sugar. This is insulin resistance. To put it bluntly, insulin does not work well. This type of insulin resistance in the body is the root cause of type 2 diabetes.

For a normal person, the food eaten is digested and decomposed into glucose. When the blood sugar rises, the pancreas begins to secrete insulin into the blood, which quickly reduces the blood sugar to the normal range. For diabetic patients with insulin resistance, due to the decreased sensitivity of the body to insulin, the same insulin cannot produce the effect of lowering blood sugar, thus forming hyperglycemia and diabetes. Insulin resistance is not only one of the fundamental causes of type 2 diabetes, it is also related to hypertension, hyperlipidemia, high blood viscosity, abnormal lipid metabolism, and is the cause of arteriosclerosis. If diabetic patients simply take hypoglycemic drugs to stimulate the amount of insulin, the final effect may not be very good. To find out the real cause of insulin resistance is to cure the root cause

Not only high-carb, high-fat, high-protein diets, overeating, and excessively greasy, sweet and spicy diets are also responsible for insulin resistance. It is precisely because of these bad eating habits that the blood is filled with toxic waste and blood pollution, which buffers and blocks the neutralization effect of insulin and blood, and the vascular channels become increasingly narrowed, resulting in hypoxia in the body cells, resulting in adverse effects on the body. The normally secreted insulin is insensitive, so that the normal level of insulin cannot stimulate the signal that induces muscle and fat cells to absorb glucose, and cannot achieve normal hypoglycemic effect. It's like scratching the itch over your boots, you cannot catch itch place, you can only scratch the itch if you take off your boots. In the same way, only when the impurities and toxins in the blood of the blood vessels are cleaned up and there is enough oxygen and vitality in the cells, insulin can play its normal function in the cells.

Therefore, while cleaning the blood toxins, it is important to increase the oxygen in the body in an appropriate amount, because the activity of the cells in the body is all regulated by oxygen.

Cell Oxygenation Is Important

Human is a living body, and the cells that make up the human body are also active. People cannot live without oxygen, and human cells cannot survive without oxygen. The enzymes in body fluid also need oxygen to activate. The human body can be energetic and perform normal functions only when there is sufficient oxygen.

The human body is composed of nearly 75 trillion cells, each of which is composed of a nucleus, cytoplasm and cell membrane. Among them, the mitochondria in the cytoplasm provide cell energy and are the power station of the cell. The sugars, fats, proteins and other substances that we eat are all decomposed in the mitochondria to produce energy, which is used by the cells of the whole body.

Mitochondria are two-layered organelles found in most eukaryotic cells. Mitochondria are the site of oxidative metabolism in eukaryotes, and the place where carbohydrates, fatty and amino acids are finally oxidized to release energy. The most important factor for substances to be fully decomposed in mitochondria is "oxygen", and the oxygen consumption of mitochondria accounts for 80-90% of the oxygen consumption of all cells. If the cells carry enough oxygen and release enough oxygen, the energy will be fully produced, the cells will be in the best operating state, the metabolism of the body will be vigorous, and the person will be healthy. However, if the oxygen carrying and oxygen release of cells is insufficient, nutrients cannot be fully decomposed in mitochondria, the cells will malfunction, and the body will have diseases.

Therefore, any nutrient that enters the cell needs enough oxygen to participate in the body's metabolism to continue life. Without the participation of oxygen, these substances entering the cells will evolve into human toxins due to insufficient metabolism, and become a killer of human health. The lack of oxygen in the cells of the pancreas causes weak endocrine function, which induces diabetes. Insufficient oxygen in the digestive tract and liver is not enough for fat metabolism, and fat residues will be deposited on the blood and blood vessel walls, leading to high blood pressure, atherosclerosis and other heart diseases.

Cell hypoxia leads to diseases. Oxygen supplementation can only relieve hypoxia, but it cannot really solve the problem of hypoxia. Only by strengthening the ability of cells to carry and release oxygen can the development of the disease be truly stopped from the source. Supplementing oxygen to cells in time and enhancing the ability of red blood cells to carry oxygen, transport oxygen and release oxygen is an important means to solve a variety of diseases. Insulin is a hormone and body fluid that contains enzymes that lower and break down sugar. The working state of the enzyme is carried out under the condition of being activated. If the hypoxia of the cells in the diabetic patient causes the cell insulin antibody, even if the insulin secretion is normal, it cannot enter the cell.

I've done many trials and with the same diet and exercise, whenever my legs are sore and people are tired, my blood sugar levels are bound to be high. When my legs are relaxed and I walk happily like stepping on a keyboard, my blood sugar level must be normal. The soreness caused by muscle hypoxia is different from the soreness after exercise. After exercise, the soreness can be relieved by using some relaxation methods, while the soreness of the legs due to hypoxia, soaking the feet, and rubbing the legs will not work. This kind of soreness will not work. It will continue for several days. Through my own practice and the experience of others, I think that there are several better ways to alleviate and solve cellular hypoxia.

Methods of natural oxygen replenishment for cells:

Abdominal breathing: Through deep breathing, the breathing volume of the lungs is enlarged, and the total amount of oxygen in the body is increased. It boosts the spirit and energy of the person

Qigong is the use of deep breathing to send oxygen into the body to operate. Qi rotates through the body, and every cell can get nourishment by oxygen.

Tai Chi: Many people use Tai Chi to lower blood sugar effectively, indicating that Tai Chi is to increase internal energy and help cells carry oxygen.

Enzymes Are Produced by the Body Fluid

Cells are the basic unit of life activities, generally composed of plasma membrane, cytoplasm and nucleus. All cells that can perform their normal functions are active, and cells that are not active and decayed are dead cells. The cell can survive because of the presence of oxygen in the cell. The purpose of human respiration is to continuously maintain life. In essence, the oxygen provided by nature is inhaled from the mouth and then decomposed into various cells. Cells survive and life can continue.

When cells perform their functions, there are many chemical elements involved, among which enzymes are the main elements for cells to function. Enzymes are produced from body fluids. All kinds of lymph fluid, pancreatic fluid, intestinal fluid and other body fluids produced in the body contain enzymes, and the enzymes secreted by different organs are different.

Organisms are composed of cells, and each cell exhibits various life activities due to the presence of enzymes, and the metabolism in the body can proceed. Enzymes are the catalysts for metabolism in the human body. Only when enzymes exist, can the human body carry out various biochemical reactions. The more enzymes in the human body and the more complete it is, the healthier its life will be. When there is no active enzyme in the human body, life ends. Most of human diseases are related to enzyme deficiency or synthesis disorders, which is what doctors call a problem with the endocrine system.

Enzymes are involved in all life activities of the human body: such as thinking, exercise, sleep, breathing, anger, joyor secretion of hormones are the results of enzyme-centric activities. The catalytic action of enzymes stimulates the body's energetic biochemical reactions, and promotes the continuous and healthy operation of life phenomena.

Humans and mammals contain 5, 000 enzymes. They are either dissolved in the cytoplasm, or associated with various membrane structures, or located at specific locations in other structures within the cell (a product of the cell), and are activated only when needed, these enzymes are collectively referred to as intracellular enzymes. In addition, there are some enzymes that are synthesized in the cell and then secreted to the outside of the cell— extracellular enzymes.

The ability of an enzyme to catalyze a chemical reaction is called enzymatic activity. Enzyme activity can be regulated and controlled by a variety of factors, so that organisms can adapt to changes in external conditions and maintain life activities. Without the participation of enzymes, metabolism can hardly be completed, and life activities cannot be maintained at all. Therefore, Chinese medicine believes that the kidney is the innate foundation, and the spleen (pancreas) is the acquired foundation, that is, the spleen (pancreas) is the core organ of enzyme secretion, which explains why the spleen (pancreas) is the biochemical source of body fluids. source.

Enzymes are fermentable, and this fermentation process is the expansion process of the active body, so that the receptor becomes vivid, fresh and vigorous. The highest peak of enzymes in the human body is the best period of human development, that is to say, it is the youth period. The enzymes in the human body gradually decrease year by year. The older the person, the fewer enzymes in the body. This is human One of the main reasons for getting old.

Enzymes do not live in isolation. Enzymes are an active body attached to body fluid. There are thousands of enzymes in the human body, all living in body fluid. When we suffer from diabetes, the body's water or body fluid is reduced, the enzymes in the body are correspondingly reduced, and the enzymes provided to the cells are also reduced. The survival rate and activity of the cells in the body are compromised, and the lack of activity of the cells also compromises the performance of their functions. These are chain reactions.

Because most of the enzymes are proteins, they are easily destroyed by high temperature, strong acid, strong alkali, etc. The cause of diabetes is the imbalance of yin fluid caused by the body's internal heat, which destroys the balance of enzymes.

The presence of enzymes confirms that the entire metabolism is carried out in the correct way, and once there is no enzyme, metabolism can neither proceed according to the required steps nor complete the synthesis at a sufficient speed to meet the needs of the cell. In fact, without enzymes, metabolic pathways, such as glycolysis, cannot proceed independently.

Enzyme Oxygen and Temperature

Supplemented enzymes are active, whereas innate enzymes in the body require activators to function. The role of enzymes in cells is a chemical reaction. To keep enzymes fully functioning in cells, oxygen must be involved, so that the activity of enzymes is stimulated by oxygen, and the combination of the two makes cells healthy, full and fresh, the human body is in a state of vitality.

A healthy cell has not only the participation of fresh enzymes, but also the participation of energetic oxygen. It can be said that the relationship between enzymes and oxygen is interdependent and supports each other. Enzyme activity and oxygen activity are indispensable for cells. In the state of hypoxia, the enzyme is in a state of lethargy, the activity of the enzyme is imprisoned, the body's metabolism is slow, and people are prone to aging. With oxygen in the cell and lack of enzymes, the cell is like an empty shell without an entity and cannot be metabolized.

Many cooked foods are kept fresh by vacuum, but why can vacuum be kept fresh? We all know this is because without air, food will not rot and deteriorate. The decay of food has a lot to do with enzymes. Under normal air circulation, the enzymes in food receive oxygen in the air, and the activity of the enzymes is stimulated. The process of excitation is also the oxidation process. Generally, the degree of deterioration and decay is determined according to temperature and time. The higher the temperature, the rate of deterioration the faster, that is to say, the enzyme activity is slightly limited at low temperature, and the enzyme activity starts to be active at room temperature. The higher the temperature, the faster the enzyme dissolves the substance. Two conditions are needed to activate enzyme activity, oxygen and temperature.

The temperature in the human body is 37 degrees, which is suitable for enzymes to exert their normal activity, neither fast nor slow. If the blood circulation of the human body is slow and the body temperature is not enough, the hands and feet are always cold, which will easily cause the enzyme activity to be inhibited. Insufficient temperature not only limits the activity of enzymes, but also leads to the decline of pancreatic function, limiting the amount of pancreatic juice secreted by the pancreas, and people will suffer from dyspepsia.

Enzymes and Cells

The importance of enzymes in the human body is the same as the role of the kidneys, the relationship between innate and acquired roots, the relationship between hardware and software.

Cell division is the basis for growth and reproduction of organisms, and one mother cell usually produces two or several daughter cells.

Enzymes are not only catalysts for metabolism in the human body, enzymes are also catalysts for growth and reproduction of organisms. It is impossible for the cells of the organism to divide and multiply without enzymes. In the middle of the summer night, people can hear the noise of corn jointing in the crop fields. This is the sound of cells dividing.

There is scientific evidence that the cells of organisms carry the code of life, and I think that the enzymes inherent in organisms also carry the code of life. Enzymes are also divided into innate enzymes brought out from the mother and acquired enzymes through food. The combination of innate enzymes and the life code in the cell strictly controls the life cycle of the organism, and the acquired enzyme stimulates the activity of the organism and maintains the metabolism of the organism.

Some sources say that the amount of human enzymes is related to lifespan. Scientific research says that the normal life span of a human body is 130-150 years old, and human beings basically cannot live this age due to various reasons. Since the lifespan of the human body is fixed, even if the extraneous enzymes in the body are supplemented sufficiently, it cannot make people immortal forever. The role of human body supplementing enzymes is to maintain good cell metabolism during the normal life span, make people healthy, reduce diseases, and be full of vitality.

We have used computers and know that a computer is composed of a software system and a hardware system. The hardware system includes a processor, a motherboard, a memory, a graphics card, a sound card, a hard disk, a main box, a monitor, a keyboard, and a mouse. The software system includes operating system and other application software. The operating system manages computer hardware resources, and at the same time allocates resources to it according to the resource request of the application.

Our human body is like a complex large-scale computer. Bones, tendons, muscles, internal organs, etc are the hardware of our human body. Water, body fluid, lymph fluid, enzymes, hormones, nerves, etc. in the water fluid in the body are the software of the human body. The role of enzymes in the human body is like the operating system of a computer, which is responsible for all the chemical decomposition in the human body, meticulous and precise calculation and participation in every work link, the decomposition, absorption and removal of food, and maintain the metabolism of cells.

Every cell in the human body has the participation of enzymes, and the cells must perform a series of metabolic functions with the participation of enzymes. Cells without the participation of enzymes have no substantive content. Therefore, the quality of cells depends on the activity of enzymes. In other words, the health of a person's body depends on the quantity and quality of enzymes in the body.

Factors Restricting Enzymes

There are a large number of enzymes in the human body, with complex structures and various types. For example, when the rice is chewed in the mouth, the longer the chewing time, the more obvious the sweetness is, because the starch in the rice is hydrolyzed into maltose under the action of salivary amylase secreted by the mouth. Therefore, chewing more when eating can fully mix the food and saliva, which is conducive to digestion.

In addition, there are various hydrolases such as pepsin and trypsin in the human body. The protein that the human body ingests from food must be hydrolyzed into amino acids under the action of pepsin, etc, and then under the action of other enzymes, more than 20 kinds of amino acids needed by the human body are selected. In a certain order, the various proteins required by the human body are recombined, and many complex chemical reactions will occur in this process.

It can be said that without enzymes, there would be no biological metabolism, and there would be no various and colorful biological worlds in nature.

Since the role of enzymes in the human body is so important, the phenomenon of enzyme deficiency in the modern human body is very common. More than half of the ten people in the population have insufficient enzyme content. There are many reasons for the lack of enzymes, such as:fierce competition in society, high psychological pressure, and irregular life, which causes the aging of its own organs, such as the aging of the spleen (pancreas), comprehensively reduces the secretion of longevity enzymes, this affects the overall premature aging of 60 trillion cells in the eight major systems of the body.

We eat food every day. The intestines are food processing plants and garbage dumps. The intestines contain a large amount of toxins, which block capillaries and reduce the absorption of nutrients by the human body. Malnutrition causes premature aging of the internal organs and even produces various types. disease. Therefore, enterotoxin is not only the main source of various diseases, but also reduces the production and survival of enzymes.

Raw food contains essential digestive enzymes, which are easily inactivated by high temperature cooking. Since most of us are accustomed to mainly cooked food, the original enzymes in the food are destroyed, and the natural enzyme reserves in the body have to be consumed. In addition, the parts with the highest enzyme content in some fruits are in the peel and stem that people do not eat, and in the unripe bitter juice, the precious part with the highest enzyme content is thrown away. This is caused by the fact that we do not know the nutritional common sense of fruits.

With the rapid development of industry and the large increase in automobiles, large amounts of exhaust gas have been emitted, and the environment has been polluted， pesticide residues and the abuse of synthetic chemical additives in foods, fast-paced lifestyles, increased work pressure, and crawling in front of computer desks excessive time, lack of exercise, etc will increase the consumption of a large amount of enzymes in the body, so that the natural enzymes in the body cannot be preserved.

When we go to the mall to buy food, the shorter the shelf life, the fresher the food, and the more the enzyme activity is maintained. Because various preservatives inhibit the activity of most enzymes and achieve the purpose of long-term preservation. The human body ingests a large number of enzyme inhibitors, such as preservatives, pesticide residues, which directly affect metabolism. Expired food cannot be eaten because the preservative expires and loses its effect, the enzymes in the food begin to work, and the cells and tissues of the food begin to deteriorate, rot and deteriorate, and produce toxic substances.

Some foods are kept fresh by vacuuming. For example, the cooked food we often buy. The Beijing roast duck we buy at the airport store is packed in a vacuum bag. Open in the summer and taste as delicious as freshly baked. Therefore, food without the participation of air will not deteriorate and rot. In other words, without oxygen, the enzyme loses its activity. In the same way, human cells also inhibit enzyme activity during hypoxia.

We want both the preservation of food and the activity of enzymes in the food. A substance may be an activator of an enzyme and a restrictor of another enzyme at the same time. These are all contradictions in life, and the human body can survive and metabolize in the mutual restraint of these contradictions.

Why Need to Add Vitamin and Mineral

The chemical nature of enzymes is a protein complex, and this protein complex often requires trace elements and vitamins as its vitality core. If the trace elements and vitamins in this enzyme protein are insufficient or lacking, the enzyme activity will be greatly reduced, or even no biological activity. Then the biochemical reactions in the body cannot proceed normally. The physiological metabolism of the human body is bound to malfunction, and many disease conditions appear.

Minerals can activate enzymes, and substances that can activate enzymes are called enzyme activators. There are many types of activators, including inorganic cations, such as sodium ion, potassium ion, copper ion, calcium ion, etc. Inorganic anions, such as chloride ion, bromide ion, iodide ion, sulfate ion, phosphate ion, etc. Organic compounds such as vitamin C, cysteine, reduced glutathione, etc. Many enzymes exhibit or enhance their catalytic activity only when an appropriate activator is present, and this enzyme cooperates with the catalytic activity. Some enzymes are inactive after being synthesized, and this enzyme is called a zymogen, which must be activated by an appropriate activator before it becomes active.

Whether it is trace elements or vitamins, the human body needs extremely little, but it is extremely important to maintain our health and life. When these micronutrient intakes are insufficient, we do not feel hungry, so we do not actively take in these nutrients, but the underlying mineral starvation in the body will persist. Over time, the lack of minerals in the body has caused the occurrence of chronic diseases to be inevitable. Some of these chronic diseases are difficult to recover or irreversible, such as diabetes and malignant tumors. And some chronic diseases can be completely recovered after supplementing the micronutrients that the body lacks as soon as possible, such as night blindness. However, blindness caused by long-term vitamin A deficiency is also difficult to recover. Every year, more than 2 million children are blinded by vitamin A deficiency in the world.

Insulin in the human body is an important enzyme. It is a protein complex synthesized by pancreatic islet cells. In addition to amino acids, it also contains trace elements such as zinc, chromium and selenium. If the human body lacks these trace elements, Then the pancreatic islet cells cannot secrete the normal function of insulin. Therefore, it is very necessary for diabetic patients to supplement vitamins and trace minerals in appropriate amounts.

The pH of Human Water

Human body fluids, like any other fluids, are divided into acids and bases. The human body's (pH value) is expressed in numbers from 0-14. pH is the abbreviation of "potential Hydrogen", which means the concentration of H in the human body. The smaller the number, the stronger the acidity. 7 is neutral, more than 7 is alkaline, the larger the number, the more alkaline.

A high pH value indicates that it has a higher ability to attract H. When the pH value is low, it shows that there is less ability to attract H. The normal pH value of human tissue should be 7-7. 4. The normal pH value of blood is 7. 35-7. 45. The pH value of blood must always be kept in a relatively stable state. If the pH value of blood drops by 0. 2, the amount of oxygen delivered to the body will be reduced by 69. 4%, resulting in hypoxia of the entire body tissue.

Normal range of human pH

Blood	7. 35~7. 45
Bone marrow fluid	7. 30~7. 50
Saliva	6. 50~7. 50
Gastric juice	0. 80~1. 50
Duodenal juice	4. 20~8. 20
Stool	4. 60~8. 40
Urine	4. 80~8. 40
Bile	7. 10~8. 50
Pancreatic juice	8. 00~8. 30

The human body is composed of 75 trillion cells, and the cells live in our body fluids. Human cells are born to operate in an alkaline body fluid environment, but they also continuously produce acid and excrete acid. Cells produce acids during operation, but these are weak acids, organic acids. Unlike acids produced by acidic foods, they are broken down into carbon dioxide and water, which are excreted from the lungs.

There is sufficient scientific evidence to show that most of the body fluids of healthy humans are alkaline, and the pH value is above 7. 0. However, from the above table, we can also see that some body fluids with large changes in pH are those that stay in the body for a long time. For example, urine and feces have a pH index that varies greatly from acidic 4. 8 to alkaline 8. 4.

Human cells operate in an alkaline humoral environment, producing weak acids. This weak acid is easily excreted by the lungs and will not cause harm to people, which is the inevitable response of cells to acid. Just as people breathe faster and pant during intense exercise, it is to speed up the excretion of the acid produced by exercise.

The second source of acid in the human body is acidic food. 75% to 90% of our diet is acidic food. Although some foods are not acidic, the ash produced by the residue after decomposition is acidic. Over time, a person's body will become more acidic. These large amounts of acidic substances must be neutralized by the body's buffer system before being excreted by the kidneys. In this process of neutralization and elimination, a large amount of minerals will be consumed.

If these acids are not neutralized, or the body lacks minerals to neutralize these acidic substances, they will burn sensitive tissues when they pass through the digestive tract or are excreted. For example, sometimes we feel pain or burning when urinating, which reminds us that the minerals in the body that are responsible for neutralizing acid are not enough. We must strengthen alkaline resources and take in enough minerals to supplement our metabolic needs. It is best to extract minerals from plants, because minerals in plants are in organic form and enter the body. The affinity with the body determines the degree of absorption and utilization by the body.

People often have the wrong view that eating more alkaline foods will reduce the acid in the body. In fact, in a normal human body, acid and alkali are always in a dynamic equilibrium state. For example, no matter what food it is, it will become acidic when eaten in the stomach, because stomach acid is a strong acid containing 0. 2 - 0. 4%

hydrochloric acid. When food enters the intestine from the stomach, it is affected by alkaline intestinal fluid and becomes alkaline. Foods with different pH levels cannot change the pH of body fluids.

The acidity and alkalinity of food is not judged by simple taste, but depends on the type and content ratio of minerals contained in food: potassium, sodium, calcium, magnesium, and iron appear as alkali after entering the human body. Phosphorus, chlorine, and sulfur become acidic when they enter the human body. For example, lemon juice is a sour food, but it is a physiologically alkaline food, because lemon juice is rich in potassium, which provides alkalinity to body fluids after being digested, absorbed and metabolized by the human body. The preserved egg is an alkaline food, but it is a physiologically acidic food.

The most direct cause of acidic constitution is the excessive intake of acidic foods by the human body, such as meat, poultry, fish, dairy products, cereals, etc. After they are digested and decomposed, leaves acidic elements such as chlorine, sulfur, and phosphorus in the body. Vegetables and fruits are alkaline foods. After they are digested and decomposed, they leave sodium, potassium, calcium, magnesium, iron and other alkaline minerals in the body.

Almost all common diseases, such as colds, lack of energy, rheumatism, skin diseases, bronchitis, osteoporosis, diabetes, and high blood pressure, are manifestations of acidic physique. Eat more vegetables, fruits, and less meat to achieve acid-base balance in the body.

Excessive beer + enzymes = pancreas self-dissolving

On July 23, 2013, the Liaoshen Evening News published a news, which was widely reposted on Weibo. Mr. Zhou, who lives in Shenyang, had a drinking party with friends two months ago. At that time, he was diagnosed with high blood lipids. However, he drank nearly 20 bottles of beer overnight because of the friendship of his friends. After returning home, he felt unwell. In the early morning of the next day, because of the unbearable pain of abdomen, he was sent to the emergency department of the General Hospital of Shenyang Military Region by his family.

When Li Hongyu, deputy director of the Gastroenterology Department of the hospital, examined him, he found that Mr. Zhou's pancreas could not be found on the CT image. Then, during the blood test, the nurse drew out a 3 ml tube of blood, which turned out to be white, this is typical lipidemia. Doctors diagnosed this as a rare form of severe pancreatitis.

The next day, Mr. Zhou developed heart, lung, liver, kidney and other multiple organ failures, and he was out of danger after being rescued. But at this time, Mr. Zhou's pancreas was basically gone, and only the outermost capsule remained. After two months of hemodialysis, treatment of respiratory distress syndrome, and puncture and drainage of ascites, Mr. Zhou was finally discharged. His pancreas also grew a part by regenerating itself.

Experts say that due to food intake, the pancreas secretes a large amount of pancreatic juice, which increases the pressure on the pancreatic duct, and the obstruction of the pancreatic duct causes the pancreatic juice that should have entered the duodenum to be blocked there. This is all strong acid. , so the pancreas is dissolved by itself!

According to the PH value of human body fluid, we know that pancreatic juice is between 8. 00~8. 30 PH value, which means that the pancreatic juice in the pancreas is alkaline. In addition to water, there are electrolytes and zymogen proteins in pancreatic juice, and electrolytes in pancreatic juice the purpose of flowing through the pancreatic duct to the duodenum is to neutralize the acidic food from the stomach and make it alkaline. Therefore, the pancreatic juice is not strong acid, but alkaline. However, the zymogen protein in pancreatic juice is activated when electrolytes and acidic foods are neutralized and converted into pancreatin, also called trypsin, which is the most specific protease.

Under normal circumstances, the trypsinogen in pancreatic cells is inactive, but under diseased conditions, the pancreatic tissue is digested by trypsin. In pancreatitis, some factors activate trypsin, which in turn activates other enzymatic reactions, has a self-digestive effect on the pancreas, and promotes its necrosis and dissolution.

Mr. Zhou himself has high blood lipids, phlegm and dampness in the pancreas, and his pancreatic function is not perfect. After drinking 20 bottles of cold beer, his internal organs contracted under the stimulation of a lot of ice water. Originally, the pancreatic juice and bile flowed to the duodenum through the common channel of the pancreas, but the channel suddenly contracted under the action of cold beer, and the pancreatic juice and bile could not flow out and accumulated in the pancreas. Alcohol is constantly stimulating the pancreas to continue to secrete pancreatic juice, which accumulates and forms pancreatic edema. The pancreas was stimulated by the accumulation of a large amount of pancreatic juice and alcohol, which can also be said to be stimulated by brewer's yeast, and activated trypsin, so a chain reaction, Mr. Zhou's pancreas was dissolved by the enzymes in the pancreatic juice.

Since pancreatic juice is not a strong acid, why does pancreatic juice act like a strong acid to autolyse the pancreas? Everything has its two sides. Enzymes are indispensable chemical elements in the human body. Without enzymes, it is impossible for people to survive. However, enzymes out of control are like a manic horse, which is extremely destructive. The human body is like a chemical factory. The daily work is to neutralize acid and alkali. Enzymes perform various decomposition tasks in the chemical factory. It can be said to decompose, dissolve, or corrode, dissolving large particles of food into fine water, making it easier for the human body to accept.

Beer yeast can stimulate the activity of enzymes in the body. In other words, Beer yeast is an stimulator of pancreatic enzymes. After a large amount of beer enters the stomach, the enzymes in the pancreatic juice in the duodenum are greatly activated under the impact of the beer's yeast. Burst of intense activity, desperate to work crazy. Enzymes act like strong acids after being activated. Appropriate enzymes can decompose food into the fine essence needed by the human body. Excessive enzymes will corrode the organs. In other words, an appropriate amount of enzyme is to maintain activity, and an excessive amount of enzyme is a corrosive agent. It seems that too much enzyme activity is not a good thing, too much digestion will directly corrode the organs.

Traditional Chinese medicine says that the human body needs a balance of yin and yang. Western medicine says that the body needs a balanced nutrition. In fact, it is for the acid-base balance of the human body. To put it plainly, it is to balance the ratio of chemical elements in the body.

Therefore, do not drink cold beer on an empty stomach, and must eat food. Don't drink a lot of cold beer at once, but drink it sparingly.

The pancreas is responsible for the biochemical body fluid and the control of water transport. When the source of the biochemical body fluid is seriously damaged, the water metabolism will be out of control. The 20 bottles of cold beer he drank cannot be excreted in the body. Later, Mr. Zhou's heart, lung, liver and other organs failed, which proved the serious consequences of edema in the body caused by the loss of water metabolism in the damaged pancreas. In the past, in China, I saw many experienced drinkers of beer or liquor, during the process of drinking, they would drink water and go to the toilet non-stop. According to these drinkers, "drink through", it is to quickly excrete the beer or liquor that has been drunk from the urine to avoid drunkenness， and virtually avoiding the possibility of edema in the body.

Enteral of Biggest Cryptorrhetic Organ

We know that the longest digestive organ is the small intestine. The adult small intestine is 5-6 meters long. We don't know that the small intestine is also the largest endocrine organ in the human body. In order to fully absorb the nutrients in the digestion as much as possible, the small intestine has greatly expanded its inner surface area through the intestinal villi structure. The small intestine is flexible, and it stretches out to a total of about 200 square meters. The food eaten is mainly completed by the absorption capacity of the small intestine. The huge surface area of the small intestine allows nutrients to be quickly absorbed within 1-2 hours.

The small intestine not only has an absorption function, but also has a secretory function - it can secrete small intestinal fluid. The secretory function of the small intestine is mainly completed by the glands (duodenal gland and intestinal gland) in the mucosa of the small intestine wall. Normal people secrete 1 to 3 liters of small intestinal juice every day.

The composition of small intestinal juice is relatively complex, mainly containing a variety of digestive enzymes, exfoliated intestinal epithelial cells and microorganisms. Among the various digestive enzymes contained, there are intestinal activating enzyme, amylase, peptidase, lipase, sucrase, maltase and lactase, etc. These enzymes play an important role in further breaking down various nutrients into final absorbable products.

The secretion of small intestinal fluid is regulated by a variety of factors, including the local stimulation of the intestinal mucosa (including mechanical and chemical stimulation) by the mass of food and its digestive products, which can cause the secretion of small intestinal fluid. These stimuli are secreted by intestinal glands through localized reflexes from plexuses within the intestinal wall. The role of small intestinal juice is mainly to further break down sugars, fats, and proteins, making them absorbable substances.

Small intestine fluid is a family member of body fluid. The size of the unfolded small intestine is so huge that no organ in the body can match it. Therefore, the small intestine can also be called the largest endocrine organ of the human body.

Cozymase Q10

Coenzyme Q10 is one of the indispensable and important elements of human life. It can activate the nutrition of human cells and cell energy, and has the functions of improving human immunity, strengthening anti-oxidation, delaying aging and enhancing human vitality.

Every cell in the human body has Coenzyme Q10, which is a pure natural antioxidant substance that helps resist bacteria and free radicals, promote cell growth and self-repair. The total content of Coenzyme Q10 in the human body is only 500-1500mg and decreases with age. The content of coenzyme Q10 in human organs reaches a peak at the age of 20, and then rapidly decreases. The decrease in the concentration of coenzyme Q10 in the heart is particularly pronounced. The 77-year-old man had 57% less coenzyme Q10 in the myocardium than the 20-year-old man.

When the content of coenzyme Q10 in the human body drops by 25%, many diseases will occur, especially cardiovascular and cerebrovascular diseases. What is even more frightening is that when the coenzyme Q10 in the body drops by more than 75%, life will be terminated. Lack of coenzyme Q10 in the human body is usually prone to heart failure, arrhythmia, myocardial infarction, stroke, hypertension, hyperlipidemia, arteriosclerosis and other cardiovascular and cerebrovascular diseases.

In order to maintain normal bodily functions, each cell must continuously produce energy. In the mitochondria of cells, fatty acids from food are oxidized to carbon dioxide and water. The energy released during this oxidation reaction is the energy required for physical activity. Coenzyme Q10 is a necessary catalyst for the oxidation reaction of fatty acids. The heart is the organ that requires the highest energy in the human body, and the content of coenzyme Q10 is also the highest in myocardial cells.

The raw materials for manufacturing coenzymes come from yeast or bacteria. In the pharmaceutical industry, yeast and its products are used to treat certain dyspepsia, and can improve and adjust the body's metabolic function. Yeast powder is rich in vitamin B complex, B1, B2, and B12, which are often lacking in vegetarians, can provide complete satisfaction in yeast powder.

The human body is like fermented steamed bread. The human body when young is like a well-fermented steamed bread, soft, sweet and delicious, and beautiful in appearance. Older people are like dead-faced steamed buns lacking yeast. They are hard and dull on the outside, hard to chew in the mouth, and difficult to digest in the stomach. The coenzyme in the human body is the bursting agent of human vitality. Without this fermentation agent of human vitality, people will naturally age and get sick.

The coenzyme in diabetic patients is more lacking than normal people. Taking coenzyme can relieve diabetes, lower blood sugar level and maintain the heart. Since yeast and coenzyme have the same function, taking yeast can also replace coenzyme to increase vitality, reduce disease and buffer aging. The digestion and absorption system of the human body dominates a person's health and lifespan, and it is the coenzyme and its family of enzymes that dominate the digestion and absorption system and life.

Massage lower Jaw Solves Mouth Dry

I have dry mouth for a long time and I want to drink water all day long. After drinking water, the feeling of dry mouth still remains unresolved. My mouth was sticky, and I rinsed my mouth with water to reduce the stickiness, but after a while, my mouth was covered with sticky saliva. Experts say: after the blood sugar of diabetic patients rises, it is easy to absorb the water in the tissues around the blood vessels, causing diabetic patients to often have symptoms of dry mouth. Although I have read a lot of explanations about diabetes in Chinese medicine, how to solve the problem of diabetic dry mouth has not been completely solved.

Later, my blood sugar level was well controlled and maintained within the normal range, but the phenomenon of dry mouth has not been resolved. A few years ago, I started to learn self-massaging acupoints to assist in the treatment of diabetes. As a result, I became interested in how to use acupuncture points to cure dry mouth. Mouth belongs to the scope of the five sense organs. I checked the acupoints on the head and the explanation materials, and selected three acupoints, namely, Chengjiang, Dicang, and Lianquan.

ChengJiang Point

Chengjiang point is the intersection point of Ren Channel and Foot Yangming Stomach Meridian, on the face, when the middle depression of the chin-labial sulcus. It has the functions of producing body fluid, constricting fluid, relaxing tendons and activating collaterals. Massage this point is helpful for diabetes.

The substance of this acupoint comes from the stomach and Renmai, and the water is passed from Dicang and Lianquan points. Therefore, like Dicang, there is water from the stomach and the same as Lianquan.

Dicang point

The Di Cang acupoint is located on the face of the human body, outside the corner of the mouth, straight up to the pupil. In the warehouse, the ground is the soil, and the spleen and stomach belong to the soil. A warehouse is a place where grains are stored.

The base storehouse receives the water from the stomach, and then passes it to the acupuncture points of Cheng- jiang, forming a water spring dominated by the water from the stomach around the lips, continuously supplying the thirst for water on the upper half of the lips.

Lian Chuen Point

Lianquan point is located on the neck of the human body, the current midline, above the throat, and the depression on the upper edge of the hyoid bone. This acupuncture point has the effect of quenching thirst.

Lianquan is an acupuncture point on the Ren pulse, honesty and no corruption, the spring is water. The Ren channel is a yin channel, a meridian that runs through the abdomen of the human body, and is also the main meridian that promotes the survival of body fluid. The Lianquan acupoint takes over the wet and hot water from   Tiantu, another acupoint on the Renmai meridian, and then dissipates heat and shrinks here, and then passes to the Chengjiang acupoint.

Dicang and Chengjiang form a supply spring for the upper half of the lips, and Lianquan acupoint and Chengjiang acupoint form a supply spring for the lower half of the lips. The upper and lower parts of the lips have their own water supply sources.

The function of Lianquan acupoints: to attract yin fluid. The function of Ren mai is to manage the yin meridian of the whole body, regulate the qi and blood of yin meridian, and it is the "sea of yin mai".

Chengjiang, Lianquan are all points on the Ren Meridian, Dicang is the point on the Stomach Meridian, They are all important acupuncture points, which have the effect of treating diabetes, diabetes, and qi and blood substances, maintaining the normal operation of the human body and attracting yin fluid. Among them, Chengjiang point carries the ground water from Dicang point of stomach meridian and the ground water from Renmai Lianquan point, and gathers in this point. The Chengjian acupoint is connected t o Dicang and Lianquan, and it is most convenient to massage the three acupoints at the same time.

Ever since I got up every morning, I used my thumb to press the Chengjiang points 100 times each at Lianquan and Dicang points, and the dry mouth disappeared very quickly. The saliva in the mouth also increased.

According to Dr. Cohen of the United States, he discovered that there are two precious proteins in saliva: epidermal growth factor (EGF) and nerve growth factor (KGF). The former is a polypeptide composed of 53 amino acids, which can promote the proliferation and differentiation of cells, replace aging and dead cells with viable cells, accelerate the healing of skin and mucosal wounds, and prevent ulcers. The latter has the function of promoting the growth of nerves, which can make the broken nerve endings grow and extend, "welding" the broken nerves, so that the injured skin can restore the sensory and motor functions as soon as possible. For this, Cohen won the 1986 Nobel Prize in Physiology and Medicine.

Saliva is a very precious fluid in the human body, which can play a role in prolonging life. Bird's nest, a precious tonic in China, is the nest where the swallow's saliva condenses. Don't underestimate saliva, and don't s pit it out casually. With normal saliva secretion, not only will the mouth not dry out, but the food we eat is very fragrant. This is the blessing brought to us by the enzymes in saliva.

Diabetes Swelling and Body Fluid Transport of Disorders

People with diabetes often experience symptoms such as weight loss and edema. Weight loss and edema are both problems in the transportation and transformation of water channels in the human body. Weight loss is caused by hourglasses in the water channels, and the water in the body is excreted from the urethra. On the other hand, edema is just the opposite. The water in the body is blocked and cannot be excreted from normal channels, so it has to accumulate in the body, the skin swells, and the internal organs swell, thereby causing local edema or systemic edema. In short, both of them are obstacles to the transportation and transformation of pancreatic water, and cannot function normally.

The kidney is a blood filter, which re-sends the filtered blood into the blood circulation track, and discharges the filtered waste water into the urethra. When a person suffers from diabetes, high-concentration blood sugar flows everywhere in the person's blood vessels, which will inevitably damage the kidneys and easily lead to kidney disease.

After illness, the kidney is ischemia, hypoxia, and the speed of filtering blood is slow. As the disease progresses, the leakage of protein gradually increases. The long-term proteinuria makes the kidney damage increasingly worse, and extracellular fluid stays in the interstitial s pace, causing edema. At the same time, the body's immune system is damaged, which causes the permeability of the capillary walls of the whole body to increase, resulting in edema caused by the water in the plasma leaking into the interstitial spaces. The edema will eventually lead to heart failure in the human body and cause death.

Low-Carbohydrate Diets with Swelling and Cardiac Failure(1)

Controlling the blood sugar level within its normal range is one of the daily tasks of diabetic patients. There are various ways to control blood sugar levels within a certain range, but controlling the amount of carbohydrates is the most effective way. Because carbohydrates are members of the sugar family, controlling carbohydrates means controlling sugar intake and directly controlling the increase in blood sugar levels. The low-carbohydrate diet was first proposed by Dr. Robert Atkins in the United States. He is an American cardiologist and nutritionist who is famous for inventing the meat-eating weight loss method.

A low-carbohydrate diet causes the body to release less insulin. When the insulin level is normal, the body starts to consume its own fat for energy, thereby achieving weight loss. Maintaining a stable insulin level not only allows the body to consume fat, but also reduces hunger and appetite. In short, the Atkins method controls insulin levels by controlling carbohydrate intake.

The American Medical Association found in a comparative study that Atkins therapy is the most effective and the longest lasting weight loss method among the four mainstream weight loss methods. The New England Journal of Medicine's research concluded that Atkins' low-carb diet can replace the low-fat diet, and the effect of controlling the balance of fat and blood sugar is more obvious.

However, there has been a lot of controversy over the Atkins plan and other low-carbohydrate diets. Many in the medical profession are concerned about the increased intake of protein and fat during the Atkins plan. In addition to cholesterol levels and heart disease, they are also worried about the impact of this diet on kidney function. An increase in protein intake can lead to an increase in ketone bodies in the kidney. In particular, the cause of Atkins's death is full of opinions. The main objection is that Dr. Atkins died of a low-carb, high-fat, high-protein diet he created.

Atkins began to gain weight in his thirties. His fat body confused him and made him determined to try to lose weight. So he continued to improve his diet and wanted to find a way to lose weight. In the end, Atkins worked out a new weight loss recipe for himself. Not only is there no bread, fruits, and vegetables in this recipe, it doesn't even include all sugary foods. According to the recipe, he can eat anything that is high in fat and high protein as he wants, such as those veal steaks that are fried to tender and dripping with oil, those fragrant bacon, and those fresh and delicious fried fish. What's amazing is that it didn't take long for him to lose weight successfully and regain his normal weight. The most important thing is that this new way of losing weight didn't make him feel any pain.

In order to promote this weight loss method, in 1972, Atkins published the first medical monograph in his doctor's career, "Doctor Atkins's New Diet Revolution", which later became popular throughout the United States. In the 1990s, obesity became a common phenomenon in the United States and the world, and weight loss has therefore become a popular topic. In 1992, he revised and republished the first book, and sold 15 million copies in one go, becoming the best-selling book in the 1990s. As a result, he gained fame and not only became the leader of the new weight-loss method, he even became the spokesperson of the new lifestyle. He set off a huge movement to subvert tradition. People abandon the traditional food bread, and start to become keen on all high-fat foods.

In the last year of his life, Atkins gained fame and fortune. He not only promoted his weight loss concept, but also promoted his weight loss products, and the latter made him a billionaire. Atkins reached the peak of the most glorious life.

However, Atkins wanted more and more. He dreams of promoting Atkins food to every supermarket in the world, and dreams that Atkins food can appear in school restaurants, nursing homes, restaurants and fitness clubs. He even said: "I hope to eventually eliminate obesity and diabetes. I believe that God also wants me to do this. "

Low-Carbohydrate Diets with Swelling and Cardiac Failure(2)

After Atkins published his first book "Dr. Atkins's New Diet Revolution" in 1972, he has been practicing the methods in the book for many years and has succeeded in losing excess weight. With the popularity of this book in the United States, he has appeared on TV many times and left many photos. Everyone can see that he was healthy during that time and maintained a proper weight.

In 2000, he suffered from primary cardiomyopathy, an incurable heart disease. This disease may be caused by many reasons. Atkins was diagnosed with a viral disease. The doctor said there was no evidence that the disease was caused by diet, and his coronary artery report showed that it was unobstructed. Patients with this disease are more prone to cardiac arrest, which is not related to diet. His doctor pointed out that, in addition to primary cardiomyopathy, Atkins' cardiovascular system is extremely healthy.

Regarding Atkins' weight, author Leith, William wrote after interviewing Atkins during a cardiac arrest: "He looks less than six feet, about 200 pounds, and he is not thin, but it's definitely not fat. " Atkins Nutrition that Atkins is a tennis player and weighs frequently. He has always been under 195 pounds and his height is about 1. 8m. Later, his wife's public medical report also indicated that Atkins weighed 195 pounds before entering the hospital.

On April 8, 2003, Atkins fell on thin, unmelted ice, hit his head against the ice, and caused brain hemorrhage. He had lost consciousness on the way to the hospital. After that, his body deteriorated rapidly and suffered extensive organ damage. During the two weeks in the hospital, his body obviously accumulated a large amount of fluid, that is, the accumulated fluid made his weight change from 195 pounds to 258 pounds. The cause of death stated in his death certificate was "epidural hematoma caused by a head bruise", not because of a heart attack as anecdotal.

Low-carbohydrate diets with swelling and cardiac failure(3)

Regardless of whether Dr. Robert Atkins died of edema or heart disease, these are all related to body fluid biochemical abnormalities and lymphatic system disorders. The essence of weight loss is to reduce water. A person's fatness and thinness are mainly related to the amount of water in the body. The water content in the body of a fat person is much greater than that of a thin person.

When people solve one problem, another problem may arise. Even though the control of carbohydrates can effectively control blood sugar and reduce weight, it does not mean that the problem of diabetes is really solved. On the contrary, there are more hidden dangers in the body.

Carbohydrates, also known as sugar compounds, are an important type of organic compound that exists most in nature and has the widest distribution. Mainly composed of carbon, hydrogen, and oxygen. Glucose, sucrose, starch and cellulose are all sugar compounds. We know that carbohydrates are an important part of the body's energy source, especially for maintaining the function of the brain. Long-term non-eating of carbohydrates will cause the imbalance of certain nutrients in the body, as well as imbalance in the production and transportation of body fluid.

Only 2% of the carbohydrates we eat every day are stored in the human body, and the rest are stored as fat in the human body in addition to being consumed as energy. Carbohydrates exist in every cell of the human body. Although carbohydrates can be converted into fats in the body, high protein and high fat meals cannot replace carbohydrates. Just like the earth, it not only has a lot of water, land, mountains, forests, and minerals, but also needs sunlight, moonlight, wind, and rain, so that everything can grow and life can continue.

Carbohydrates, proteins and fats are the three basic substances in the biological world, providing the main energy for the growth, movement and reproduction of organisms. In the short term, a low-carb, high-fat, and high-protein diet will indeed lead to weight loss and control of blood sugar, but this high-fat and high-protein diet requires the human body to consume more resources such as minerals and trace minerals, vitamins and various enzymes are used to digest and decompose. In the long run, it will damage the vitality of the human body, resulting in the loss of the innate immune function in the body, and the acquired immune disorders.

The human body lacks the participation of carbohydrates, so it has to consume inherent natural minerals and enzymes to maintain the body's metabolism and operation, and gradually consume these inherent human resources.

Dr. Robert Atkins fell on thin ice and injured his head. Within two weeks of being admitted to the hospital, he had accumulated a large amount of fluid in his body, and his weight had changed from 195 pounds to 258 pounds. Obviously, the water accumulated in the body of Dr. Atkins after the injury could not be absorbed and excreted well, and the lymphatic system imbalance caused edema in the body, and he died of a hematoma. That is to say, Dr. Atkins's blood circulation and lymphatic circulation system malfunctioned. It was precisely because of the long term consumption of high-fat and high-protein that his immune system was greatly damaged during his lifetime. The imbalance will form a large area of edema in the body, and the paralysis of the immune system makes the body unable to save itself, resulting in death.

From the example of Dr. Robert Atkins, I believe that a high-fat, high-protein, low-carbohydrate diet is not advisable, and lowering blood sugar should not be based on superficial results. The treatment of diabetes should be considered from the conditioning of the entire body. To control the blood sugar level of diabetes, we must strictly abide by scientific laws, adhere to the principle of nutritional balance, maintain the balance of yin and yang in the body, and maintain a balance of pH and alkalinity. It is absolutely not possible to go from one extreme to another.

Diabetes, Pancreatitis Cancer with Body Fluid(1)

Diabetes and pancreatitis are both pathological conditions of the endocrine and exocrine functions of the pancreas. The incidence of pancreatic cancer in people with chronic pancreatitis and diabetes is higher than that in the normal population. Pancreatic cancer is a malignant tumor arising from the pancreas. Pancreatic cancer is usually the most malignant tumor among the common tumors, and also has the highest mortality rate.

Generally speaking, cancer is the continuation of chronic diseases. Patients with pancreatic cancer have a history of pancreatitis or diabetes. Therefore, chronic diseases and long-term inflammation are both a cause.

We know that many celebrities have pancreatic cancer, such as Italian tenor Pavarotti and Hong Kong artist Shen Dianxia are obese pancreatic cancer patients, which means high protein, high fat, high-calorie foods can have some adverse effects on the occurrence of pancreatic cancer. The late Apple co-founder Steve Jobs suffered from pancreatic cancer because of a severe nutritional imbalance in his body caused by staying up late and his eccentric diet.

Jobs was a vegetarian. Not only that, he did not eat any parts that could hinder the growth of plants. He also went on a diet and only drank juice during his illness. In the movie "Jobs", the actor Ashton Kutcher revealed that he had been in the hospital because of his habit of imitating Jobs, and he was miserable. "Simply drinking fruit juice can

really cause serious problems, "Kutcher said. "I suffer. The pancreas test data is completely disordered. " Overeating can cause pancreatic dysfunction. Dieting on a vegetarian diet can also cause pancreatic secretion disorders. This is one of the main reasons Jobs got pancreatic cancer.

Some people say that the cause of Steve Jobs' cancer is not his vegetarian diet. People in the computer industry have basically been exposed to carcinogenic and harmful chemicals, which have different effects on the body. But another Apple founder, Steve Wozniak, who started his business with Steve Jobs, 's favorite foods are typical American pizza and hamburgers, which are completely different from Jobs' eating habits. The fattened Wozniak is 4 years older than Jobs and is still alive.

Choosing a vegetarian diet is an individual right, and we have no right to interfere. But I'm writing about a diabetes regimen and am very curious about Jobs' strange diet, and diabetics are more likely to get pancreatic cancer than non-diabetics. Therefore, by discussing this issue, I have a clear understanding of the progress of diabetes, and I also want to communicate with the majority of diabetes friends.

The material composition in our body is like the epitome of the material in nature, and it needs balanced nutrition to meet the needs of the body to function well. I personally think that the biggest disadvantage of vegetarians is that they have abandoned the fat and protein in the three major sources of human energy, and the only protein taken in by the body is also plant protein, which is far from meeting the metabolic needs of human cells. At the same time, it also destroys the balance of the human body, causing defects in human cells.

Protein is an indispensable component of the structure of all cells and tissues. It is the most important material

basis for human life activities. In the human body, its total amount is second only to water. Protein is composed of different amino acids, some of which can be synthesized by the body itself, called non-essential amino acids, and there are about eight kinds of amino acids that must be supplied by food, called essential amino acids.

The intake of protein nutrients by the human body is not only about the quantity, but also its type and quality. The nutritional value of protein mainly depends on the digestibility and the type and combination of amino acids contained in the protein. Any protein that is easily digested, absorbed and utilized by the human body has high nutritional value. Animal protein contains high-quality protein better than soybean protein, and vegetable protein is difficult to digest due to the surrounding fibrous film, so animal protein is easier to digest and absorb than vegetable protein.

Therefore, it is not advisable for vegetarians to completely abandon meat. A vegetarian diet not only causes the body to not get enough fat, but also reduces the absorption of protein.

From the perspective of western medicine, nutrition and immunity are closely related. Vegetarians cannot get all the nutrients needed by human cells, and their own immunity is weak, and they cannot withstand the invasion of foreign viruses and bacteria.

Diabetes, Pancreatitis Cancer with Body Fluid(2)

Ancient Chinese medicine in China has always attached great importance to the role of qi and blood, and believed that qi and blood are insufficient for all diseases.

There are many reasons for the loss of qi and blood. One is that the body is tired to a certain extent and has to start overdrafting the blood and body fluids of the human body. However, our body has a strong compensatory ability and can continue to work in the case of physical losses, that is, to maintain normal operation by overdrafting the body's blood and body fluids.

Second, a strict vegetarian is actually a person with insufficient qi and blood. Because vegetarians blindly insist on being vegetarian and refuse to eat animal fats, the nutritional basis of the three major energy sources of the human body lacks two. In the long run, the human body lacks the necessary nutrients of fat and protein to maintain normal work, and the malnourished body nourishes the malnourished cells, resulting in cell defects.

Third, under high tension and pressure for a long time, the nerves are tense, resulting in disorders of the endocrine system, insufficient secretion of body fluids, decreased immunity, and poor gastrointestinal absorption.

And Steve Jobs accounted for these three points. Workaholics, out-and-out vegetarians, and the sense of mission of the industry have kept him under tremendous pressure.

The endocrine system is an important regulatory system of the body. It complements the nervous system to regulate the growth and development of the body and various metabolisms, maintain the stability of the internal environment, and influence behavior and control reproduction.

Certain nerve cells in animals can secrete some biologically active substances, which can regulate the functions of other organs through blood circulation or local diffusion. These biologically active substances are called neurohormones, and the nerve cells that synthesize and secrete neurohormones are called neuroendocrine cells. Neuroendocrine cancer can occur in the entire neuroendocrine system, but the most common site of involvement is the pancreas. And Jobs suffered from neuroendocrine cancer in the pancreas, which is located on the islet cells of the pancreas. Because the islet cells belong to the pancreatic endocrine, it is called neuroendocrine cancer, not the pancreatic cancer.

When Jobs was 30 years old, symptoms of neuroendocrine system disease appeared. A report on Jobs's quirk at a conference in 1987: "His hands are inexplicably pale yellow, and they are constantly moving. " Medically said, Certain liver diseases, gallbladder diseases and blood diseases often cause symptoms of jaundice. And Jobs's hand has been moving because of a problem with the nervous system in the body, which led to the loss of control of the hand nerves. This was the initial symptom of Jobs's neurosecretory system malfunction- jaundice and shaking hands. It can be said that 10 years after Jobs started a vegetarian diet at the age of 20, his body began to develop defects and eventually developed into fatal pancreatic, it is called Neuroendocrine carcinoma.

Steve. Jobs is a person with very strong willpower. He has always inspired himself: "To live, you must change the world. " His life and passion like a roller coaster have made a legend, a very creative corporate leader, and he pursues perfection and the unstoppable passion has revolutionized the six industries of personal computers, animated films, music, mobile phones, tablet computers and digital publishing. In the process of achieving success, as a manager of an industry, Jobs can be described as painstakingly dedicated to his life.

As the career continues to grow and succeed, what everyone sees is an extremely aggressive, irritable and exhausted Jobs, but they don't know that this is an external appearance of his internal disease. The cry of illness did not attract Jobs's attention, nor did it attract the attention of those around him. Everyone thought it was a character problem of Jobs. In fact, these symptoms are caused by diseases in Jobs's body, and he can't control his emotions at all. Most people suffering from endocrine diseases are prone to irritability and anger. This is because the hormones in the body are out of balance, which makes the patient's mood easily out of control.

It was Jobs who had extraordinary willpower and conviction to overcome many physical inconveniences, which delayed the disease in the body for many years and finally broke out. At the same time, it also made him miss the best self-adjustment period. Every one of us lives with cancer cells in our lives, but some people spend their lives safely, and some people cause cancer for various reasons. Anything can be transformed within a certain period of time. Nothing in the world is immutable. Invariance is relative, and change is absolute.

After contracting cancer, Jobs reflected on himself. He attributed his illness to early hardware hand-made exposure to harmful chemicals. However, his mood has not been consciously controlled, and his diet has not been consciously improved. The endocrine system directly controls and regulates the nervous system, so he must rest. But how can Jobs calm down? Changing the world does not include changing himself.

Jobs' diet is the exact opposite of Dr. Robert Atkins. The former is a completely vegetarian and resolutely rejects animal fat; the latter is a complete carnivorous, with high-protein and high-fat as a staple food, the essence of which is from an extreme going to the other extreme, failure to respect science and the laws of metabolism of the human body results in disorders of water and fluid in the body, lack of body fluid, and thus diseases. It is the human diet that causes these cell defects. The food eaten every day severely changes the human body's function and destroys the human body's immune system. All food that exists in nature is a gift from heaven, which has been set by the Creator a long time ago. One must not favor one another, and use subjective consciousness to forcefully replace the needs of the body. Balanced nutrition is the key to maintaining various metabolisms of the human body.

Why pancreatic cancer is the most malignant tumor among the common tumors, and also has the highest mortality rate. This is because the pancreas is the biochemical source of body fluid, and it is the general arrangement of water transport in the entire human body. The hormones secreted by the endocrine system also belong to body fluid, and thus also belong to the pancreas. One can imagine the extent and severity of pancreatic disease. It is like the host computer of the computer suffers from disease and crashes. Secondly, water circulates in the body，there is water everywhere in the body, even in the bones. The pancreas, which is the source of biochemical body fluid, has cancer. The cancer cells spread very quickly and widely as the liquid flows down from the source.

Cancer does not form in a day, cancer is the evolution of chronic diseases. Facing diabetes and chronic pancreatitis seriously, actively repairing the pancreas, the biochemical source of body fluid, creating favorable conditions for the endocrine system and nervous system to maintain various metabolisms.

The kidney is the congenital foundation, and the pancreas is the acquired foundation. It can be said that all diseases in the body are related to body fluid. Water can make boats walk, can also capsize.

The Role of Body Fluid in the Immune System

The human body has three lines of immune defense. The first is composed of skin and mucous membranes outside the body. They can not only prevent pathogens from invading the human body, but their secretions (such as lactic acid, fatty acid, acid and enzymes, etc.) have a sterilizing effect.

The second line of defense is the bactericidal substances in body fluids-lysozyme and phagocytes. The first and second lines of defense are natural defense functions gradually established by humans in the evolutionary process. They are characterized by being born in humans, not against a specific pathogen, and have a defense against multiple pathogens. Therefore, Called innate immunity.

The third line of defense is mainly composed of immune organs (tonsils, thymus, lymph nodes, lymph glands, bone marrow and spleen, etc.) and immune cells (lymphocytes, phagocytes) with the help of blood circulation and lymphatic circulation. The third line of defense is the acquired defense function that the human body gradually builds up after birth. It is characterized by the fact that it is only produced after birth and only acts against a specific pathogen or foreign body, so it is called acquired immunity. After the pathogen has invaded, the lymphocytes are stimulated, and the lymphocytes produce a special protein called an antibody that resists the pathogen. Substances (such as foreign bodies such as pathogens) that cause the body to produce antibodies are called antigens. We were vaccinated against the smallpox virus when we were kids, using the pathogen to make antibodies against the smallpox virus.

The immune organ of the third line of immune defense in the body functions through the blood and lymphatic circulatory system, and is under the jurisdiction of the spleen. The spleen is the largest immune organ in the human body. The spleen is an important filter in the blood circulation. It can remove foreign bodies, germs, and aging and dead cells in the blood, especially red blood cells and platelets.

Diabetic patients have insufficient nutrient absorption and lack of body fluids in the body, which directly affects the body's immune system and weakens its function. That is to say, the ammunition prepared in the munitions depot is not enough to withstand the aggression of foreign enemies. In the early stage of my diabetes, because of poor blood sugar control, I would catch a cold immediately when I went out, and my body's resistance was very weak.

The lymphatic system protects the normal circulation of blood and is the patron saint of blood. If there is a problem with the lymph, the blood will be damaged by the virus and cause various blood diseases. The human body cannot operate without water. Body fluid is the essence of water in the human body. The strength of the immune system depends on adequate body fluid support and good water operation. Therefore, diabetic patients should not take it lightly, thinking that everything will be fine if blood sugar is controlled, and they should pay close attention to the operation of body water. Only when the water is running normally and the body maintains a balance, the blood sugar level can truly remain stable and normal.

Lungs and Body Fluid

"Nei Jing" says, "All qi belong to the lung. " Therefore, the cultivation of qi deficiency, the smooth adjustment of qi inverse, the discharge of turbid qi, and the irrigation of clear qi can all be achieved by regulating the function of the lung. "

A substance can have many manifestations, including liquids, solids, and gases. The same is true for the water in the human body. This is the law of nature. As a natural person, the law of survival and metabolism in our body is also inseparable from the constraints of nature. The water in the human body, the blood and lymph flowing in the blood vessels are liquid, and the blood stasis is solid after exposure to cold and dampness and lag.

Ancient books say that the liver hides the yang god, and the lung hides the yin god. The yang yin souls are hidden in the body fluid, the yang soul is hidden in the liver in the form of body fluid turned into gas, and the soul is hidden in the form of body fluid turned into liquid in the lung.

Insufficient lung fluid, liver fire is easy to prosper, people are easy to get angry, liver fire is too big, the production of body fluid that damages the spleen, and the function of the spleen is impaired, which affects the kidneys.

Body fluid is distributed and transported in the body by qi, which is like steam going up, and liquid is going down. kidney water upload to purge the heart fire, this form of kidney water's transmission is that qi goes up. Only qi can go to high places. Once the kidneys are weak, the power to transmit upward will not be enough, and the kidney water will not be able to moisturize the fire of the heart, irritability and insomnia caused by the fire of the heart, then the heart is restless, and the qi is easy to be scattered everywhere, causing qi stagnation and blood stasis.

Heart dysfunction in turn affects the function of the lungs. To nourish the lungs, we must first calm the irritability, replenish qi and blood, go to bed early, drink plenty of soup, and replenish yin fluid.

Tap the Pericardial Meridian to Enhance Water Transport

The normal pericardial cavity contains 25-30ml of fluid (up to 50ml). Any reason the amount of fluid in the pericardial cavity increases. If it exceeds 50ml, pericardial effusion will appear.

Hydropericardium is the flow of fluid into the pericardium, where it accumulates and cannot be excreted. Hydropericardium is a manifestation of the failure of the body's drainage system. Hydropericardium is caused by various causes of the heart, and it is also related to the decline of the spleen's ability to transport water. The health book says that massaging the pericardial meridian can reduce or remove hydropericardium.

Why does knocking on the pericardial meridian can eliminate pericardial effusion. The pericardium referred to in Chinese medicine is a thin film on the outside of the heart, which can take on behalf of the heart and suffer from evil, that is, when an external evil invades the human body, it takes the place of the heart to withstand the invasion.

Modern people's unbalanced diet and inconsistent lifestyle habits make blood cholesterol and fat increase abnormally. When the amount of cholesterol in the blood is too much, it will gradually stick to the blood vessel wall, resulting in narrowing of the blood vessel and poor elasticity. When the blood flow is not smooth, it is more likely to induce serious complications such as myocardial infarction and stroke.

But tapping or rubbing the pericardium can speed up blood flow, peel off the cholesterol attached to the blood vessel wall, and then excrete it from the body. When the pericardium accumulates fluid and fat is gradually eliminated, the heart's pulsating power will increase.

The pericardium meridian is massaged along the meridian. It is not necessary to find the correct acupuncture point. Just press it little by little along this line. Each point is based on pain. The massage is basically from the chest to the hands. The key is that the point that is pressed can reach the heart all the time. When pressing each point, the force penetrates inward, so it takes a long time and the technique is not very heavy, so that you can get qi..

The heart function becomes stronger, nourishes the spleen, and strengthens the water transport capacity of the spleen (pancreas). The natural world cannot do without water, and the human body cannot do without water. Water plays an irreplaceable role in biological evolution and survival. The health of the human body and water are inseparable. Keeping the balance of water and liquid in the human body preserves health.

God of Water and Vulcan

In ancient Greece, the legendary Oceanus, the god of water, gave birth to all the rivers on the earth and three thousand sea nymphs. Therefore, many cities in ancient Greece had altars to worship the god of water Oceanus.

The god of fire in Greek mythology is Hephaestus, one of the twelve gods in Greece, and the Roman name is Vulcan, the son of Zeus and Hera. He was the ugliest god, and he was lame, but he married Aphrodite, the goddess of love and beauty. He is the god of fire and the blacksmith of the gods, with high skill, making many weapons, tools and artworks. Apollo drove the day car, Eros's golden arrow, and the silver arrow were all made by him.

Gonggong, is the god of water in ancient myths and legends who controls floods. According to the ancient Chinese book "Shan Hai Jing", it is said that Gonggong has always been incompatible with

Vulcan Zhu. Due to the "incompatibility of water and fire", there was a earth-shattering battle. In the end, Gonggong failed and had to collide Bu Zhoushan, make heaven and earth tilt.

Both water and fire are the most important elements in nature, and human beings cannot survive without water and fire. Water and fire are opposites and unified. When water and fire are in a balanced state, they are unified and harmonious. Once there is a deviation, they are opposites. The same goes for the water and fire in our bodies. The fire in the human body has heart fire, liver fire and spleen fire.

The god of water in our human body is the pancreas, which is in charge of the shipping of the waterways and the metabolism of water in the human body. Since she is a water god, she has to live in water, and she is very free in water like a fish.

The liver is a hot-tempered fire god that controls the source of fire in the body. People often say that anger can hurt the body. However, Vulcan loses his temper regularly. For example, if the liver eats some food that is easy to get angry, feels thirsty and has no water supply, stays up all night without rest, does not eat enough or eats too much, etc, he will lose his temper , will also open the city gates to let in toxins, and not work well, causing other organs to be ischemia, without any awareness of the overall situation. The best way for Vulcan liver is to drink and eat in moderation, and ensure enough sleep time, so that there is no chance for him to get angry, he will perform hematopoietic work obediently.

The pancreas constantly secretes various pancreatic juices every day to provide it to the small intestine and digest the various foods we eat. The pancreas secretes so much pancreatic juice every day that it can't even move. The small pancreas of a normal person can secrete 1 to 2 liters of pancreatic juice every day, which is 10-14 times that of its own. The secretion is so strong that it is amazing that the work intensity of the pancreas can be imagined. The pancreatic secretion of pancreatic juice needs to be continuously provided with water resources to protect it. Once the body's water is insufficient and the pancreas cannot get enough water to supplement, the pancreas will dry up, just like the dry cracks of the land. The god of water is no longer a free fish, but a stiff dried fish. By the way, isn't the shape of our pancreas just like a fish? The Creator is really too clever.

In order to balance the water god and fire god of the body and maintain uninterrupted coordination work, we must drink enough water to ensure that both the water god and fire god have the right amount of water to maintain. Minimize the conflict between water and fire, eat less barbecued food, roasted seeds and nuts, don't lead to fire, and keep body fluid sufficient. We know, since ancient times, there has been a saying that water and fire are incompatible. This is not a fake. Ancient people are wise. The natural world is incompatible with water and fire, and the human body is incompatible with water and fire. It is the same truth. The wisdom of health is to balance the water and fire in the body and coexist peacefully.

The Relationship Between Water and Kidney

The blood in our body is filtered by the kidneys, and the body produces a variety of waste products in the metabolic process. Most of the waste products are filtered through the glomerular blood, and the secretion of the renal tubules is excreted in the urine by adjusting the acid-base balance to maintain the stability of the internal environment. The kidneys also have endocrine functions, erythropoietin, which stimulates bone marrow hematopoiesis.

The kidney contains active vitamin D3, which regulates calcium and phosphorus metabolism. The kidney is also the site of degradation of endocrine hormones such as insulin. When kidney function is insufficiency, endocrine hormones such as insulin will go wrong, causing metabolic disorders. The kidney itself can also cause water metabolism disorders, the blood cannot be purified well, and the waste dirty water cannot be normally excreted in urine, leaving it in the body and causing edema throughout the body. Diabetic kidney disease is one of the complications of diabetes.

The workload of the kidneys is huge. Each kidney has more than 1 million nephrons, and each nephron is like a small high-efficiency filter, which never stops washing our blood, recovering beneficial substances, forming urine and eliminating waste or toxins from the body. The kidney is like a huge sewage treatment plant composed of millions of small filters. It can be called a miraculous environmental protection plant in the body.

Scientific research shows that: the blood of the whole body passes through the kidney nearly 20 times per hour.

That is, every 4 to 5 minutes, all the blood in the human body flows through the kidneys and is filtered, and the metabolic waste in the blood becomes urine and excreted from the body. Renal blood flow accounts for about 1:4 to about 1:5 of the whole body blood flow. The glomerular filtrate in the nephron produces about 125ml per minute, and the kidney filters and cleans nearly 200 liters of blood every day.

Kidney problems, first of all, the water metabolism in the body is also disordered, edema is an obvious symptom of kidney disease.

The environmental protection of such a huge internal environmental protection factory is very important. Chinese medicine believes that the kidney is the innate foundation. If we want to be healthy, our innate foundation must be maintained and adjusted. Try not to make our body too tired, pay attention to our work and rest time, ensure that we have enough sleep, be in a good mood, and have a light diet. Do not eat excessive amounts of high-protein and high-fat foods, which will bring unnecessary extra burden to the kidneys and cause the kidneys harm. Keep enough drinking water every day to avoid too thick blood and keep our urine transparent. The kidneys are well maintained, which will greatly help cure diabetes.

Gestational Diabetes and Body Fluid

Many women are in good health and do not have any symptoms of diabetes. However, the state of hyperglycemia appeared after pregnancy, most of which did not attract their attention, or even if the hyperglycemia occurred, they did not know. In recent years, the number of pregnant women suffering from gestational diabetes has gradually increased. Many of my female colleagues have experienced high blood sugar levels after pregnancy. Fortunately, family doctors in Canada are responsible for correcting the deviations of pregnant women in time. Avoiding the development of type 2 diabetes, making blood sugar return to normal.

There are nothing more than two factors that cause gestational diabetes. One is that pregnant women will experience severe nausea and vomiting in the early stages of pregnancy. Pregnant women's nausea and vomiting can affect their normal diet intake. In severe cases, dehydration, electrolyte imbalance, acid-base imbalance, nutritional deficiency, weight loss, etc, can occur. Severe vomiting can spit out bile and even cause mucosal hemorrhage.

We know that the human body is composed of cells, and water and electrolytes are important components of cells, which are widely distributed inside and outside the cells, participate in many important functions and metabolic activities in the body, and play a very important role in the maintenance of normal life activities. The dynamic balance of water and electrolytes in the body is achieved through the regulation of nerves and body fluids. Electrolytes are minerals and salts, and people obtain these by consuming food and beverages.

Because some women have too intense pregnancy reactions, nausea and vomiting are severe, they vomit what they eat, and even drink water, which leads to a decrease in electrolytes and electrolyte disorders. Inability to perform normal metabolic functions, gestational diabetes is formed. Some pregnant women who experience severe vomiting in early pregnancy should go to the hospital for medical treatment as soon as possible, and take necessary medical measures to increase maternal nutrition and maintain normal maternal and fetal development.

The second is that some pregnant women have no pregnancy reactions after pregnancy, and their appetite is particularly good. Their diet has increased a lot compared to before pregnancy. Sudden increase in food volume has caused an excessive burden on the digestive and absorption system in the body and occupies a large amount of digestive enzymes. At the same time, these unconsumable nutrients are stored in the body and deprived of many internal resources, disrupt the original endocrine system, cause metabolic disorders in the body, and form gestational diabetes.

The older generations say that pregnant women should eat more to increase nutrition. One person eating is equivalent to two people consuming food. The more they eat, the better the development of the baby in the belly. In fact, this is a misunderstanding. It is true that pregnant women need to increase nutrition. However, you must not eat without restraint. You must scientifically adjust your diet according to your physical condition, maintain the balance of various nutrients in the body, allow the fetus to develop normally in the mother's body, and maintain the mother's normal metabolism.

Why does electrolyte imbalance cause diabetes? This is because electrolytes are an important part of the human pancreas. When electrolytes are disturbed, the function of the pancreas will change, and normal pancreatic juice will not be produced, which will cause gestational diabetes.

Electrolyte disorders can also be said to be endocrine disorders. Generally speaking, the human endocrine system secretes various hormones, together with the nervous system, it regulates the body's metabolism and physiological functions. Under normal circumstances, various hormones are kept in balance, but this balance is disrupted due to pregnancy, resulting in endocrine disorders. Therefore, the mother needs to rebalance the endocrine system and nervous system, so that the hormones can function normally in a state of mineral balance.

Hormones are produced by the endocrine system and belong to the body fluid family. The synthesis of body fluid and the metabolic regulation of the nervous system are inseparable from minerals. Protecting human mineral resources is to protect our health, to scientifically understand the components of our human body, and why people get sick, which parts of the body appear and what pathological conditions correspond to the problems, timely adjust the balance of yin and yang in the body, acid-base balance, how to finding a balance point and so on, these are all conducive to promoting our physical health.

We know that the fetus develops in the amniotic fluid in the mother's womb, and the amniotic fluid contains some minerals, such as sodium, organic matter, and hormones. There are a certain amount of antibodies in the amniotic fluid, so the amniotic fluid has a certain lytic effect, which can reduce the infection of the fetus in the uterus. Amniotic fluid also belongs to the body fluid family of the human body. Gestational diabetes can cause excessive amniotic fluid in the mother's body. Too much and too little amniotic fluid will have an adverse effect on the development of the fetus.

Chapter 6

AVOID DIABETIC COMPLICATION

Diabetes itself does not directly affect people's normal activities. It is its complications that cause death. Therefore, we must be vigilant and prevent its many complications.

Diabetic complication is a common chronic complication, which is transformed from diabetic lesions, and the consequences are quite serious. Podiatry (foot gangrene, amputation), nephropathy (kidney failure, uremia), eye disease (fuzziness, blindness), cerebrovascular disease, heart disease, skin disease, venereal disease, etc are the most common complications of diabetes. The main factor leading to the death of diabetic patients.

The occurrence time of various chronic complications of diabetes generally starts after 5 years of diabetes. The time and severity of their occurrence is directly related to the quality of blood sugar control, blood lipids, and blood pressure.

Even though we diabetics can successfully keep our blood sugar levels within the normal range in various ways, that doesn't mean we can take it lightly. After all, we diabetics have impaired pancreatic islet function, so preventing and treating diabetic complications will accompany us diabetics throughout our lives.

For people with type 2 diabetes, they may have had diabetes for many years when they were diagnosed, so we should check the occurrence of chronic complications every year from the time of diagnosis of diabetes, and predict our physical condition in advance, early treatment and prevention of possible diabetes complications. At the same time, develop good living habits, actively use traditional Chinese medicine massage on meridian points to dredge and adjust diseased or easily diseased parts, take a certain dose of vitamins and minerals, balance the pH in the body, and prevent problems before they occur. Do not have diabetes complications for life.

Reason of Diabetic Complication

Chronic complications of diabetes are the most worrying consequences of diabetic patients, and they are also the core and focus of diabetes treatment. However, because traditional diabetes treatment focuses on the control of blood sugar levels, diabetic patients have always regarded lowering blood sugar levels as the only indicator of whether blood sugar is normal. As a result, the complications of diabetes have not been effectively controlled. Diabetes is based on the pathological basis of blood sugar and blood viscosity being too high and the cells lacking trace elements, so the complications of diabetes always occur around vascular diseases.

As long as a little observation is needed, the causes of these complications of diabetes can be found. In fact, they are all atherosclerotic lesions of the corresponding organs. The difference is that kidney, eye, and foot diseases are mainly caused by tiny blood vessels, while brain and heart disease are caused by large blood vessels. blood vessels, but its pathological basis is atherosclerosis. The direct cause of arteriosclerosis is not the level of blood sugar, but is related to the level of blood lipids in the blood, the viscosity, the adequacy of trace elements in the body, as well as moisture, hypoxia, waste cells and free radicals.

Therefore, when we diabetic patients control the blood sugar level by various means, we should not be paralyzed and think that if the blood sugar level is stable, diabetes will not harm the body. It is necessary to make the three highs, namely high blood sugar, high fat, and high blood pressure, return to the normal range, eat a balanced diet, and keep the body in a weak alkaline state while meeting the body's needs for various nutrients. Only when the body reaches an acid-base balance can the internal environment remain stable, thereby truly preventing diabetes complications. In addition, it is necessary to strengthen the immune system of the body. When the body is strong, the self-healing ability will be strengthened, and the body will gradually recover to a healthy level.

Incidence of Diabetic Complication

In 2010, according to the statistics of the American Diabetes Association (ADA), the risk of complications in patients with diabetes for more than 3 years was more than 46%; the probability of complications in patients with diabetes for more than 5 years was more than 61%; those with diabetes have a 98% chance of developing complications. Diabetes is not terrible, but the complications caused by diabetes can make patients deadly. The mortality rate of diabetes complications is higher than that of cancer.

Among diabetic complications, ischemic heart disease is the leading cause of death in diabetic patients, accounting for 60% to 80% of deaths in diabetic patients. Cerebrovascular disease causes approximately 10% of deaths, and its death rate is twice that of non-diabetic patients. Diabetic nephropathy generally accounts for 10% to 30% of the total deaths. The younger the age at onset, the higher the proportion of deaths caused by diabetic nephropathy.

According to statistics from the World Health Organization, diabetes has now become the third most serious disease that endangers human health after tumors.

Relevant statistics also show that 30% to 40% of patients will develop at least one diabetic complication 10 years after the onset of diabetes. The prevalence of diabetic neuropathy in the course of diabetes is 5 years, 10 years, and 20 years later, it can reach 30% to 40%, 60% to 70% and 90%, respectively. After the course of retinopathy is 10years and 15 years, 40%-50% and 70%-80% of patients will be complicated by the disease. Approximately 10% of patients will develop severe visual impairment 15 years after onset, and 2% of patients will be completely blind.

Microalbuminuria is a precursor of diabetic nephropathy. The incidence of microalbuminuria can reach 10%-30% and 40% after 10 and 20 years of the disease course, and 5%-10% of patients will deteriorate into end-stage renal disease after 20 years. 40% of diabetic patients with onset in adolescence will develop severe kidney disease by the age of 50, requiring hemodialysis and kidney transplantation, otherwise they will only face death.

In addition, the risk of cardiovascular disease in diabetic patients is 2 to 4 times higher than that of the general population, and the age of onset is earlier. Due to vascular and neuropathy in diabetic patients, it often leads to foot ulcers and amputations.

Of course, there are also diabetic patients who live over a hundred years old. For example, Chen Lifu from Taiwan got diabetes at the age of 58, because he learned how to protect his body, thereby reducing the harmful effects of diabetes in the body to zero, and there will be no complications of diabetes throughout his life. Therefore, people with diabetes can live a long life, mainly depending on how we deal with the punishment and warning given by the body. It is not terrible to have diabetes. The terrible thing is to continue to adhere to bad habits and ignore the wake-up call from the body. As long as we get rid of bad habits, our body will adjust itself accordingly and gradually transform into a healthy track.

Therefore, the key to prevent diabetes complications is to increase the blood production rate, reduce the high blood lipids and blood concentration in the blood, detoxify and remove dampness, clean the blood, develop good living habits, and increase the body fluid production rate. Only by nourishing the yin fluid can we maintain the whole life.

Diabetic Oculopathy

Diabetes can cause a variety of eye diseases, such as corneal ulcers, glaucoma, vitreous hemorrhage, etc, but the most common ones that have the greatest impact on vision are diabetic retinopathy and cataracts. Diabetic eye disease is one of the most common chronic complications. It is the arteriosclerosis of the capillaries of the eye, which can make the patient's vision loss and eventually lead to blindness. The blindness rate is 25 times that of normal people. The most important cause of blindness in the world is diabetic eye disease.

The eyes are the first of the five senses, an important organ of the human body, and the window of the human soul. They are essential to people's work, study and life. Eyes are the only way to the light. With eyes and good vision, we live in a bright world and see all the creatures and plants that nature has given us. Can feel more of the beautiful side of the world.

October 10 is "World Sight Day", to highlight the importance of protecting eyesight and remind people to prevent eye diseases and avoid blindness. In order to protect our eyes, diabetic patients must not only control blood sugar, but also control blood pressure and blood lipids to prevent the development of vascular arteriosclerosis.

Living in Canada, there are few social activities and entertainment activities. In addition to doing housework after work, the rest of the time is to watch news and entertainment programs online, and to contact the society and see the world through online media. Over time, I noticed that my vision began to blur and diminish, and there was a loose black cloud floating in front of my eyes. When I closed my eyes, the black floating clouds disappeared, and when I opened my eyes, they appeared again, and the black clouds fluttered quickly with the movement of my eyeballs. For a while, my eyes hurt so much that I couldn't read books or watch news online. I was afraid of light and shed tears. I was worried that the complications of diabetic eye disease were starting to look for trouble, so I checked the online information and found that it was a pre-symptom of diabetic cataract.

So I went to see a specialized ophthalmologist. After the doctor gave me some mydriatic medicine, she used an ophthalmoscope to directly check whether there was any disease in the retina of the fundus. Fortunately, the doctor told me that everything in my fundus was normal and there was no disease. I think it is very likely that my work environment and my long time online are caused by visual fatigue, which is also a trigger for the occurrence of diabetic eye disease cataracts.

However, the monotonous life in North America makes me rely on online communication, and I usually like to use the computer to write articles. The only way is to eliminate eye fatigue and strengthen the resistance of the eyes in time to increase the blood supply to the eyes.

Few eye massage points I chose:

Cuanzhu acupoint: In the depression on the inner edge of the eyebrows. Frequen-tly pressing this point can relieve common eye diseases such as wind and tears, eye congestion, and eye fatigue.

Jingming acupoints: Futaiyang bladder meridian Shu points, located outside the inner canthus of the eye, half aminute away from the inner corner of the eye on both sides of the bridge of the nose.

Use your fingers to press on the acupuncture points and squeeze, move up and down, you can feel a dull pain inthe deep part of the nose. Often massage this point to relieve eye fatigue.

Yuyao acupuncture point: located on the forehead, with pupils straight up and in the eyebrows. Massage this point is helpful for red eyes, swollen eyes, drooping eyelids, myopia, acute conjunctivitis, facial nerve palsy, trigeminal neuralgia, etc.

Chengqi acupoint: Located on the face with the pupil straight down, between the eyeball and the infraorbital rim.

This point is one of the important points in the treatment of eye diseases in acupoint therapy. It can prevent various common eye diseases such as red eyes, swelling and pain, tearing, night blindness, keratitis, optic nerve atrophy, eye fatigue, wind and tearing, presbyopia, cataract, etc. Of course, other related acupoints are needed to be treated together to achieve significant results.

Temple point: The temple point is in front of the auricle, on both sides of the forehead, above the extension line of the outer corner of the eye, and in the depression about a horizontal finger backward. Massage this point can relieve headache, eye disease, toothache and facial pain.

A few years ago, when I was at work, I accidentally hit the corner of the table with my eyes, smashed the glasses, and blood flowed out, blurring my eyes. At that time, I covered my injured eye with one hand, and blood flowed out from between my fingers. My heart was trembling, and there was only one thought, my eyes were pierced by the lens, and I must be blind. My colleague drove me to the hospital to see a doctor to wash the wound. The red and swollen eyes were full of scars and kept bleeding, which was horrible to see. Fortunately, the eyes can see objects after cleaning, thank God, the eyeballs are not punctured by the lenses.

Then I went to see an ophthalmologist, and the eyeball and fundus were examined with special equipment. The doctor said that I was lucky and almost stabbed the eyeball. However, the impact force of the corner of the table on the eyeball is very large. The eye pressure of the hit eye is very high, it is dry and tingling, and it is impossible to look at the lights or surf the Internet. The doctor said that if the eyeball is hit, it will take a long time to recover, so don't worry. During that time, in addition to taking eye drops, I used a hot towel to compress my eyes every morning and before going to bed at night, and insisted on massaging the acupuncture points around my eyes and extending the massage time. In this way, my eyes slowly recovered, my eyes were afraid of seeing light, my eyes were dry, and the problems of high intraocular pressure were also resolved. Half a year later, even the scar across the eyelid disappeared.

At first, I felt sore when I massaged the Zanzhu acupoint. I touched the acupoint with my fingers and felt that there are many particles under the skin of the acupoint. The book said that this is caused by the blockage of the meridian of the acupoint. This acupoint has been blocked for a long time, and other acupoints such as Yu Yao and Qingming are also sore. With the improvement of the eye feeling, these acupoints are slowly massaged and do not feel pain.

In the prevention and treatment of diabetic eye disease complications, I take the following measures:

Visit a specialist ophthalmologist every year to check whether the retina of the fundus is in good condition.

Massage the acupuncture points around the eyes every morning. When you feel tired at work or surfing the Internet, massage the Seimei acupoint immediately to relieve fatigue.

Eat a handful of wolfberry every day. Lycium barbarum can nourish the liver and kidney, and improve eyesight.

Take one vitamin A tablet per day. Vitamin A is also known as retinol. Vitamin A can assist in the treatment of eye diseases, including diabetic eye disease.

Take mixed vitamin B, vitamin E, vitamin C daily. These vitamins can scavenge free radicals in the body and increase the body's immunity.

Eat chicken liver once a week or two to nourish blood and improve eyesight. Due to the high cholesterol in animal liver, it cannot be eaten regularly. As a result, there has been no lesions on the bottom of the eyeball so far.

Diabetic Cardio-Cerebrovascular Disease

Diabetic cardiovascular and cerebrovascular disease is one of the important complications of diabetic patients, and its incidence and mortality are high. Cardiovascular and cerebrovascular disease has become the main cause of death in diabetic patients, with a mortality rate as high as 12% to 28%. The incidence of diabetic cardiovascular disease is 25% - 35%, which is 2 - 3 times that of non-diabetic patients. The incidence of diabetic cerebrovascular disease is 20-30%, which is 4-10 times that of non-diabetic patients. Its high morbidity and mortality seriously threaten human health, so the prevention of diabetic cardiovascular and cerebrovascular diseases is very important.

Why is diabetes and cardiovascular and cerebrovascular diseases so closely related? Because diabetes is an endocrine disease with glucose metabolism disorder as its main manifestation. The main reason is the absolute or relative lack of insulin secretion by the pancreatic β-cells of the patients, causing disorders of sugar, fat and protein metabolism, which not only increases blood sugar, but also converts glucose into fat. The fat is excessively oxidized and decomposed into triglycerides and free fatty acids, especially the increase in cholesterol is more significant, forming hyperlipidemia, and accelerating the arteriosclerosis of diabetic patients.

According to reports, the incidence of arteriosclerosis in diabetic patients is 10 times that of normal people, and the age of onset is early and the course of the disease progresses rapidly. The lesions are mainly located in cerebral arteries, coronary arteries and lower extremity arteries. Due to arteriosclerosis, the elasticity of the arteries is weakened, and the intima of the arteries is rough, which is easy to cause platelets to adhere to the arterial wall, so cerebral thrombosis is prone to occur.

According to statistics, 80% of patients with cerebral infarction have coronary heart disease, angina pectoris, myocardial infarction, and cardiac insufficiency at the same time. When the heart suffers from cardiac insufficiency, myocardial ischemia, frequent premature beats, atrial fibrillation, and atrioventricular block, it can reduce the cerebral circulation blood flow. In addition to the original cerebral arteriosclerosis, it increases the risk of cerebrovascular accidents. Therefore, heart disease is often a risk factor for diabetic cerebrovascular disease.

Ischemic heart disease, also called coronary heart disease, is a disease caused by insufficient blood supply to the heart. It is mainly caused by atherosclerotic plaques on the inner walls of the three coronary arteries that supply blood to the heart, and these arteries are blocked. When the heart is ischemic, it not only causes its own disease, but also affects its blood supply to the brain, causing cerebral infarction.

Due to the impaired pancreas function of diabetic patients, the lack of absorption and digestion capacity, it is unable to provide good nutrients to the body, which is the main cause of ischemic heart disease. Therefore, in order to reduce and eliminate diabetic cardiovascular and cerebrovascular complications, under the condition of ensuring normal blood sugar levels, diabetic patients must actively provide themselves with food that increases blood. Only when the heart has sufficient blood and its own resistance is enhanced, can it be able to remove the hardened plaque on the blood vessel wall. Detoxification and dampness, balanced nutrition, and adequate sleep are all good ways to reduce arteriosclerosis.

High blood pressure and high blood lipids are the enemies of the heart and blood vessels of diabetes. The increased blood viscosity of diabetic patients affects the speed of blood flow, which is also an important factor.

The initial cause of my diabetes was the evolution of longterm hyperlipidemia. When I first suffered from diabetes, my blood lipids and blood pressure were high, and my blood lipids were several times the normal value. The doctor prescribed me a blood lipid-lowering medicine, which is a small pill a day, which I take before going to bed. After taking medicines and taboos, blood lipids gradually reached normal values, and blood pressure gradually dropped. It seems that the three sisters with high blood lipids, high blood pressure, and high blood sugar are like shadows, and they are all companions wherever they go.

Because I have a history of three highs, when treating diabetes, I pay more attention to controlling hyperlipidemia and hypertension. And began to pay attention to develop good habits, such as, used to like to bathe and wash hair before going to bed. After reading the knowledge of health care, I know that it is easy to catch a cold when I wash my hair before going to bed at night, and the wind can easily invade from the acupoints on the head and the gaps in the hair to cause headaches, colds and other diseases. Now I don't wash my hair before going to bed, my head is heavy and the headache is gone. I like to eat snacks. After I have diabetes, I can't eat sugary snacks. I have to eat some dried fruits, peanuts, and melon seeds. However, these snacks are high in fat and can't be eaten too much. For a while, I ate too much peanuts, and the test results showed that the triglycerides exceeded the standard again. I immediately started to stop eating peanuts. After insisting on getting up in the morning and drinking fruit vinegar, triglycerides came down. Now I dare not eat too much dried fruit, eat a little every day.

For a long time, my heart would occasionally beat sharply when it was still, and I felt chest tightness and breathlesswhile drinking water at night. Looking at the information, it is said that this is the phenomenon of premature heart beats, which is an early heart disease. Drinking water and chest tightness is caused by the accumulation of water in the heart. It is also said that people with bad hearts have stripes on their earlobes. I looked at my ears in the mirror, and there were literally stripes on the lobes. This shows that there is something wrong with my heart. It is probably the hidden danger left by the high blood lipids at the beginning. Although the blood lipids are now back to normal, the hidden dangers left by the high blood lipids have caused certain cardiovascular blockages. So, in addition to eating black fungus regularly to remove the oil from the blood vessels in my body, I started to massage and tap the acupoints on the heart meridian according to the steps of health care knowledge.

The specific measures I have taken are:

Strictly control blood sugar level. Fasting blood glucose is maintained at around 6. Insist on measuring blood sugar with a pocket blood glucose meter every day without interruption.

Do golden rooster exercises independently every morning. Close my eyes and one foot independently, practice the balance of the brain, prevent dementia and brain diseases.

Do back-to-wall exercises every morning. Let the acupuncture points on the entire back wake up from sleep, quickly restore vitality, open up many acupuncture points and meridians on the back, let the blood flow unimpeded, and provide enough nutrients for the body.

Tap the acupuncture points on the Heart Channel every day. For example, Neiguan, Quze, Laogong, Ximen, Tianquan.

Take a few slices of garlic and ginger every day. Garlic is a natural scavenger of human blood vessels, and ginger is a natural scavenger for blood vessels. Help reduce blood pressure.

Keep walking. Keep walking 5 days a week, 1 hour a day.

Keep eight glasses of drinking water every day. Get up in the morning and drink the first glass of water to dissolve the viscosity of blood at night, speed up blood circulation, and maintain normal metabolism in the body. After drinking water, do wall-to-wall exercises, so that water can be flushed in the intestines, and the intestines can be cleaned very well, thereby keeping the intestines and stomach clean, increasing the absorption function of the intestines and stomach and the body's immunity.

When the blood sugar level is stable for a long time, increase the blood and body fluid food to improve the self-repair ability and increase the body fluid to improve the water metabolism ability.

Insist on soaking feet or steaming legs in hot water every day to detoxify and promote blood circulation. The feet are the roots of human beings. Only when the roots are raised, the branches and leaves will flourish.

Results: So far, blood sugar, blood lipids and blood pressure have remained normal. Premature heart beats and chest tightness never appeared again.

Diabetes and Hypertension

Hypertension is the most common chronic disease and the main risk factor for cardiovascular and cerebrovascular diseases. Hypertensive patients are prone to complicated heart, brain and kidney diseases, such as stroke, myocardial infarction, heart failure and chronic kidney disease. Diabetes and hypertension have commonalities in terms of etiology, influence and harm. Therefore, diabetic patients often suffer from hypertension at the same time, and hypertensive patients are also diabetic patients, so they are collectively referred to as diabetic hypertension.

Diabetes and high blood pressure are both related to high blood lipids. These two diseases basically start with high blood lipids and gradually evolve into them. Diabetes is easy to cause kidney damage, and diabetic kidney damage can cause blood pressure to rise. In addition, diabetic patients have high blood sugar, high blood viscosity, damaged blood vessel walls, and increased vascular resistance are all factors that can easily cause high blood pressure.

Salt will increase the risk of cardiovascular disease. Most hypertension patients have heavy tastes and love to eat salty foods. Therefore, to prevent diabetes and hypertension, we must first change our eating habits, reduce the intake of salt per meal, and eat light food. Not exercising is also a major cause of hyperlipidemia, high blood pressure, and high blood sugar. Therefore, we must exercise actively, reduce stress, treat the disease optimistically, be friends with the disease, do what you like, relax, and blood pressure will naturally not be high, thus avoiding the possibility of complications of diabetes and hypertension.

Vegetables to Lower Blood Pressure

Celery: rich in protein, carbohydrates, carotene, B vitamins, calcium, phosphorus, iron, sodium, etc. The leaf stems also contain medicinal ingredients such as apigenin, bergamot lactone and volatile oil, which can lower blood pressure and lower blood lipids. , The role of prevention and treatment of atherosclerosis.

Radish: sweet in taste and cool in nature. It can eliminate stagnation, resolve phlegm heat, disperse blood congestion, relieve alcohol toxins, lower blood lipids, and soften blood vessels. Regular eating can prevent coronary heart disease and arteriosclerosis. Radishes can be used as a vegetable to lower blood pressure and reduce the symptoms of hypertensive patients.

When I first got diabetes, I didn't know how to treat the disease correctly. I couldn't control all aspects of my body well. My blood sugar was high and blood lipids were high. For a while, the high blood pressure reached 160, and the low pressure was more than 90. My head is bloated all day, I feel irritable and get angry easily. Later, I learned some health care knowledge, understood the structure and operation of the body, and gradually adjusted it. Now my blood pressure has remained normal. Like young people, the high pressure is 110-120, and the low pressure is about 75. No headache, no dizziness, no irritability.

Diabetic Ketoacidosis

Ketoacidosis is one of the acute complications of diabetes, which is caused by a severe lack of insulin in the body. When the patient is severely deficient in insulin, the disorder of glucose metabolism is aggravated sharply. At this time, the body cannot use glucose, so it has to use fat for energy, and fat burning is incomplete, resulting in serious secondary fat metabolism disorder. When the decomposition of fat is accelerated, the production of ketone bodies increases beyond the level that the tissues can use, and the accumulation of ketone bodies in the body causes blood ketones to exceed 2 mg%, and ketosis occurs.

In order to control blood sugar levels, low-carbohydrate diet therapy has been implemented over the years. The low-carb diet was first proposed in 1972 by Dr. Atkins in the United States in "Dr. Atkins's New Diet Revolution. " Advocating a high-protein and high-fat diet to replace carbohydrates to lower blood sugar and lose weight has been popular for a long time, and many famous people have followed suit. However, both high-protein and high- fat foods are acidic substances, and long-term consumption will inevitably damage the body's function. This is an obvious consequence.

Ketone bodies are the product of fat catabolism and are only formed in the liver, not the product of hyperglycemia. Ketone bodies are a form of energy output by the liver. Consumption of carbohydrates will not cause an increase in ketone bodies, but excessive intake of high protein and high fat and fatigue will induce and produce excessive ketone bodies in the body. China's" Manual on Energy Conservation and Emission Reduction for the Whole People" calls on people to eat more vegetarian food and eat less meat, which is not only good for health, but also reduces carbon emissions.

Ketone bodies are acidic substances that can cause polydipsia and polyuria, fatigue, loss of appetite, nausea, vomiting, headache, drowsiness, irritability, rotten apple smell in the breath, dehydration in severe cases, reduced urine output, and poor skin elasticity. Sunken eyeballs, lower blood pressure, and even coma are life-threatening.

In the early years of my diabetes, the smell in my mouth when I woke up in the morning was filled with the smell of apples. During that time, I preferred a high-fat diet, because of my own disease, insufficient insulin and lipase enzymes in the body to break down and digest sugar and fat result in an excess of ketone bodies in the body. If I knew at the time that the high ketone bodies in the body were caused by the excessive intake of fat, I would timely replenish the lack of water in the body, speed up the excretion of ketone bodies, and adjust the diet structure, reduce the intake of fat and protein, and eat more vegetables, this does not happen. Fortunately, I did not repeat the previous binge eating, just a little bit on a high-fat and high-protein diet, in order to lower the blood sugar level, otherwise there will be serious consequences.

It can be concluded that the risk of ketosis in diabetic patients is significantly higher than that in normal people, and a low-sugar and high-fat diet can increase the production of ketone bodies. The best way to prevent ketone body acidosis is to have a balanced and varied diet, and drink 7-8 glasses of water a day.

Diabetic Nephropathy

Kidney damage caused by diabetes, namely diabetic nephropathy, is one of the most common complications of diabetes, with an incidence of about 34. 7%, second only to cardiovascular and cerebrovascular diseases. The kidney is a very important organ in our body. The kidney has three basic functions:

The kidneys can produce urine and excrete metabolites. Our human body produces a variety of waste products in the process of metabolism. Most of the waste products are filtered through the glomerular blood, and the secretion of the renal tubules is excreted in the urine.

Maintain fluid balance and acid-base balance in the body. Through glomerular filtration, renal tubular reabsorption and secretion, the kidneys excrete excess water from the body, regulate the acid-base balance, and maintain the stability of the internal environment.

Secretory function. Secretion of renin, prostaglandin, kinin. These hormones regulate blood pressure, promote erythropoietin, and stimulate bone marrow hematopoiesis. Many endocrine hormone degradation sites - such as insulin, gastrointestinal hormones, etc. These hormones change when the kidneys are insufficiency, causing metabolic disorders. It can be seen that the kidney plays an important function in maintaining the stability of the body's environment.

Diabetes patients usually have weak kidney function. The kidneys do not like the eating habits of big fish and meat all day long. This is equivalent to making the kidneys work overtime every day. Excessive workload will damage the function of the kidneys and are prone to disease.

The organs of the human body are interdependent, and one of the links has a problem, and other functions must be affected. If the kidney of a diabetic patient has problems, it will also be accompanied by problems such as liver, high blood pressure, and cardiovascular and cerebrovascular problems.

Diabetics must control their blood sugar well and not add extra burden to the kidneys. Good blood sugar control can halve the incidence of diabetic nephropathy. While controlling our blood sugar, we must pay attention to diet control. To prevent diabetic nephropathy, it is necessary to treat the kidneys well and cater to the tastes of the kidneys.

I used to have a bad problem with my diet. I like to put too much salt every time when I cook vegetables. If the vegetables are weakly fried, I will feel tasteless. This may be the real cause of high blood pressure. After paying attention to my eating habits, I should try to cook lightly, eat less salt, less oil, and use less seasonings for cooking, so that the original taste, blood pressure gradually becomes normal, and the head is not heavy. The feeling of putting on the curse disappeared. The blood pressure is normal, and the kidneys have reduced the burden and become more relaxed. Of course, I was a little uncomfortable at the beginning of the change. I am used to eating heavy-tasting meals, and light-tasting foods can't stimulate appetite. But for good health, bad things must be corrected. Now, I'm used to eating light food instead of salty food.

The general principle of prevention and treatment of diabetic nephropathy is to eat more light, digestible, nutritious, and vitamin-rich foods, eat less seafood, and do not smoke or drink alcohol. Eating too much protein and salt will increase the burden on the kidneys.

1. To prevent diabetic nephropathy, treat the kidneys well and eat foods that the kidneys like.

The kidneys like to eat black foods. Chinese medicine says that black foods are good for the kidneys, such as black beans, black rice, and black fungus.

(1) Keep drinking enough water every day. Keep the body full of water and full of cells, which helps the kidneys to detoxify and detoxify.

(2)   Detoxify regularly.

(3)   Strictly control the intake of salt

(4)   Eat less or avoid greasy and fried foods, and appropriately control the intake of high protein.

2.   To prevent diabetic nephropathy, we must treat the kidneys kindly and do what the kidneys like.

Massage the acupoints to improve the function of the kidneys. Zhaohai, Gongsun, Yongquan, Taixi, Fuliu and other acupoints strengthen the kidney.

3.   Keep warm. The kidneys love warmth and are afraid of cold, so we must protect our waist and keep our kidneys in a warm state.

4.   Eat blood-rich foods. The liver is strong, the blood supply to the kidneys is sufficient, and the kidneys also increase horsepower and become stronger.

5.   Hit the wall with our back. The yang qi in the body rises by hitting the back against the wall. There are Shenshu acupoints on the back, the back is warm, the waist is warm, the kidneys are warm, and the internal organs are warm. The blood circulation throughout the body is smooth.

6.   Try to keep calm in everything, and naturally we will be stable.

7.   Don't be tired, stay up late, try to reduce the burden on the kidney.

Diabetic Neuropathy

The probability of neuropathy in diabetic patients is very high, and it is difficult to cure it. Because of the different physical conditions of diabetic patients, the degree of diabetic lesions is also different. Some diabetic patients have good blood sugar control, and diabetic neuropathy may also occur. Some diabetic patients have poor blood sugar control, but no diabetic neuropathy occurs. This is all related to genetics. However, the main reason is that the lack of minerals in the body causes cell dysfunction.

Diabetics suffer from poor digestion and absorption and lack of minerals in the body, which can easily cause metabolic disorders in the body. The nerve cells in the body transmit minerals to the outside. On October 7, 2013, Professor Thomas of Stanford University. Thomas Sudhof won the Nobel Prize in Medicine. His award-winning achievement was to study the way of information transmission in the human brain 25 years ago, and to study how nerve cells transmit information to other nerve cells through calcium ions. (His results can help understand what kind of genetic mutations can cause neurodegeneration, such as schizophrenia and autism.)

Neuropathy in diabetic patients is mainly caused by cell dysfunction caused by lack of minerals in the body, The research of Thomas Sudhof confirmed that the nerve cells of the human body transmit information to each other through calcium ions.

Nowadays, people do not sleep well. In addition to other reasons, there is another main reason for the lack of calcium in the body. Calcium can regulate nerve cells. Without calcium, the nerve cells of the human body will become unstable, and many diseases related to nerve regulation will occur. The main reason for the poor sleep of the elderly is the lack of calcium, because the bones of the elderly lack calcium and osteoporosis, which causes poor sleep. Young people can also cause calcium deficiency in their bodies due to fast growth or bone damage.

Diabetic patients have weak absorption and digestion due to their own diseases, and the food they eat is not well absorbed and then excreted. As a result, there is a lack of nutrition and a lack of minerals and vitamins in the body.

Calcium is a major element in the body, and the demand is large. Whether it is a diabetic or a normal person, a long-term lack of calcium can lead to neuropathy and metabolic diseases.

Although diabetics can live like normal people with good blood sugar control, it does not mean that we have to work as hard as normal people. After all, the physical strength and endurance of diabetic patients are not as good as those of normal people, and they are easily injured if they are not careful. Since I got diabetes, my hands are often numb and my limbs are weak. Even in summer, my hands are numb, and I often have diarrhea. When I came to Canada, because of the nature of my work, I had to keep working with my hands. I repeated the same movements every day. My wrists were easily injured, and my fingers were numb, inflexible, and stiff. In severe cases, the arm cannot be raised and cannot be combed normally. After reading the knowledge about diabetes, knowing that this is one of the complications of diabetes, diabetes has affected my body and nerves.

During that time, not only the nerves of the arms and hands had problems, but my fingernails also became very easy to crack. Often the nails cracked accidentally, so I cut all the nails short. But it still can't stop the cracking. During the period of nail cracking, sleep is not good, often insomnia, insomnia all night and all night, all methods are exhausted, still can't fall asleep, obviously very sleepy, just can't fall asleep. These symptoms are reminding me of my calcium deficiency. But I don't know it at all, and I don't have any common sense of health care.

People need calcium supplementation in middle age, especially women, lack of calcium, bones are prone to osteoporosis. The lack of calcium in nerve cells is equivalent to lack of communication and contact with each other, which results in dysfunction of neuroregulation. What's more, I am a diabetic and I am more prone to mineral deficiency in my body. I don't want to become an old lady with bones full of hornet's nests, the nerves in my hands and feet are atrophied, and I stay in bed all day long. So, I started taking calcium tablets to supplement myself with calcium. Since calcium supplementation, my sleep has improved and my arm nerves have also improved. Since then, I have learned the importance of calcium, and I have continued to supplement calcium without interruption over the years. Later, I added magnesium and zinc, these two minerals are to maintain bones, nerves, and assist calcium metabolism together.

Later, I looked at the information and said that there was an old man who turned his wrists and ankles every day. He was still in his eighties and was still full of energy. He was not deaf or dazzled, and rarely got sick. There are many meridians and tendons on human wrists and ankles. Meridians are the channels of the human body. Tendons are the ligaments and tendons on the human body. These two important parts of the human body have many confluences at the wrist and ankle. Rotating the wrists and ankles can unclog the meridians well. Ancient Chinese medicine believes that the liver governs the tendons. Repair the liver by conditioning the tendons. The function of the liver is strengthened, and the body's detoxification function, digestive function, and hematopoietic function will be significantly improved.

Ever since, I followed the old man's practice, turning a few hundred times a day. On the way to work every day, I walk and turn my wrists, which is not boring at all. After turning, I feel relaxed at the extremities, and the stiffness disappears immediately. Every night before going to bed, massage the Yongquan acupoints to massage the Dijin (the lower end of the Yongquan acupoints) incidentally. This is the best blood and liver nourishing medicine. I believe in the magical theory of the meridian of traditional Chinese medicine with a long history in China.

Since I started massaging the acupuncture points on the meridians and turning the tendons of my wrists and ankles last year, this summer, I took off my gloves. Every day I go to work with bare hands, and there are no large areas of small blisters on the back of my hands. This shows that the meridian theory of traditional Chinese medicine is correct, the blood vessels of the whole body are unblocked, and the lesions will gradually disappear naturally.

My treatment protection method:

1. Rotate the tendons of the wrist and ankle to increase tenacity and immunity.

2. Insist on using hot water to wash clothes, hands, and vegetables all year round. Keep your hands and feet warm.

3. Massage meridian points. (mentioned above)

4. Adhere to calcium and magnesium supplements every day to strengthen bones, assist and increase the conduction of nerve

cells.

Diabetic Foot

Diabetic foot is a serious complication of diabetes. It is one of the important reasons for the disability and even death of diabetic patients. It not only causes suffering to patients, but also severely affects and burdens patients, their families and society. In view of this, International Diabetes The theme of the Alliance's 2005 Diabetes Day is "Diabetes and Foot Care" to call on the whole society to pay attention to diabetic feet.

Diabetic foot is caused by neuropathy in diabetic feet that reduces the protective function of the lower limbs, and large blood vessels and microvascular diseases make arterial blood flow insufficient, resulting in microcirculation disorders and ulcers and gangrene. The foot is the direct bearing part of the human body's weight, and it is also the most easily injured part of diabetic patients, which causes the incidence of diabetic foot to increase year by year.

Diabetic foot disease is the main cause of lower limb amputation in diabetic patients. Of the approximately 150 million diabetic patients in the world, 15% to 20% may develop foot ulcers or gangrene during the course of their disease. The amputation rate of diabetic foot disease is 15 times that of non-diabetic patients, and about 50% of the annual amputation patients are diabetic patients. Statistics provided by the American Diabetes Association (ADA) show that 86, 000 patients in the United States will lose their feet or lower limbs due to diabetes and become disabled every year. The treatment of diabetic foot ulcers is costly. Holzer's health insurance survey of the 7 million diabetic patients database in the United States indicated that the cost of direct diabetic foot ulcers in two years was US$16 million, and the average cost of each foot ulcer was US$4595. The incidence of diabetic foot disease in China has been increasing year by year.

The symptoms and signs of diabetic foot vary according to the course of the disease and the severity of the disease. In mild cases, only slight pain in the feet and ulcers on the skin surface. Moderate patients may have deeper penetrating ulcers with soft tissue inflammation. In severe cases, ulcers are accompanied by soft tissue abscesses, bone tissue lesions, localized gangrene of toes, heels or forefoot, or even whole foot gangrene.

External causes: 1. Scratching the skin due to itching between the toes or feet. 2. Collapse, blister burst, burns. 3. Injuries, collisions and wear from new shoes, etc.

Intrinsic causes: 1. Diabetic neuropathy. 2. The moisture in the body is high. 3. High blood lipids and high blood viscosity.

At first, my diabetic symptom was a large C-type blood mark on the ankle, which couldn't heal. The scab formed from autumn to the end of the spring of the second year, and the self-healing ability was very poor. I didn't know why my skin healed so badly at the time. I just felt very tired all the time. I was tired without doing anything, and I didn't have any strength in my whole body. This is an early warning of diabetes, reminding me from the feet.

Since understanding the serious consequences of diabetic feet, I have always paid great attention to protecting my nerves and feet, but the key is to keep the blood sugar level within the ideal range. Only when the blood sugar level is stable can other indicators be adjusted accordingly.

My approach is:

1. Insist on taking vitamin B1, because it has the effect of stabiliz-ing and regulating nerves.

2. Rotate the left and right ankles 200 times a day to dredge the bones and meridians. There are arteries and 12 meridians passing through the feet. Rotating the ankle is beneficial to the dredging of blood and each meridian.

3. Soak my feet with hot water every night to remove dampness and detoxification.

4. Try to wear comfortable and loose shoes, so that there is a prop-er space for my feet in the shoes.

Over the years, my feet have been in good condition, the skin is tight, neither dry nor swollen, and there are basically no cracks and calluses on the heels. Even if the foot is accidentally injured occasionally, it can heal quickly, and the wound healing ability is very strong.

Diabetic Dermadrome

Diabetic skin disease is the most common complication of diabetes. The incidence is very high, accounting for about half of diabetic patients. The incidence is very high. Almost one in every two diabetic patients will have diabetic skin disease. This not only affects the normal life of diabetic patients, but also causes great harm to our health.

Why are diabetics so prone to skin diseases? In life, some people around us will heal themselves very quickly if their skin is injured, while some people are hard to heal if their skin is injured, and the affected area is constantly red and swollen. Diabetes patients are most afraid of skin injuries. Once injured, it is difficult to heal. These people whose skin is difficult to heal have blood problems, causing bacteria to multiply in tissue cells, causing local infections and blocking the healing of cell tissues.

The medical professiong enerally refers to the skin diseases of diabetic patients as "diabetic skin diseases", including many kinds of diseases, which can be divided into three categories: One type is skin diseases caused by abnormal intermediate metabolites produced in the body of diabetic patients, such as skin infections, skin itching, and xanthomas. The occurrence of these diseases is directly related to the hyperglycemia and hyperlipidemia caused by diabetes. When the diabetes is controlled, these lesions will be relieved.

The second category is related to the chronic degeneration of diabetes, such as diabetic skin diseases, erythema and necrosis, diabetic skin bullae, sclerosing edema, diabetic neurological diseases and so on. The pathogenesis of this type of disease is that diabetes causes microvascular disease, resulting in reduced blood supply to the skin, and damage to the dermal connective tissue and other adnexa associated with vascular disease. This type of disease occurs slowly, and it is difficult to treat.

The third category is skin diseases associated with diabetes but not related to metabolic disorders or degenerative diseases, such as progressive necrosis of diabetic lipids, granuloma annulare, and vitiligo. These diseases are more common in people with diabetes, but the medical community has not yet figured out the relationship between them and the pathogenesis of diabetes.

Chinese medicine believes that the lungs control the skin. Through its transport function, the lung can distribute the nutrients of wei qi and qi, blood and body fluid to the whole body, nourish the skin and fur to maintain its normal physiological function, so the function of the fur is dominated by the lung qi, that is to say, the skin on our body any problems with hair will be directly or indirectly related to the lungs.

From the perspective of traditional Chinese medicine, diabetes is caused by the lack of water due to injury to the yin. Therefore, diabetic patients lack the water to moisturise the skin and hair, the soil will dry and crack due to lack of water, and the same is true for the human body. From the point of view of Western medicine, the sugar content of the skin of diabetic patients is higher than that of blood sugar, and once damaged, it is easy to cause infection and difficult to heal.

Diabetes patients have poor microvascular circulation, which leads to poor local cell function. Peripheral nerve endings are prone to inflammation, which can easily lead to abnormal hands and feet, and skin itching. Diabetes patients have high levels of sugar in their blood, and various bacteria can easily invade and cause infections. Generally, diabetic patients seldom sweat because of reduced sweat secretion, and are prone to dry skin and pruritus. The skin is easy to dry, so apply some moisturizer immediately after taking a shower or hands to keep the skin moisturized.

There are various causes of skin infections, and they are usually cured quickly. Only when the blood sugar level is not well controlled will the disease worsen. In other words, only when the blood sugar level is normal, the soil for the growth of germs and bacteria is changed, and the inflammation gradually disappears.

Chapter 7

Self Test Blood Sugar

Adherence to blood glucose monitoring in diabetic patients is an important part of self-supervised treatment. Through self-monitoring of blood sugar, we can grasp the level of blood sugar in time and adjust blood sugar in time. For active diet control, active control of the appropriate amount of exercise and medication is a very important means.

Diabetics are unlikely to go to the doctor every day and ask the doctor to follow behind to supervise us. Going to see a doctor requires special guidance from experts. Special equipment is used to detect the problems that need to be improved in the patient's body and the stage of the patient's physical condition. After knowing the stage of the disease and the need to adjust the treatment, the role of the patient itself becomes more important. Although self-monitoring of blood sugar is only the blood sugar of a patient at a certain point in time, it is of great reference value for adjusting daily life.

Blood Sugar Level

The sugar in the blood is called blood sugar, and in most cases it is glucose. Most of the energy required for the activities of tissues and cells in the body comes from glucose, so blood sugar must be maintained at a certain level to maintain the needs of various organs and tissues in the body.

The fasting blood glucose concentration of normal people in the morning is 3. 9 – 6. 1 moles of blood glucose, and the blood glucose plasma is 3. 9 – 6. 9.

When the fasting blood glucose is above 5. 6 moles and the plasma blood glucose is 6. 4 moles, a glucose tolerance test should be done.

Fasting blood glucose is greater than 6. 7 moles, and plasma blood glucose is greater than 7. 8 moles. Diabetes can be diagnosed by repeating the measurement twice.

One hour postprandial blood glucose 6. 7 – 9. 4 moles, not more than 11. 1 moles (200 mg)

The blood sugar is less than 7. 8 moles two hours after a meal. Three hours after the meal, blood sugar returned to normal.

If the blood glucose concentration exceeds 8. 9 to 10 moles, a part of the glucose will be excreted in the urine, which is diabetes. A blood glucose concentration lower than3. 8 moles is called hypoglycemia. When hypoglycemia occurs, the brain tissue first responds to hypoglycemia, manifesting as dizziness, palpitations, cold sweats, and hunger. If the blood sugar continues to drop below 2. 6 moles, hypoglycemic coma can occur.

Sugar is one of the essential nutrients for our body. People consume grains, fruits and vegetables, which are converted into simple sugars (such as glucose, etc.) through the digestive system, enter the bloodstream, and are transported to the cells of the whole body as a source of energy. If it cannot be consumed for a while, it is converted into glycogen and stored in the liver and muscles. The liver can store 70-120 grams of sugar, which accounts for about 6-10% of the liver's weight. The glycogen that cells can store is limited. If too much sugar is ingested, the excess sugar will turn into fat.

When the food is digested, the stored glycogen will become a normal source of sugar and maintain the normal concentration of blood sugar. During strenuous exercise, or if there is no supplementary food for a long time, glycogen will also be consumed. At this time, cells will break down fat to supply energy. 10% of fat is glycerol, which can be converted into sugar. Other parts of fat can produce energy through oxidation, but its metabolic pathway is different from that of glucose.

The human brain and nerve cells need sugar to survive. When necessary, the human body will secrete hormones to destroy certain parts of the human body (such as muscles, skin and even organs), and convert the proteins into sugar to maintain survival.

The sugar needed by all cells of the human body is transported by the blood, so it is important to maintain the proper concentration of sugar in the blood.

Under normal circumstances, the blood glucose concentration fluctuates slightly throughout the day. Generally speaking, the pre-meal blood sugar is slightly lower and the post-meal blood sugar is slightly higher, but this fluctuation is maintained within a certain range. The fasting blood glucose concentration of normal people fluctuates between 3. 9~6. 1mmol/L (70~110mg/dl). The blood sugar is slightly higher 2 hours after a meal, but it should be less than 7. 8mmol/L (<140mg/dl). Because the production and utilization of blood sugar in normal people is in dynamic balance, it can maintain blood sugar relatively stable, neither too high nor too low.

Experiments show that when blood sugar is only at 90-95 mg/dl can the body maintain normal activities, at around 70 mg/dl, people will feel hungry, tired, and tired. When it reaches 65 mg/dl, we will be hungry. If we don't take measures, your blood sugar will continue to decrease, and you will experience dizziness, weakness, heart rate disturbances, weak legs and even vomiting, which is the so-called hypoglycemia.

The movement of human brain and nerve cells requires sugar to provide energy, not fat or protein. When the blood sugar drops slightly, the mind becomes confused and unresponsive. When the blood sugar drops below the normal value, people become irritable and moody.

Cells use glucose without the effect of insulin. When the blood glucose concentration is too high, the pancreas will increase the secretion of insulin, and the blood sugar will decrease accordingly, so insulin is also called hypoglycemic hormone.

If we consume too much sugar for a long time, the pancreas will become fatigued due to the large amount of insulin secreted. If it goes on for a long time, it will lead to decline. It will not be able to provide the required insulin at any time, and the blood sugar level will not be effectively controlled, resulting in high blood sugar. Allowing the development of high blood sugar can lead to diabetes. Diabetes has become the third "health killer" after cardiovascular and cancer.

The side setting range of the blood glucose meter is [0. 5~27. 7 mmol/L (10~500 mg/dL), the normal blood glucose range is 3. 5 mol-6. 2 mol).

Glucose from glucose millimoles (mmol/L British standard) to glucose g/dL (mg/dL American standard) conversion table chart

mmol/L	mg/dL	mmol/L	mg/dL	mmol/L	mg/dL
2. 8	50	9	162	19. 0	342
3. 0	54	9. 4	170	20. 0	360
3. 3	60	10. 0	180	20. 8	375
3. 6	65	10. 5	190	21. 0	378
3. 9	70	11. 0	196	21. 5	387
4	72	11. 1	200	22. 2	400
4. 4	80	12. 0	216	23. 0	414
4. 7	85	12. 5	225	23. 5	423
5	90	13. 0	234	24. 0	432
5. 5	100	13. 9	250	25. 0	450
6	106	14. 0	252	25. 5	459
6. 7	120	14. 4	260	26. 0	468
7	126	15. 0	270	26. 4	475
7. 2	130	15. 6	280	27. 7	500
7. 5	135	16. 0	288	30. 0	540
7. 8	140	16. 6	300	33. 3	600
8	145	17. 0	306	36. 1	650
8. 3	150	17. 5	315	38. 8	700
8. 9	160	18. 0	325	40. 0	720

Causes of blood Sugar Fluctuations

There are many reasons for blood sugar fluctuations.

(1) Climatic factors: Cold stimulation can promote the increase of adrenaline secretion. The liver glycogen output increases, and the muscle's glucose uptake is reduced, which makes the blood sugar increase and the condition worsens. The summer is hot and sweaty, so we should pay attention to replenishing water in time, otherwise the blood will be concentrated and the blood sugar will increase.

(2) Blood sugar can rise after catching a cold.

(3) In patients with trauma, surgery, infection, fever, severe

trauma, vomiting, insomnia, anger, anxiety, irritability, fatigue, acute myocardial infarction and other stress conditions, blood sugar can rise rapidly and even induce diabetic ketoacidosis.

(4) When the blood sugar level is not truly stable, the diabetic patient reduces the amount of the drug by themself, resulting in an increase in blood sugar.

(5) Sudden changes in the working environment and living environment cause temporary adverse effects ofthe body.

(6) Excessive intake of high-fat foods will cause the pancreatic islets to fail to secrete insulin well, which will increase blood sugar.

(7) Long-term constipation can lead to metabolic disorders, unfavorable blood circulation, and affect blood sugar.

(8) Insufficient drinking water can cause metabolic imbalance and affect blood sugar.

Blood Glucose Test Record

Speaking of blood sugar testing, very few people with diabetes can persevere in testing every day. Most of them find it troublesome, afraid of pain, and some are not used to it. Self-testing blood sugar involves pricking our finger with the special needle that comes with the blood glucose meter, just like being bitten by a wasp. However, self- monitoring of blood glucose is one of the essential links in the treatment of diabetes. It is impossible for doctors to follow every diabetic patient. The main treatment depends on the diabetic patients themselves. As the saying goes, a long illness becomes a good doctor. Diabetic patients know their own physical condition best, and most doctors listen to the patient's own narrative when they consult. In a sense, diabetic patients are their own best doctors. Therefore, daily adherence to self-monitoring of blood glucose is a necessary course for diabetic patients.

Since I was diagnosed with diabetes when I went abroad for medical examination in 1999, I bought a blood glucose meter for self-monitoring. In the initial blood glucose test, I simply recorded the blood glucose level and then threw it away. Later, although I kept recording the blood sugar level, I didn't record the food I ate. Checking the records could not find the reason for the increase and decrease of blood sugar. It did not provide any more useful help for grasping the trend and law of blood sugar. Later, I improved the way of recording, recording the food I generally ate, my schedule, and exercise routine every day. In this way, with the facts, I have a good grasp of the rise and fall of blood sugar levels, and it is very convenient to self-adjust and strictly prevent the development of the disease.

Adjust the Drug According to the Level of Blood Sugar

2000 was the beginning of diabetes. I took the Chinese patent medicine Xiaoke Pills brought in China, and my blood sugar level remained stable.

Because I believe in traditional Chinese medicine, I refused to take western medicine to lower blood ugar. In 2001, 2002, and 2003, I took homemade Chinese medicine soup for lowering blood sugar. My blood sugar level was high and sometimes low. I often felt hungry, ate too much, and did not grow meat. I am in poor physical condition, often sick, dizzy, heavy feet, and weak. My own immunity is very poor, and a little wind will cause a cold when I go out.

In 2004 and the first half of 2005, I insisted on doing exercises and food therapy in the gym every day. I did not take medicine. The fasting blood sugar level in the morning remained stable below 6 moles, and my body was less sick.

In 2006, due to the night shift, the blood sugar level has been fluctuating around the normal value, and the flat conductors often get inflammation and catch colds.

In the summer of 2007, when I returned to China, I did not control my diet. I ate too much high-protein and high- fat food, which caused the blood sugar level to soar. The highest fasting blood sugar level in the morning reached 18 moles. After returning to Canada, I insisted that I did not take hypoglycemic drugs, thinking that as long as I controlled my diet, my blood sugar would naturally drop. Who knew that this time the diet control method would not work, and the blood sugar level would not drop to the normal value for a long time. However, it was much lower than the blood sugar level tested during my return to China, so I was not in a hurry.

During that time, China said Guyuan Ointment was a magical, universal food, so I returned to Canada and I ate homemade Guyuan Ointment every morning. Because Guyuan Ointment contained red dates and longans, the sugar content was large, so I tested it every time. The blood sugar levels are higher. And I believe that diet therapy is better than medicine. The doctor also said that as long as the blood sugar is kept stable, there is no problem even if the blood sugar level is a little higher, and the body will automatically adjust and accept it. I don't know about the development of diabetes. I am confused about what the doctor said is right, so I use the body's nourishment as the main excuse, and I haven't deliberately lowered my blood sugar to an ideal value for a long time.

In the second half of 2008, I told the doctor that my blood sugar was higher than normal for a long time. If this continues, it is likely to cause diabetes complications. So my family doctor prescribed the western medicine Mepyrida, mainly to reduce my postprandial high blood sugar. I take two mepyrida (glipizide) pills a day, one in the morning and one in the evening, and I continue to take the Guyuan Ointment. Since Mepyrida can reduce blood sugar by preventing the intake of food, after taking Mepyrida, the food is not good, I don't eat much, and my weight has plummeted.

During a break at work in 2009, I chatted with my colleague about diabetes. He said he also had this disease. I asked him what medicine he was taking. He told me that it was the medicine his wife had chosen for him. It was a diabetes medicine. The effect is very good. So I stopped taking Mepyrida (glipizide) and switched to taking Diamicron(Gliclazide). This medicine has small particles and has little side effects on the stomach. Take 2 pills hypoglycemic medicine each day. The blood sugar level began to drop, soon reached the normal value, and has been very stable. Moreover, the sweet taste of eating food in the past has been restored.

Everyone's physical fitness is different, and the pathology that causes diabetes is different. When taking hypoglycemic drugs, we must find a hypoglycemic drug that suits our condition to minimize the damage to our body. I obviously feel uncomfortable in my stomach, and I have to keep taking it every day. Not only does it cause damage to other organs, but it also doesn't help much in stabilizing blood sugar levels in the long term. Since then, Diamicron (Gliclazide) has been my first choice for drug adjuvant therapy.

After my blood sugar stabilized for a long time, I started to subtract the amount of medicine. Originally, I took 2 pills a day, but I changed to 1 pills a day. One pill per day can still keep the blood sugar level stable within the normal range, so I want to stop the hypoglycemic drugs and use a combination of exercise and massage acupoints to replace the hypoglycemic drugs. Since the summer of 2011, I have been walking for about an hour a day, taking half a hypoglycemic drug every night, and my blood sugar level has remained good. Starting from November 30, 2011, I stopped taking drugs and used morning and evening acupoint massage instead of hypoglycemic drugs, and blood sugar levels remained within the normal range.

After stopping the drug for more than a year, in order to move towards a deeper treatment of diabetes, in the spring of 2013, I started to replenish qi and blood, detoxify and remove dampness, and started taking medicine again, but this time I did not take medicine because of high blood sugar. I was taking precautions. Take the initiative to take medicine. In order to improve the body's fitness and immunity, so as to be able to clean up blood stains and garbage in the blood vessels, and prevent the cardiovascular and cerebrovascular complications of diabetes, I began to eat more red dates, black rice, glutinous rice, red beans and longans, etc. Taking medicine can keep blood sugar levels within the normal range. Keep walking every day and take half a pill at night to achieve my goal. In the summer, I started to invigorate body fluids, eat white fungus, longan and other yin-reinforcing foods with high sugar content, supplement my pancreas with nutrients, and take half a pill each morning and evening, and still keep my blood sugar level within the normal value.

If I follow the previous practice, I will not take medicine, and let my blood sugar level be 6-7 moles or 8 moles. But now I won't. I must keep my blood sugar level within the normal value, because it's unsafe if the blood sugar level exceeds 7 moles. Over time it will cause damage to the microcirculation, so there should be no fluke. My experience is that if the blood sugar level is between 6 mol and 7 mol, the body will still feel tired and lack of energy. Only when the blood sugar level is kept below 6 mol and between 5 and 6 mol, the body will feel relaxed.

Stabilization of Blood Sugar Level, Confidence in Increasing Adjuvant Therapy

In 2013, the body's immunity was greatly improved by replenishing qi and blood, detoxification and dampness, and nourishing body fluids. The pancreatic islets seemed to release more insulin, which promoted a significant increase in sugar tolerance. With the same dosage of medicine and the same diet, the blood sugar level does not rise but drops in winter. Since January 2014, the blood sugar level will sometimes even drop below 5 moles. Facts have proved that the methods of replenishing qi and blood, replenishing body fluid, dispelling dampness and detoxification, and cleaning blood vessels are correct.

Keeping exercise is very important for diabetic patients. Although the body fluid produced by the pancreas is yin fluid, the pancreatic islets are lively and active, like a child, sitting for a long time, the pancreatic islets are prone to drowsiness, becoming lazy and passive. , Lose its due function. For 3 years, I walked every day for at least 5-6 days a week, and I walked for about an hour every day, all year round.

I started recording blood glucose test values in 2006. I opened the previous test results and compared the current test results. Now my blood sugar is regular. Even if the blood sugar level is higher than the warning line on a certain day, I can immediately know what caused it. It is possible that many sugar friends, like me, have gone through many twists and turns in the process of treating diabetes, from the earliest ignorance of diabetes to the expert in self-treatment of the disease. In fact, the process of self-treatment of diabetes is a blind person touching the elephant, learning and accumulating experience bit by bit, until we gradually establishes a set of best treatment plans for our disease.

As long as we take disease seriously and live in harmony with it, there is no fortress that cannot be conquered. Our body is like a child, what you feed, the body reflects back to you. Therefore, the daily diet is very important, scientific collocation, and 7 kinds of nutrients are balanced. When we talk to the body in a pleasant way, the body is relaxed and happy, and the spirit is full. When we exercise with our bodies, our bodies are happy, full of vigor, and our steps are light. When each of us can create such a human environment with our hearts, in a harmonious big family, what opinions will the internal organs make trouble with?

To be kind to the disease is to be kind to ourself, to our family, to the society, and to be kind to our own life.

In July 2013, due to staying up late at work and hurting my yin, my mouth began to become dry and cracked, water came out, and the corners of my mouth were so painful that it could not heal for a long time. Blood sugar is easy to rise during the period of July, August, and September with a little carelessness, and the blood sugar level is unstable. At the same time, I have used raw potatoes, carrots, and apples to squeeze the juice every morning for the past few months. Potatoes are very effective in curing the liver and also good for the pancreas. Because the body's various vitamins and minerals have been supplemented, the chapped lips have not improved for a long time. I believe this is not the deterioration of diabetes, but the potato juice is helping the pancreas to heal and heal itself.

Because potato juice contains a lot of starch, that is, it contains a lot of sugar, in order to reduce the blood sugar level to the normal range, I added half a pill, one pill a day, twice in the morning and evening. And began to drink white fungus soup, because white fungus is the best ingredient for yin, the pancreas should like it, and the sugar content of white fungus is lower than potato juice. Red dates have been eating, and the body will be vigorous only when there is sufficient blood.

The cracks in the corners of the mouth lasted for more than two months, and the cracks leaked water, and after drying, there were still crystalline grains. This was repeated many times, my lips were dry and cracked, and the corners of my mouth were open. I put some petroleum jelly on my lips to ease the pain of the cracks. According to the data, summer is the season for nourishing the spleen (pancreas). With the experience of nourishing the liver during the Spring, I am not at all panicked about the long-term cure of chapped lips. Instead, I prayed in my heart and silently blessed my pancreas to bravely challenge her disease.

Sure enough, in the autumn, the chapped lips healed unconsciously, the function of the pancreas was stronger than before, and the sugar tolerance was stronger than before. In the past few months, my lips have never been chapped. When I go to work, I am not sleepy anymore, my eyes are energetic, my legs are easy to walk, especially when I walk uphill, I don't feel strenuous at all.

Years of blood glucose records have proven that as long as we treat our bodies well, there will be good returns.

The treatment process of diabetes is a process in which each patient self-recognizes their body. Because everyone's physique is different and the cause of the disease is different, the treatment methods are also different. Doctors only follow conventional methods to treat, and do not have a thorough understanding of each patient's specific condition. Through the comparison of daily diet, exercise volume, climate, mood, sleep and other factors, we can record blood glucose test results on time, and treat our diseases with our heart, it is a positive way to promote the transformation of the disease to the better.

In recent years, through daily testing, I have found a lot of reasons for the rise and fall of blood sugar, and made adjustments in a timely manner.

For example, one day due to excessive eating during the day or too much sugar in the food caused blood sugar to rise, so adjust the food in time on the next day, eat less staple food, or eat less food with high sugar content, try to eat something containing foods with low sugar content.

For another example, if one day does not eat more foods with high sugar content during the day, the blood sugar is still high the next day. Why is this? And through several tests and comparisons, to find the cause of the increase in blood sugar.

1. Blood sugar fluctuations caused by eating too much meat.

2. Blood sugar fluctuations caused by insomnia.

3. Fluctuations in blood sugar caused by fatigue.

4. Bad mood can cause blood sugar fluctuations

5. Everyone has different reactions to different foods. For example, if someone eats cucumber, the blood sugar will not increase but decrease, but if I eat cucumber, the blood sugar will definitely increase. I have tried it many times.

6. Improper exercise can cause blood sugar fluctuations.

In short, through blood glucose monitoring, we have found some patterns, basically mastered the various states of our body in the comprehensive adjuvant treatment, and maintained the stability of blood sugar, thereby reducing and eliminating the occurrence of complications.

Chapter 8

DIABETIC HEALTH - CARE

The "Victoria Declaration" issued by the World Health Organization at the International Heart Health Conference held in Victoria, Canada in 1992: Health is golden. If a person loses his health, then everything he originally had and what he is creating will be zero!

The declaration stated: "The main problem at present is to build a healthy golden bridge between scientific evidence and the people, so that science can better serve the people. This healthy golden bridge has four cornerstones, they are: reasonable diet, moderate exercise, and quit smoking, limit alcohol, mental balance. These four cornerstones constitute a healthy lifestyle, which can reduce high blood pressure by 55%, stroke by 75%, diabetes by 50%, tumors by one-third, and average life expectancy by more than 10 years. And it doesn't cost much, the health method is very simple, and the effect is very good.

As the saying goes, one-third of the disease, seven of nourishment. Traditional Chinese medicine emphasizes health preservation, not only on the material to replenish qi and blood, but also on energy health preservation, that is, the strength of a person's energy determines the ability to heal diseases..

After the diabetic patients control the blood sugar to be stable, they mainly focus on health preservation to improve the function of the body and increase the strength of the energy field in the human body.

When the overall condition of the body is improved, with a strong physique, local problems will gradually heal themselves.

It is easy to maintain health, but it is often interfered with by some bad things, and the determination is not strong enough to control oneself. As the saying goes, habit becomes natural. Diabetics are the easiest to maintain health, why do I say that? Because diabetes is a strict inspector, if we are lazy, dereliction of duty, staying up late, gluttonous, overworked, etc, the diabetes inspector will immediately punish us, and the blood sugar level of the next day will be displayed immediately, reminding us to be vigilant. Take the initiative to correct their mistakes. Therefore, with the strict control of the diabetes inspector, diabetic patients must strictly observe good living habits if we want to maintain a stable blood sugar and restore a healthy body. Unless there is a sugar friend who doesn't cherish their own bodies and their own lives.

I have always been grateful for diabetes. If it weren't for diabetes, I still don't know how to protect my body, nor would I understand so much health knowledge. With diabetes by my side to supervise me, health care is a daily homework. I can't say that I am 100% consciously complying with the requirements of diabetes for patients, but I can comply with more than 95%, leaving only a little room for myself to be presumptuous. Hey, this is my little secret. It's not an exaggeration to satisfy your mouth for delicious taste occasionally. However, while relieving my greed, I will take hypoglycemic drugs to escort me and measure my blood sugar in time. In case the blood sugar level exceeds the standard, I will immediately adjust my diet and resolutely prevent high blood sugar from staying in the body for more than 24 hours.

I have always been grateful for diabetes. If it wasn't for diabetes, I still don't know how to protect my body, and I would not know so much health care knowledge. With diabetes by my side to supervise me, health care i s a necessary home work every day. Now I can't say that I am 100% consciously complying with the requirements of diabetes patients, but I can achieve more than 95% compliance, leaving only a little space for myself. Hey, this is my little secret, it's not an exaggeration to occasionally satisfy my mouth's need for deliciousness. However, I will take anti-diabetic drugs to protect my cravings, and measure blood sugar in time. If the blood sugar level exceeds the standard, I will immediately adjust the diet structure, and resolutely do not allow high blood sugar to stay in the body for more than 24 hours.

The Role of the Five Elements in the Body

Gold, wood, water, fire, and earth constitute all things in the universe. As long as the five elements are balanced in the universe, the weather will be smooth in nature, and all things will grow and coexist peacefully. The relationship between the five elements is that water produces wood, wood produces fire, fire produces soil, earth produces gold, and gold produces water. If the five elements are unbalanced, there will be accidents in nature, such as floods, droughts, hurricanes, mudslides, sandstorms, tsunamis, earthquakes and other natural disasters. The five elements have formed a restrictive relationship: water overpowers fire, fire overpowers gold, gold overpowers wood, wood overpowers soil, and earth overpowers water.

Both Chinese medicine and religion regard the human body as a microcosm of the natural universe, that is, everyone who has practiced knows the small universe of the human body. They believe that the structure of the human body is the same as that of the natural world. The five internal organs, lungs, liver, kidneys, heart, and spleen in the human body correspond to the gold, wood, water, fire, and soil in the natural world. The relationship between these five elements is the same as in the natural world. When the five elements in the human body are in balance, the five internal organs are healthy, the physique of the human being is strong, human immunity is strong. On the contrary, if the five elements in the human body lose their balance, the five internal organs will cause disease, human health will be harmed, and the human body's immunity will decline.

In Chinese medicine, the lung is gold, liver is wood, kidney is water, heart is fire, and spleen is soil.

The earth is the big thing, and the five internal organs and the spleen are the mother. The lung is the heaven of the five internal organs, the spleen is the mother of qi and blood, and the kidney is the root of life.

The spleen (pancreas) corresponds to the stomach. It is a relationship between an outer and inner husband and wife. If the spleen is not good, the stomach is not good, and if the stomach is not good, the spleen is not good.

Kidney belongs to water, spleen belongs to soil, and soil restrains water, that is, spleen soil can restrict kidney water. If spleen soil is normal, it can prevent kidney water from flooding.

Heart and lung: Heart governs blood, lung governs qi.

The heart governs the blood, and the small intestine is on the outside and inside, and the tongue is opened. The liver governs the tendons and the gallbladder, and opens the eyes to the eyes. The spleen controls the muscles, the limbs and the stomach are on the outside and inside, and it opens up to the mouth.

The lungs dominate the skin and fur, are in line with the large intestine, and open to the nose.

Liver and Kidney: Kidney stores essence and liver stores blood. Liver blood needs to be nourished by kidney essence and kidney essence needs constant replenishment of liver blood. The two are interdependent and breed each other.

Kidney and Lung: From the aspect of water and fluid metabolism, the meridian of the kidney is connected to the lung, and manages the three energizers. The three internal organs of the lung, spleen and kidney are closely related to the normal activities of water and fluid metabolism in the whole body. If one of the organs fails to function properly, it will cause water retention and edema.

Among the five internal organs, the spleen is the mother of hundreds of bones, therefore, strengthen the spleen and the soil, and the stomach will help. From 9:00 am to 11:00 am, it is the best time to nourish the spleen (pancreas). Gently massage the spleen and stomach and the corresponding acupuncture points to improve the digestive function of the spleen (pancreas) and stomach.

The color and five flavors of food correspond to the five elements like the zang-fu organs. Black enters the kidney, white enters the lung, green enters the liver, red enters the heart, and yellow enters the spleen. The five flavors are that the liver likes sour, the fire likes bitter, the spleen (pancreas) likes sweet, the lung likes spicy, and the kidney likes salty. However, the five flavors corresponding to these five viscera are not the more the better, but the moderation. Because the nutrients of the five-color foods are different, they learn from each other's strengths and complement each other, and provide the nutrients needed by the body in a balanced and sufficient manner. Foods of different colors have a relationship with the internal organs of the human body. After understanding the taste of the five internal organs, if we find problems, we can adjust them in time and supplement them.

The five internal organs in the body also correspond to the five sense organs. For example, the liver corresponds to the eyes. Generally, dry eyes are caused by insufficient blood in the liver. The heart corresponds to the tongue. Observing the tongue can reveal the degree of heartburn. The spleen (pancreas) is the mouth, and the health of the spleen can be understood from the saliva in the mouth and the degree of dry mouth. The lungs correspond to the nose, and respiratory diseases are generally lung problems. The kidney corresponds to the ear, and tinnitus is an obvious symptom of kidney deficiency.

The heart corresponds to joy, and the heart cannot be too happy and sad. As the saying goes, overexcitement can damage the heart. The spleen (pancreas) viscera corresponds to sorrow. People who are too worried can easily damage the spleen (pancreas). The lungs correspond to grief. Grief can easily lead to the accumulation of qi in the lungs, and the blocked qi cannot form normal breathing communication with the outside world, which damages the lung function. The kidneys correspond to terror, and excessive fright will damage the kidneys.

The Most Important Thing Is to Clear Blood Vessels, Remove Dampness, Detoxify and Lower Lipids

People with type 2 diabetes are basically high in blood lipids, and are accompanied by high blood pressure. The initial cause of the disease is basically high blood lipids in the body and acidity of the body, which leads to pancreatic islet fatigue and failure.

Nowadays, the treatment plan for diabetics is basically the same. Taking medicine, controlling diet, and exercising are all auxiliary to lower the glycemic index to meet the basic needs of the body. However, the toxic substances left in the human blood vessels have penetrated into the deep layers of the blood vessel wall, which is still a hidden danger of causing diabetic heart disease. Therefore, in a stable situation, insisting on cleaning the blood vessels in the body, removing dampness and detoxification, and minimizing the damage of toxic fat to the human body are the primary treatment tasks for our diabetic friends.

There are many ways to clean blood vessels, mainly food cleansing. If we get up in the morning, mix it with a little vinegar or baking soda and drink it in plain water. Eat vegetables and fungus food. Vegetables include onion, garlic, ginger, okra, burdock and so on. There are fungi, black fungus, seaweed, mushrooms and so on. These foods have to be changed every day, and the blood vessels will gradually change. When the blood vessels are unblocked, the elasticity is restored, and the blood flow increases, I will feel the changes in my body. For example, I feel that I am not so easily tired, my chest is no longer tight, and my heart does not have premature beats.

Replenishing blood is very important for clearing blood vessels. Only when there is sufficient fresh blood in the blood vessels can they have the ability to clean themselves. Actively maintain and clean up blood vessels' dirt, detoxify and remove dampness, and clear obstacles to the recovery of the pancreas.

Reactivating the islets is the fundamental task of improving diabetes. Taking medicine, controlling diet, and exercising all assist in lowering the blood glucose index to meet the needs of the body. Reactivating pancreatic islets is the ultimate goal pursued by diabetic patients. Dredging, clearing blood vessels, removing dampness and detoxification is to create good conditions for the recovery of pancreatic islet function.

Replenishing Qi and Blood is a Daily Task

Food is the easiest way to replenish qi and blood. We have to eat food every day to provide our body's needs, but our body is a very honest friend who can accept whatever we eat, without adulteration at all. If we eat high-fat fish chicken and duck meat all day, our body will definitely produce three highs, damage blood vessels and liver, and develop into many serious diseases. Therefore, we must treat our bodies well, let this friend who has been with us all our lives happy, energetic and loyal to its duties, and let the whole body function well.

Food is divided into attributes, and there are many natural blood-enriching foods around us. Eating these natural foods to replenish the qi and blood in our body is the best way of nourishing, without any harm to the five internal organs. As the saying goes, medicine tonic is not as good as food tonic. Pay attention to the proper nutrition in the daily diet, and increase the qi and blood food reasonably, which has a certain effect on improving the immune system of the body and assisting in the treatment of diabetes.

In general, beef, mutton, chicken, pork, pork liver, pig blood, red beans, glutinous rice, red dates, soybeans, crucian carp, carp, quail, rice eel, shrimp, mushrooms, black sesame seeds, walnut meat, longan meat, etc. Although the consumption of red dates and longan can quickly replenish qi and blood, due to the lack of insulin in the body of diabetic patients, in order to avoid fluctuations in blood sugar levels, we should be supplemented after the blood sugar level is stabilized, and not excessive.

I have not taken hypoglycemic drugs for several years. Since I started to replenish qi and blood in the past two years, I have eaten red dates every day. Red dates are sweet and the sugar content is not low. To be on the safe side, I started to take hypoglycemic drugs again. To keep blood sugar steady. I think that simply lowering blood sugar is not the goal, but the key is to increase the qi and blood to increase the immunity of the body.

Since replenishing qi and blood, my physique has strengthened day by day, I have gained weight, and my immune system has also become stronger.

Balanced Nutrition, Scientifically Matched

Water, protein, fat, carbohydrates, minerals, vitamins, cellulose are the seven major nutrients that maintain human survival. We need to diversify our diets so that we don't have nutritional imbalances due to partial eclipses. The diet I adopt is to supplement food according to the seven major nutrients that the human body needs. I don't have a partial eclipse and eat everything. However, there are main and secondary foods. Some foods can be eaten more, and some foods can be eaten less.

Take appropriate amounts of various vitamins and minerals to supplement the deficiencies in the body.

The seven major nutrients in my body are maintained as follows: Eight glasses of water a day to ensure adequate water supply in the body. Protein-one egg a day, a variety of high-quality beans every week. Fat - Eat moderate amounts of meat dishes, such as chicken, duck and fish, but control my intake. Carbohydrates-Basically mixed rice made from brown rice and rice for two meals a day. Minerals - Provided in water and various foods, supplemented with appropriate amounts. Vitamins -extracted from food, supplemented with appropriate amount. Fiber - Eat several different vegetables that contain fiber every day.

Nutritional Diversity

The nutrition required by the human body is diversified, which is why health care workers advocate a balanced diet. It is best to eat all kinds of food, and the diet should be diversified, so as to avoid partial eclipse, resulting in some kind of nutrient deficiency or insufficiency.

The whole process of human life is inseparable from nutrition, and the human body without nutrition will wither. Reasonable nutrition, for adults, can maintain the lasting vitality of life and delay the body's aging process. For diabetics, reasonable nutrition is a good foundation for curing their illness. With a reasonable supply of nutrients, the body can get sufficient energy to repair the damaged parts of the body and restore its normal functions.

I basically eat everything, not picky eaters. In addition to trying not to eat fried food, the favorite Sichuan hot pot is basically not eaten, and white sugar and brown sugar products are resolutely avoided. Adjust the diet structure according to the seven nutrients the human body needs. There are beans every week, rice is eaten every day, meat, fish, and shrimp are eaten in small amounts every day. The amount of vegetables is the champion on the dinner table. Eat more crude fiber, Eat porridge. In the case of ensuring a balanced diet, add some vitamins and minerals in moderation.

I basically eat whatever I want, and I don't have a limit, but I don't eat too much, because I have developed a habit that I will automatically stop eating when I'm seven or eighth full. Therefore, the stomach is rarely full. After getting up in the morning, drink a glass of warm water, exercise, and then eat breakfast. The lunch was eaten in two parts, and the dinner was once. Have some almonds and dried fruits in the evening.

Excessive Eating Hurts the Body

I watched a health program not long ago, and a teacher said that if you have a good appetite, eat more, you can increase the nutrition in the body. It seems that the more food you eat, the better, the body will be nourished and healthy. Is it true that the more food you eat, the better your body will be? From the perspective of health preservation, this view seems unscientific.

A healthy person does not need a lot of food every day. According to the dietary guidelines for Chinese residents, cereals should eat 250g-400g per day; vegetables and fruits should eat 300g-500g and 200g-400g per day; fish, poultry, meat, eggs, etc. Animal food, should eat 125g ~ 225g per day (fish and shrimp 75g ~ 100g, livestock and poultry meat 50g ~ 75g, eggs 25g ~ 50g);should eat milk and dairy products equivalent to 300g of fresh milk every day, and soybeans and their products equivalent to 30g to 50g of dry beans; cooking oil and salt, no more than 25g or 30g of cooking oil per day, and no more than 6g of salt.

In fact, the food that most of us eat every day exceeds the standards given by health care experts. Some people eat the same amount of food for a whole day in one meal, even more. Eating is a kind of enjoyment, especially the overwhelming feeling of eating in the mouth and tasting on the taste buds, it is really wonderful. The appetite is too good, which is not necessarily a good thing for our body. Exuberant appetite is an abnormal phenomenon. Like other desires, it can damage our body. Everything has an amount and a degree. If it exceeds this amount, it changes from a good thing to a bad thing.

Illness comes from the mouth. This is not false. The main source of diabetes is caused by eating, and the consequences of excessive meals. Most people can't control their mouths. It is a common problem that people love to eat. Some people around me said that if you want to limit your food, what's the point of being alive? It can be seen that a large part of the meaning of living is related to eating. I don't want to control my diet. It's better to eat whatever I want. But if I eat too much, my body can't bear it, and the blood sugar level rises, and it is me who suffers. In the early years of diabetes, my blood sugar level became unstable due to my inability to control my mouth and other reasons, and I quickly lost weight. Now as long as we follow the dietary guidelines to control our diet, we will gradually develop good eating habits.

Excessive food in the human body will overload various organs, just like a donkey pulling mill, the original physical energy can only pull 1000 laps, an additional 1, 000 laps, a total of 2, 000 laps of physical energy consumption, make the donkey feel very Tired, like this every day, the donkey will be exhausted all day, and eventually become exhausted because of exhaustion. When food enters the esophagus, the digestive system in the body starts to operate busy. The entire digestive system, intestines and stomach, pancreas, liver, and kidneys all participate, releasing hundreds of enzymes, even thousands of enzymes and coenzyme chemistry. Participate in the decomposition, absorption and transportation of elements. In the process of digesting food, all kinds of stored energy in the body will be consumed. A large amount of food will cause certain resources in the body to deplete, and people will inevitably get sick. It can be said that the people who destroy the internal resources of the human body are ourselves. For the health of the body, we must control our own mouths.

If everyone can follow the daily dietary standards per person in the Chinese Dietary Guidelines, I believe that more than half of diabetic patients can maintain a stable blood sugar level without taking medicine.

Moderate Exercise

Life lies in exercise, but exercise must be moderate, not all exercises are suitable for diabetic patients. Diabetes patients should choose appropriate exercise methods according to their actual conditions and develop good exercise habits.

People with diabetes must exercise according to their actual situation, and the amount of exercise is not the bigger the better. I have experienced that whenever I finish exercising, my whole body feels comfortable, relaxed, not fatigued, does not affect work and life, and I am in a good mood, and the blood sugar level will definitely decrease the next day. If after increasing the amount of exercise, the body feels tired, the calf feels sore and weak, and the blood sugar level will definitely rise the next day.

Once, I saw an introduction on the Internet that doing 300 squats can lower blood sugar levels, so I immediately learned to do 100 squats. At night, my legs are sore and weak, soaking my feet in hot water doesn't help, and doing qigong doesn't help either. The next day my blood sugar level rose, my legs felt very tired when I walked, I had no strength, and my calf was bulging. , without physical strength, I felt like I was sick, and my blood sugar level remained high for several days. Doing a new exercise should be done step by step, slowly increasing the amount of activity, and suddenly increasing the more difficult exercise, which will cause knee joint and thigh injury, consume physical energy, and disrupt blood sugar metabolism.

It seems that excessive exercise is not only not helpful to the body, but it is easy to deprive the body of oxygen, resulting in a decline in immunity. After receiving the lesson, the exercise methods I choose from now on are more suitable for me, and I won't make myself very tired.

The exercise that suits me for a long time is walking. I walk about an hour a day on average, and the effect is pretty good. Everyone has an exercise that suits their own body. As long as they can achieve physical exercise and enhance their physical fitness, there is no need to imitate others. Walking is also aerobic exercise, and I can walk with my arms and take a deep breath. I can also practice looking around with both eyes, and I can exercise my whole body. Also, I like to do simple qi gong. It works well to stretch my arms and stretch my muscles when I'm tired.

Appropriate exercise can increase the oxygen in the body and enhance one's physical fitness and endurance. People with diabetes must exercise, but do not choose intense exercise, which will cause excessive physical energy consumption, excessive sweating and cause hypoglycemia. Gentle and moderate exercise is necessary for diabetics, and it is also a good way to assist in the treatment of diabetes.

Congee and Soup Good for Nourishing Stomach and Enriching Blood

Chinese people pay attention to food culture, the word food, drinking is the first, followed by food. Our ancestors are telling us that to nourish our body, we must first drink as the main ingredient. Drinking is drinking water, drinking soup, and drinking porridge.

Drinking soup is also a good way to nourish the stomach and blood. Drinking nutritious soup to nourish the stomach and nourish the body is a direct and convenient benefit to the body, which is conducive to the digestion of the intestines and stomach. The nutrients in the soup will be directly absorbed and converted into nutrients needed by the body. Bone soup, ribs soup, beef soup, fish soup, mutton soup, chicken soup, etc are the best sources of high protein, vitamins and minerals.

Soup is a good way to tonic. Drink some soup before meals to lubricate the mouth and esophagus, which can prevent dry and hard food from irritating the mucous membrane of the digestive tract, facilitate the dilution and stirring of food, and promote digestion and absorption. At the same time, it can also increase satiety and reduce food intake. Drinking soup after a meal will dilute the chyme that has been well mixed with the digestive juice, which will affect the digestion and absorption of food.

Through the test, drinking soup does not affect the fluctuation of blood sugar level at all, because drinking soup can reduce the consumption of meals, but it is helpful to control blood sugar level.

At the same time, the nutrients in the soup can be quickly absorbed directly by the stomach, and the warm soup except for nutrients it can also warm the stomach and nourish the stomach, which is deeply loved by the stomach. Every time after drinking the hot soup, I feel my stomach feels very comfortable and my whole body is warm, and my head sweats slightly. The soup should be light and not too oily.

Boil fresh fish head soup, fresh fish soup, beef soup, and chicken soup basically without seasonings, only a little salt and ginger, the original soup has the original flavor. The substances that nourish qi and blood are all melted into the soup, which has a good tonic effect. Drinking soup can better absorb the nutrients in food. Therefore, drinking more soup can increase nutrition in the body.

Eating red dates, citron, yam, and barley porridge are good blood-enriching foods. I have tried to increase the consumption of porridge without taking medicine, which will affect blood sugar fluctuations. Every time I eat porridge, blood sugar will definitely increase the next day, and even exceed the normal value of blood sugar most of the time. This is because the body increases the absorption of blood sugar, which is an increase in nutrients. Therefore, when I eat porridge that nourishes qi and blood, I must take half a sugar-lowering tablet to keep my blood sugar level stable.

Diabetics with weak gastrointestinal function, poor absorption, dry skin, and insufficient body fluid should drink porridge and soup. This is the most effective way to replenish qi and blood to moisturize the body while ensuring the stability of blood sugar level.

At first, I didn't dare to drink soup or porridge, thinking that it would increase blood sugar levels, so I controlled my diet and carbohydrates all the year round, and didn't dare to eat foods that replenish qi and blood. As a result, the body does not get adequate nutrition, lacks physical energy, and people are also listless and always feel very tired. Later, I started to drink porridge and soup, my nutrition increased, my physique changed, my weight also increased, and my complexion became rosy.

Quit Smoking and Limit Alcohol

Smoking is harmful to the human body without any benefit. It can cause chronic bronchitis, lung diseases, and increase the risk of heart disease and high blood pressure.

Appropriate drinking can promote blood circulation. Excessive consumption will be detrimental to the health of the five internal organs, affecting digestion and absorption and the metabolism of nutrients, as well as having a greater negative impact on the treatment and rehabilitation of various diseases.

I don't smoke or drink, so these two are not harmful to my body. However, friends with diabetes who smoke and drink, please cherish your body, drink less and quit smoking.

Points Enriching Blood

Massage acupuncture points can replenish qi and blood, which is a health care method that I have learned over the past ten years.

From the point of view of modern medicine, qi deficiency and blood deficiency are caused by insufficient biochemistry and operation of human energy. The spleen in Chinese medicine is responsible f or the biochemical qi and blood of the human body. Pishu acupoint is an acupoint on the bladder meridian of Foot Taiyang, where the spleen's essence is infused into the back, and is directly connected to the spleen. Therefore, stimulating the Pishu acupoint can quickly restore the spleen's qi and blood biochemical functions. Chinese medicine believes that the stomach meridian is the meridian with the most qi and blood. Stimulating the Zusanli point of the stomach meridian can stimulate the biochemistry and operation of qi and blood. There has always been a folk saying that "Often moxibustion at Zusanli is better than eating old hens", which shows how important Zusanli is to a strong body.

In addition to stimulating Pishu points and Zusanli, it strengthens the function of the spleen and stomach. I also used massage points such as Qihai, Xuehai, Taixi, and Taichong. Qihai and bloodhai, as the name implies, the qi hai is the sea of qi, and the bloodhai is the sea of blood. These two acupuncture points are very important for replenishing qi and blood and have an inescapable responsibility. Think about it, if the sea of qi and blood are sufficient, there is no need to worry about the qi and blood provided to the body.

Back bump method. The Pishu point is on the back, and it is impossible to massage it with our hands unless we have the help of a doctor. We can massage ourselves by using the back bumping method, and we can take care of the acupuncture points on the entire back.

Massage Qihai can be connected with massaging the entire abdomen, such as Shenjue, Guanyuan and other important acupoints. Massage once a day before going to bed and after waking up, each time the left and right hands are stretched and overlapped and massaged in a clockwise direction for two hundred times, and then the right and left hands are overlapped and massaged in a counterclockwise direction for two hundred times. Over the long term, it not only increases Qi, but also enhances the absorption of the small intestine and the excretion function of the large intestine.

The massage of other acupoints is the same as the previous one. Acupuncture point massage requires persistence. If we insist on it every day, we will see the effect after a period of time.

Going to Bed Early Is Important for Blood Sugar Stability

As the saying goes, work only after taking a break. After resting, the body has the opportunity to replenish nourishment and repair damaged parts.

Yin deficiency-night is the best time to replenish yin deficiency.

Sleep is very important for diabetic patients. The human liver's hematopoietic function can produce blood between 11 o'clock and 3 o'clock in the evening. Resting during this time period will promptly replenish a certain amount of blood to the body.

Strictly observe work and rest time. Do not stay up late, and ensure a normal sleep schedule. It is best to go to bed before 11 o'clock and no later than 12 o'clock. Night is the best time to nourish yin. According to the Book of Changes health regimen, the Liver Meridian is on duty from 1:00 to 3:00 when it is ugly. The liver needs to detoxify and make blood, all of which must be carried out at this time. Therefore, three in the middle of the night is also the time to sleep. It is best not to indulge in playing games and drinking alcohol during this time. People who are used to working and studying at night are all bad habits. At this time, the human body needs to rest, and our liver still has to work. Most people with liver disease are people who like to stay up late, because the liver needs to make blood in the middle of the night and clean up the toxins from the blood. If we don't give it a chance to repair and maintain health, the human body will inevitably get sick.

Diabetic patients are mostly deficient in Qi and blood. In order to have sufficient blood to maintain the virtuous circulation of the body, it is necessary to sleep in time when the liver is detoxifying and hematopoietic, so that the body has a good rest and replenishment process. There was a period of night shift, and I didn't go to bed until after 2:30 every day. In the morning, my body's biological clock woke me up naturally. Basically, I didn't get enough sleep every day. In this way, if the blood production is not enough in the long run, it is easy to lack qi and blood, which will bring unfavorable factors to the disease. Usually, when I don't get enough sleep at night, my blood sugar must be high the next day.

Take a hot bath before going to bed to help relieve fatigue, dredge the meridians and blood vessels, and improve the quality of sleep.

Before going to bed, keep a calm state of mind, abandon distracting thoughts, and enter a state of rest.

Maintain normal calcium in the body. Lack of calcium can also affect sleep.

Eat less dinner, but don't skip dinner. An empty stomach before going to bed can also cause insomnia.

Diabetics Should Pay Attention to the Combination of Work and Rest

Since I got diabetes, I get tired easily, and my face always looks very tired and can't lift the energy. A colleague of mine also suffers from diabetes. His mental state is the same as mine. He seems to be very tired and weak. I have observed other people with diabetes and they are also very prone to fatigue and poor energy.

As the saying goes: Overwork leads to illness, people are in a state of fatigue for a long time, the resistance will decline, and various diseases will come to the door. Nowadays, with the rapid development of economy, while people store wealth, they are also accumulating fatigue, damaging their health, and even overdrafting their own lives. So, cumulative fatigue equals chronic suicide.

Diabetes has poor body constitution and is prone to fatigue itself. In order to control blood sugar, some sugar friends consume low calories every day, and accordingly, it is difficult to obtain sufficient nutrients. in the body. Excessive dieting will aggravate the fatigue of diabetic patients. Therefore, diabetic patients should scientifically calculate the daily calories required according to their own specific conditions(including gender, age, weight, labor intensity, etc.), and formulate a reasonable diet treatment plan, so as to ensure the necessary nutritional supply, It does not increase the blood sugar excessively, causing a series of problems.

In fact, this ideal state is very difficult to achieve. Because any kind of food maintains its unique nutrients, such as fruits are generally rich in minerals and trace elements. However, diabetic patients can only eat fruits after their blood sugar is stable. Even if the blood sugar is stable, they still eat a very small amount of fruit selectively. This makes it difficult to get the unique nutrients in the fruit like normal people.

But even if it is difficult, it can still be done. Diabetics know their own body best, and as long as they have confidence, they can always find a solution. My approach is to first take medicine to lower the blood sugar level, stabilize the blood sugar level in the normal range, then increase the amount of food we eat.

If friends with diabetes want to maintain adequate physical strength and reduce the occurrence of fatigue, they must not be overworked, maintain a good rest, and ensure adequate sleep time. Having a high quality of sleep is very important for diabetics to stabilize blood sugar.

If I do not sleep well, my blood sugar level will definitely rise, so I try to maintain 7-8 hours of sleep a day.

Diabetics are best not to walk with weights. Because weight-bearing walking consumes a lot of oxygen and energy, rapid physical energy consumption and hypoxia are also an important cause of fatigue.

Diabetes patients should ensure adequate intake of nutrients. It is best to make the daily carbohydrates accounted for about 30-40%, protein accounted for about 15%, fat accounted for about 15%, vegetables and fruits accounted for about 30%-40%. Carbohydrates are an important source of increasing physical fitness. Diabetics must not give up carbohydrates in order to lower blood sugar levels, causing physical exhaustion.

Diabetes self-care is very important. Diabetics should learn to relax and learn to adjust. This is the key to self-care.

Anger Is the Biggest Stumbling Block to Health

Professor Irma, a physiologist at Stanford University in the United States, once made a very famous experiment. He collected the breath that people exhaled when they were angry, sad, and troubled, and then input them into a bottle of potion. The potion in this bottle the color will change, the qi in anger can turn the potion into purple, the qi in sorrow can turn into gray-white, and then the purple water will be pumped out and hit the mouse. The mouse will shrink and die within a few minutes. This clearly tells us that we are actually secreting toxins when we are angry and confront others.

According to Professor Elma's research, the energy consumed by a person for three minutes of anger is the same as the energy consumed after running three kilometers. Therefore, when a person gets angry, he becomes fatigued, and immediately after fatigue, his hands and feet become numb. Because fatigue consumes energy, peripheral circulation is not good, which will cause numbness in the hands and feet. Many of us have this experience. When we are angry, our hands and feet are cold, our face is blue, and our body keeps shaking. Why is this happening? Because of anger, qi and blood stagnate, and big anger damages the liver.

Anger can instantly change the normal working state of the human body, and it is very lethal. Anger is not only the creator of disease, but also a guide for cancer. People who are angry every day have their nerves tense, and the anger in their hearts dominates everything. Such people will soon send themselves to the final nursing home to be company with God. Even if you can't go to the holy place, the rest of the day will be like years. Not only is it painful, it also brings troubles and many inconveniences to the family and the people around you.

Life is often unsatisfactory, and few people are really not angry. The key is that some people are good at controlling their emotions, and some are good at relieving conflicts, thinking twice before acting. And some people know that anger is bad for their health, but they can't control their anger when it's critical. If we want to have a good mood, we must learn to be good at controlling our emotions and maintain a peaceful mind.

There are nothing more than two types of anger. One is external factors. For example, the main reason for our anger in life is that we like to punish ourselves for other people's mistakes, which is not worth it. The other is internal factors, anger is to compete with oneself, to be angry with oneself, it is a bad gas generated from one's heart.

My experience is that if I want to vent my anger, I'd better shift my goal, think about other things, and try to dispel the anger in my heart. The biggest disadvantage of being angry is that it is not good for our body. If we are angry, others don't know, and even if they know, they won't replace us.

Someone has made a good analogy. If a perfect life is 100, then health is 1, wealth and money are the two 0s behind. The formula: 1 + 0 + 0 = 100, that is, health + wealth + success = 100. If the 1 at the front is tuned, that is to say there is no health, the two 0s at the back are nothing, because without health, wealth and success become worthless.

Think about it, without health, everything is lost. Is there any reason why we can't remove the stumbling block that hinders health, anger?

Psyche Health -Care

Mental health is also psychological health. From ancient times to the present, Chinese medical health experts have paid attention to "chi". It is brought about by the human body, and is the energy needed by the human spirit.

"Chi" is the energy required by the non-material body and the spirit, that is the energy required by the human spirit body. We heard such a legend, a child was crushed under the wheel, and a weak mother actually lifted the car with her weak arms. You must know that the weight of the car is dozens of times the weight of the mother, and she actually exploded super energy in an instant and lifted the car. It was the great mother's love that inspired the super energy in her body. There are also many cases of people bursting out with dozens of times more energy than they usually do. This super energy is the "Chi" hidden in the human body.

In the body's health maintenance, "Chi" is a kind of healing energy. If this energy can be stimulated, its effect is often more significant than that of any medicine. "Chi" belongs to the spirit body and needs to emerge and erupt in a peaceful state of mind and a high-level spirit. Meditation, qigong all stimulate the potential energy in the body. Diabetics cultivate this potential, relying on an indifferent heart. A person who can be indifferent and clear will be able to achieve peace and achieve far without being happy with things. Don't feel sorry for yourself. With health, you can add any zeros after health. Without health, no matter how many zeros there are, there is nothing. So, with health, there is everything.

When the body reaches a tranquil state of mind, the body's autoimmune ability, self-repair ability and self-healing ability are in the best state, so as to exert the best performance, so that the internal organs of the body reach a harmonious and peaceful state. Yin and Yang balance, the virtuous cycle takes over the main body, the body's disease begins to retreat, and the white flag surrenders. This principle is what Chinese medicine says, the heart governs the spirit. The mind governs the body. Once the heart is calm, the mind will be balanced, and the physiology will be balanced. Diseases will not occur, and even if there is a disease, it will quickly heal itself.

Spiritual health should learn to taste happiness. What is happiness? Different people have different definitions of happiness. Happiness is a feeling, a subjective feeling of a person, and a beautiful emotion that emerges from a person's heart. Many people are looking for happiness, and true happiness comes from our own hearts. Happiness is all around us, and only by learning to be content can we feel happiness. We must learn to taste the joy that various small things bring to us, and the little joys will make up our happy life.

Maintaining peace of mind is a good life attitude in life, and it is also a state of mind necessary for spiritual health.

Every morning I get up and smile at myself in the mirror. It is a happy smile, so I have a good mood from the morning.

Keeping the Body Warm Is a Prerequisite for Flowing Qi and Blood

Human body temperature is always maintained in a very narrow temperature range, if it exceeds 37 degrees 5 and falls below 36 degrees, it is considered to be sick. In cold weather we help our bodies gain and maintain a certain temperature by dressing more and eating warm and high-calorie foods. When the climate is hot, we eat cool foods and use air conditioners to regulate our body temperature.

It is very important for diabetics to keep the body warm. When the body is warmed, the qi and blood will run easily in the body. I am a person who is afraid of the cold, and I usually wear more clothes than others. When my body is warm, my hands and feet will not be cold anymore.

Both cold and hot weather will directly affect blood sugar fluctuations in the body. Weather changes can also affect the blood sugar stability of diabetes. The weather is hot and rainy, especially in the days before the climate change, I will feel it, and it will directly affect the fluctuation of blood sugar. For example, sometimes I can't fall asleep for no reason at night, and the climate changes on the second or third day. It changes to rain and snow, or the temperature drops and winds. The hot weather in summer affects sleep and feels irritable. If I do not sleep well, I will find the problem by measuring my blood sugar the next day.

In winter, the cold weather outside makes our blood vessels constrict. One year in January, the temperature here once dropped to minus 35 degrees, and the wind felt almost minus 40 degrees. I wore two sweaters that day, two woolen hats, an extra-long down coat, a pair of cotton pants, two pairs of gloves, and a long scarf wrapped around my face and mouth, leaving only one pair of eyes to see the way. I walked in the snow for 45 minutes, and I did hand exercises while walking to keep my hands from freezing. Since I came out of a warm room, my whole body was still warm, and my hands and feet were constantly moving. nor feel cold, when I got to work, my whole body was hot and sweaty. But it was different when I got off work at night, because I waited more than 10 minutes for the bus to arrive at the stop sign on the side of the road. The cold of the snow took away all the heat from my body, and my whole body became icy. This small experiment shows that wearing the same clothes, walking in the severe cold and standing still have a big difference in the supply and consumption of heat to the human body. Later, I tried my best not to walk outside in cold weather, because an excessively cold climate is not good for diabetics after all.

Eat hot food to keep the body warm, and eat ginger to speed up blood circulation. People with cold hands and feet generally have poor blood circulation. Eating more ginger will promote blood circulation and smooth blood. Ginger is best eaten in the morning and noon. The ancients have a saying that "Eating ginger in the morning is better than ginseng soup; eating ginger at night is better than arsenic". In the morning, the yang is raised, and ginger is eaten to strengthen the spleen and warm the stomach; in the evening, the yang is to be closed, and the yin qi is enriched outside, so you should eat more food that clears heat and lowers the qi and eliminates food, which is convenient for resting at night.

The lower limbs and feet of diabetic patients are prone to chills because of poor microvascular circulation. There are many acupuncture points on the feet of the human body, which are also the gathering places of various meridians. The lower limbs are cold and the blood circulation is not smooth, which also blocks the movement of the meridians. In addition to doing foot massage to promote blood circulation in the lower limbs, I wear knee pads all year round on my leg joints and wear leg covers on my calves to warm up my legs and feet. The lower limbs and feet are warmed, the blood circulation in the body is better, the meridians are unblocked, and the blood sugar level is easy to stabilize.

Stay Room and Avoid Heat Toxins in Summer

In the hot summer, try to avoid going out in the house as much as possible. It is hot outside by the high temperature of the sun. The cement road generates huge geothermal heat and enters our body through our feet, which produces a lot of internal heat and internal poisoning, which is very easy to cause blood sugar fluctuation.

After May, the climate in China starts to become very hot. There are many high-rise buildings in China's cities. Under the scorching sun, the cement and asphalt roads exude a huge enthusiasm, which can literally bake people. When I returned to China the year before, I often walked outside due to shopping and errands. Within two days, my gums swelled up, and many blisters appeared on the soles of my feet. The body absorbed a lot of heat poison from the ground through the soles of my feet. Since there are cement roads everywhere, the toxic substances in the human body cannot find a vent through which the earth and gas can communicate, and the toxic gas has to be excreted from the human body. If you are in a large area of land, people are between heaven and earth, and they are connected to each other, and the meridians of the human body can reduce the damage to the body through soil detoxification.

The highest summer climate in Canada is only 20 degrees, which lasts for about two weeks. However, due to the strong ultraviolet rays in the air, the sun shines on the body hot, and the shade and the sun have very different temperatures. Therefore, you should wear a hat or use an umbrella to shade your body when you go out to avoid direct sunlight. which may lead to the accumulation of heat poison.

In the Canadian summer, the highest temperature is less than 30 degrees, and the time lasts for about three weeks. However, due to the strong ultraviolet rays in the air, the sun shines hot on the body, and the shade and the sun have completely different temperatures. Therefore, we should wear a hat or an umbrella to shade our body when we go out. We can avoid direct sunlight, causing heat toxin accumulation in the body.

In summer, diabetic patients tend to accumulate heat toxins in our bodies and need to drink some tea for clearing fire and detoxification frequently.

The Best Way to Nourish the Spleen and Stomach

1. Avoid Uncooked and Cold Food

Chinese medicine believes that the spleen (pancreas) and stomach are both the biochemical sources of qi and blood, which means that the qi and blood of the human body is transformed from food by the spleen (pancreas) and stomach, so the spleen (pancreas) and stomach are the foundation of the acquired.

The pancreas and stomach are organs that like warmth. To nourish the pancreas and stomach, we must first respect the characteristics of the pancreas and stomach, and provide warm food. Often eating cold food, the elasticity and softness of the stomach become worse and worse, and finally the stomach becomes rigid and inelastic, which cannot provide good nourishment for the whole body. The pancreas cannot get enough nutrients from the stomach, and the function gradually declines, and the disease begins.

In the early days of the illness, I didn't know how to take care of my body. The newspaper said that eating bitter gourd could lower blood sugar, so I brewed bitter gourd tea every day. After drinking it for a long time, the blood sugar dropped, but the digestion ability of the stomach seems to be getting worse and worse, often it seems that something is blocked in the stomach, there is always hot air coming out of the mouth. So I thought it was stomach heat, I tried desperately to drink bitter gourd tea to reduce the fire, and took Sanhuang Jiedu Pills. The symptoms were not getting better, and the smell in my mouth was not good. Later, after reading the health care book " It is better to seek medical treatment than to seek oneself ", I realized that bitter gourd tea is not something that everyone can drink casually. People with a cold constitution like me drink bitter gourd tea and the body becomes colder and colder, which makes the body not only unable to repair itself Instead, it entered a vicious cycle. Since then, I never drink bitter gourd tea.

There are reports that eating raw vegetables is more nutritious than fried dishes. A lot of nutrients in cooked dishes are lost, and eating raw vegetables can absorb more nutrients. So, I started to eat raw vegetables, such as tomatoes, parsley, large peppers, lettuce, broccoli and other dishes. At first I felt that the taste was good. After a few days, the stomach began to resist, and the lettuce that was eaten messed up in the stomach. , So that the stomach begins to feel uncomfortable, swollen, and tight. Therefore, I quickly stopped eating lettuce to increase nutrition. After all, it is not a herbivore. People still need the help of fire. Eating cooked food is the most basic way of eating that humans have maintained for thousands of years.

My physique requires the best to eat cooked food and eat hot food. There may be many diabetic patients like me, and they will do experiments on themselves immediately after hearing about health care knowledge, regardless of whether it is beneficial to their condition and body. Therefore, we cannot hear any information and adopt it without analysis, but should deal with it according to our own physique and illness.

However, sugar friends with good stomachs, it is another matter. Eating raw vegetables and fruits in moderation can increase the activity of enzymes and increase vitamins

Eating cold food is not good for the heart. It is reported that someone ate iced watermelon after heart surgery and died. It was because the stomach and the heart were very close. The iced watermelon caused the blood vessels of the heart to suddenly cool and stop flowing. It is not only the food that heart disease is most afraid of, but also diabetic patients should avoid eating cold food to avoid clogging of blood vessels in the body due to the cold, which will cause new troubles in the process of curing diabetes.

2. Avoid Cold Water or Juice

Drinking raw cold vegetable juice and fruit juice is popular on the Internet, saying that it is great for the body, so I blindly imitated it. After getting up early, I used a juicer to mix various fruits and vegetables together to make the juice, and drank it on an empty stomach. A large glass of ice-cold juice water. It is very comfortable to drink cold water in the hot summer weather.

However, cold water is not good for people with weak spleen and stomach, it will only stimulate the stomach, because people with weak spleen and stomach have insufficient blood supply and belong to a cold constitution. Drinking cold water and eating cold rice is equivalent to adding cold to cold. The healing didn't do any good, it went in the opposite direction, and as a result, my stomach started to feel sick again. With the lesson of drinking bitter gourd tea, I immediately stopped drinking cold fruit juice, The fruit taken out of the refrigerator is soaked in hot water before eating, or in the morning, an apple or other fruit is cut into several pieces and eaten in hot milk. Slowly, my stomach does not feel uncomfortable. Now, my face is starting to brighten up. I firmly believe that the stomach is slowly regaining its elasticity, and it is again fulfilling its duties earnestly and providing sufficient essential nutrients to the spleen.

Some time ago, it was popular on the Internet to mix potatoes, carrots, and apples into juice. It is said to be able to prevent and treat many diseases. Because of the previous lesson of drinking fruit juice in the morning, I did not immediately follow suit, because my physique is not suitable for drinking cold juice. For me, drinking a glass of plain water after getting up in the morning is the best way to thin blood. However, potatoes have obvious anti-swelling and anti-inflammatory effects. Even if I drink potato juice, I will add hot water to it, so that I don't make my stomach feel cold when I drink it.

Avoid or Minimize Fried and Hard Food

Fried food is crispy and fragrant. Not only Asians love fried food, but also almost every nation in the world has its own preference for fried food. The famous foreign fast food KFC sells French fries and chicken nuggets, with branches all over the world. The deep-fried foods Chinese people like include deep-fried dough sticks, fried spring rolls, fried glutinous rice cakes, fried stinky tofu and so on. During the Chinese New Year, each family will have fried meatballs, which symbolizes reunion. When I was a child, my mother often fried all kinds of small snacks for us to eat, such as twists and sweet noodles. Fried food is really fragrant and tempting.

Long-term consumption of fried food by adults is not only detrimental to health, but also causes cardiovascular disease, and even cancer in severe cases. First of all, oil repeatedly frying food at high temperature produces a lot of carcinogens, and these carcinogens enter our body through the fried food we think is delicious. Secondly, fried food is very difficult to digest, especially for people with poor gastrointestinal function, it is best not to eat fried food. Third, fried foods are high in calories, and frequent consumption will cause high blood lipids, high blood pressure and high blood sugar.

Our human stomach is soft and like soft and easy-to-digest foods. Eating hard food will harm the function of the stomach. Diabetes patients have poor pancreas and stomach function, and more attention should be paid to protection. Hard foods are not easy to digest, bring weight-bearing burden to the stomach, and easily damage the gastric mucosa. I have this experience. If I eat beef that is not digestible, my stomach will feel uncomfortable and even hurt. So now I cook meat, which is basically boiled and rotten, easy to eat, and easy to digest and absorb by the stomach. I used to like to eat meat, but now I control the amount of meat I eat every day, a little at a time, so that my nutrition is taken care of and my stomach can easily accept it.

Avoid Sweet Food

Sweets are the nemesis of diabetes, which is the food that every diabetic suffers from. However, the delicacy of sweets in life is too tempting for one's appetite. Every time I pass by the pastry shop, the creamy coconut sweetness exudes from all kinds of pastries floating on the face. I couldn't stop drooling from the corners of my mouth. I used to like to eat cakes, chocolates, cookies, egg rolls, ice cream, glutinous rice wine, hi, so many sweets are my favorites.

Not eating sweets is a very painful thing, especially when people around us are eating sweet desserts that exude appetizing milk, coconut, chocolate and other sweet desserts, it is true for me who loves sweets. Is a very painful thing. There is nothing more cruel than restricting the food you love. But, who calls me a diabetic? Why did I not know how to cherish my body before? Since our body does not allow us to eat sugar, we must restrain ourselves in order to restore our health.

Many sweets are made of white sugar and honey. After eating, blood sugar will rise straight. Diabetic patients lack insulin and cannot adjust sugar automatically. This is very certain. There is a pastry reception at the company meeting, and my colleagues usually bring some homemade desserts to share. Every time I encounter this situation, I keep swallowing and try to restrain my desire to eat desserts. Colleagues also sympathized and understood my situation. After a long time, everyone knew that I was a diabetic, so they took the initiative not to let me taste desserts. Under the control of self-discipline, I myself have become accustomed to watching other people eat sweet pastries without being tempted.

Over the years, I have strictly restricted white sugar, brown sugar, and chocolate. Don't eat at all. Don't drink sugary drinks at all, basically avoid eating sweet cakes, just occasionally eat a small piece of cake that is not too sweet, only a few times a year in total.

Basically, the dishes in the restaurant are filled with sugar, because the dishes are more delicious when they are fried with sugar, especially the meat dishes. I try not to buy dishes sold in restaurants. If I eat with colleagues or friends in restaurants, I can take half a tablet of hypoglycemic drugs in advance to prevent blood sugar from rising.

Diabetics should strictly limit the intake of white sugar, brown sugar, honey, jam, desserts, chocolate, sugary drinks and sweet juices, because most of these foods contain more glucose, sucrose, and higher calories, which will be obvious after absorption raise blood sugar.

Most nut foods are also high in calories, such as peanuts, melon seeds, walnuts, almonds, etc. Each 100 grams contains about 40-50 grams of fat. Regular consumption of blood lipids will increase, which will affect the fluctuation of blood sugar level, so it must be strictly control intake. I am a snack lover, and I want to eat snacks and grind my teeth when I am free. This is a habit that has been cultivated for many years, and it is also a problem of women's love of snacking. Since I got diabetes, all pastries and sweets have been declined, and even fruits are not eaten as I want. In desperation, I had to choose dried fruits such as peanuts, melon seeds, walnuts and almonds. I know that these dried fruits have a high heat content, but I can't stop being greedy. I have to control the amount and interval of food every day, and keep exercising to consume calories in the body and prevent the accumulation of fat from forming potential vascular problems.

Learn Food Exchange Algorithm

If you can't resist the deliciousness of sweets, you can eat a little bit to satisfy the taste. Generally, eating a small piece of cake and reducing the staple food will not affect too much blood sugar fluctuation. Unless I eat very sweet chocolate cake, I must take medicine to remedy it.

Although diet control is the basic treatment of diabetes, diabetic patients are not not allowed to eat sweets at all, but should be decided according to the calories of the food. If you eat pastries, reduce the amount of rice accordingly. The sugar content of carbon compounds in rice is generally very high, and the sugar content in 100 grams of rice is 60-70%, which is why it is necessary to control the diet. If you eat cakes that are not too sweet, you can reach the original stable blood sugar level by reducing the amount of rice consumed accordingly without increasing the amount of medicine.

Knowing the sugar content per hundred grams of various foods can help us better grasp our daily diet and freely control the conversion between various foods, not only can we control the sugar in food well. We can also eat a small amount of our favorite sweets.

Maintaining a Good Mood and Reducing Stress Are the Internal Motivation to Treat Diabetes

Modern life is stressful, people are running around and working hard every day, and their mental state cannot always relax well. The spirit and mood of diabetic patients are very important. Poor spirit and mood will directly affect the fluctuation of blood sugar in the body.

Keep a normal heart. The temptation of material to people is too great. There is an old Chinese saying that people die for money, and birds die for food. From birth, modern people are faced with a long-term struggle process. This process was initially designated by their parents and then made by themselves. In order to achieve better results in a highly competitive society, people's nerves have been tense, struggle, struggle, work hard, and work hard.

Of course, if a person does not have the spirit of struggle, nothing can be accomplished. However, the goal of hard work is far from one's own ability, and it is impossible to achieve it. It is necessary to revise the goal to meet one's own ability and achieve the goal through hard work. In spite of difficulties and mental pressure, we must not be pessimistic emotionally. Optimism is the driving force for success.

All kinds of pressure are not easy for normal people to step through, and for diabetic patients, it is a big mountain pressing on the top of their heads. After all, most of it is material temptation.

We are born naked, and we are naked when we go. In fact, people's needs for life are very low. We can survive if we have enough food, dress well, and have a place to live. More material enjoyment is to be seen by others, and it is all about vanity. People's comparison psychology is more than self-needs. If people can maintain a normal mind, then they will not live very tired, at least not mentally tired. After the mental pressure is relieved, the body will really relax and the occurrence of diseases will be reduced.

When illness comes, pessimism is useless, pain is useless, and an indifferent attitude cannot solve the problem. Only by facing positively, optimistically, reducing stress, and maintaining a good mental state are the internal driving forces for the treatment of diabetes and the key to curing diabetes.

Don't compare everything, do what you can. Maintain an optimistic and cheerful attitude towards life. Tolerance replaces complaining, generosity replaces retaliation.

Learn to balance the mind quickly-transfer method, dispersion method. When we diabetics encounter problems and cannot avoid them, we are stressed and depressed. We must quickly find a way to resolve them. That's how I am. When I feel down or encounter something unpleasant, I will feel chest tightness and I can't be interested in anything. I know that this situation is very detrimental to my condition, so I try to find ways to transfer the low mood, such as reading books, watching TV dramas, and walking outside. As soon as my thoughts shifted to other things, my emotions shifted, and my heart soon calmed down and my worries were forgotten.

In addition, do not concentrate on doing a mental task for a long time. Diabetes patients have poor autonomic control, too concentrated, and the brain is too nervous, which will also cause psychological stress and cause insomnia. Break down the main things or work, do some every day, and do some other things at the same time, so that there will be no neurological disorders.

Overcome Obsessive-Compulsive Disorder

Modern people are more or less obsessive-compulsive. Some things can obviously be done slowly, but must be done immediately. Some things can be done in batches, but must be done all at once. Some things are beyond your power, even if you are desperate to do it. And so on, forcing yourself, adding pressure to yourself. Those who are light, the mental burden will increase, the physical strength will be exhausted, and they will also suffer from mood disorders and physical diseases. In severe cases, life-threatening.

I used to go to the supermarket after get off work, and I always had to buy two large bags of various vegetables and other food, even the rice was carried back on my shoulder. Obviously knowing that walking home with such a heavy load for half an hour will make me very tired, but the psychological obsessive-compulsive disorder is causing me to force myself to do superpowers. I usually take things at home. I used to hold one or two cups in one hand, but I want to hold 4 or 5 cups in one hand. I ran two trips to get things, but I solved it in one trip. At work, I also move very fast, as if I can't slow down. With many such things, I let myself into an involuntary self-obsessive-compulsive state.

For a period of time, the brain will involuntarily repeat a certain musical interlude or a certain lyric, or go out a few steps and come back to see if the switch of the electric stove is turned off. The filled-in form was put in an envelope, so I reopened it again for fear of being left behind, and so on. This situation lasted for a while. I knew that there was a problem with the control of the nervous system. Obsessive-compulsive disorder is also a diabetic neurological complication.

First of all, I slow down my movement frequency, work rhythm, do not force myself to do overloaded things, let my brain relax. Secondly, taking vitamin B1 can increase the self-regulation ability of the nervous system. Slowly, the singing in my brain disappeared, and I no longer cared whether the door was locked and double-checked the filled form.

Diabetes patients should try our best to maintain stability, slow down, overcome anxiety and irritability, and calm down, and the internal functions of the body will be stabilized, so that blood sugar fluctuations can be well controlled.

Keep Eight Glasses of Drinking Water Every Day to Keep the Cell Tissue Fresh and Full

When it comes to drinking water, some diabetics are a little taboo, because the symptoms of diabetes are more than three and one less, and one of them is drinking more water. Therefore, some diabetics try not to drink water as much as possible, which seems to be reduced by more than one. In fact, it is not the case. Pathological drinking more water and normal drinking water are two different things. We cannot greatly reduce the amount of drinking water or not drink because of the symptoms of drinking too much water. It is precisely because of lack of water in the body and insufficient body fluid that diabetic patients will feel thirsty, and it is necessary to ensure sufficient water supply in the body.

From the perspective of human weight, most of the human body is made of water. Water accounts for 70% of the human body's weight, and the baby's body contains 80% of water. The water content in human blood accounts for 83%, water accounts for 76% in muscles, 80% in the heart and lungs, 83% in the kidneys, 68% in the liver, and 75% in the brain. Even the bones that appear to be strong have more than 20% water.

Water is the first element of human life. It is the first of the seven nutrients (water, protein, fat, carbohydrates, minerals, vitamins, fiber) of the human body. Water nourishes every cell wall and fills every cell. Without water, any part of the human body cannot survive. It can be said that the credit of water in the human body is irreplaceable.

Water is circulated and flowing. We drink about one and a half liters of water every day. Another liter of water is obtained from the food we eat. The human body needs 2. 5 liters of water every day to maintain normal metabolism and eliminate it. Urine is about 1. 5 liters, another liter of water evaporates from sweat and breath, and a small amount of water participates in the excretion of feces.

The metabolic wastes in the body are mainly processed by the liver and kidneys. The kidneys are most importantly responsible for mediating the balance of water and electrolytes in the body, metabolizing wastes generated by physiological activities, and excreting them in the urine. However, when it performs these functions, it needs enough water to assist.

High blood sugar increases the viscosity of the blood. Thick blood means that the tissues are deprived of oxygen, which leads to an increased rate of glucolysis and excess lactate production. This lactate is returned to the liver and kidneys for resynthesis into glucose. Such a vicious circle is extremely detrimental to the liver and kidneys, and also affects the aggravation of diabetes.

Water not only dilutes the viscosity of blood, but also brings a lot of oxygen.

Solution: Develop the habit of drinking plenty of water to dilute the urine and allow the urine to be discharged quickly, which not only prevents stones, but also helps to lighten the urine when taking too much salt, thereby protecting the kidneys. Some people use beverages instead of water. This method is wrong. The beverages contain a lot of chemical components and sugars, which are extremely detrimental to the recovery of diabetes.

Water assists and excretes waste from the body. The human body produces about 11 liters of water every day, of which the salivary glands supply 1 liter to moisten the mouth and activate the digestive system. The stomach produces 1. 5 liters of digestive juice, and the pancreas, liver, and intestines produce about 5 liters of water. All of this fluid flows through the small intestine, and if not reabsorbed, eventually reaches the large intestine, where it is excreted in feces used to make semi-solids, or back into the body through the intestinal wall.

Water can radiate heat and regulate body temperature. Chemical activities are carried out everywhere in the human body, and the heat generated by muscle activity when we are engaged in physical work or sports is enough to burn us. However, the water that infiltrates and penetrates the cell tissue can immediately absorb the excess heat generated in the body.

Water lubricates and protects joints, it also lubricates eyes and protects skin smoothness and full of elasticity.

The water in the human body is constantly circulated and exchanged between various organs and various systems. In a day, up to 200 liters of water is filtered out of the blood vessels and sent back into the blood by the kidneys. We usually say that blood is the most important liquid, however, water that flows, lubricates, clears heat, dissolves various substances and carries the various molecules that nourish us, is the real liquid that life depends on.

When the human body loses 10% of body weight, dehydration occurs, oliguria occurs, the heartbeat increases, and blood pressure drops. When water loss accounts for 15-20% of body weight, it will be life-threatening.

How important is water for the human body to maintain life, how can the body lack water? Sugar friends must drink eight glasses of water a day, and don't pretend to think that controlling drinking less or not drinking water is controlling diabetes.

Since insisting on drinking eight glasses of water every day, the cells in the body are nourished by sufficient water, urination is normal, and the blood viscosity is greatly reduced. In the past, every time I measured blood sugar, I squeezed hard for a long time before a little blood came out. Now, as long as the needle is pierced, the blood will come out immediately from the eye of the needle. Also, the most noticeable change is that my skin is more radiant than before.

Eat a Light Diet and Eat Less Salt to Reduce the Burden on the Kidneys

Everyone knows that eating too much salt can cause high blood pressure, but we just can't control our mouth in our daily life. In the past few decades, I used to eat heavy flavors. I put a lot of salt in my stir-fry. I like to eat Sichuan hot pot, which is spicy and flavorful. It always feels that salty food is easier to eat than light food, and it tastes good, and we can eat more. Unknowingly, all kinds of super-salty foods entered my body every day, slowly causing vascular diseases, such as high blood pressure, high blood lipids, and high blood sugar.

In order to control blood sugar, not only to control high-fat, high-protein intake, but also to control salt intake. Be sure to get into the habit of eating bland food. Eat a small amount of salt every day, mainly light dishes, and the taste will become light after a long time.

Eating less salt directly reduces the burden on the kidneys. The kidneys are the innate nature of humans and the organs for human beings to store sperm. They are very important organs for human life. When the kidney function is strong, the kidney's detoxification ability will be strong, and then the liver will be strong. When the liver is strong, the heart will be strong. A strong monarch can speed up the recovery of diabetes.

Salt is an important culprit that increases the burden on the kidneys. 95% of the salt in the diet is metabolized by the kidneys. Too much intake will increase the burden on the kidneys. In addition, the sodium in the salt will make the body water difficult to excrete, which will further increase the burden on the kidneys, resulting in decreased kidney function.

The scientific daily salt intake should be controlled within 6 grams, of which 3 grams can be obtained directly from daily food. Therefore, it is best to keep the food within 3 to 5 grams when seasoning.

Don't Overeat High-Protein Foods

Protein is one of the indispensable nutrients for the human body, but excessive consumption of protein will burden the liver and spleen. Excessive consumption of protein is a source of toxins in the body.

Excessive protein is not only a source of toxins, but also disrupts the osmotic balance of cells. Osmotic balance refers to the balance of fluid pressure inside and outside the cell membrane. When the balance is disturbed, water enters the cell, in addition to trying to restore the balance, it will also dilute the excess protein in the cell. Dilution is a physiological response to cope with excess substances in cells, just like drinking water will dilute the blood. Although adding water can restore the osmotic balance, it can also cause edema. Therefore, it is not advisable to eat excessive high-protein foods to replace carbohydrates, and it is easy to cause edema in our body.

In order to metabolize protein and deal with acidic waste, the body must consume a lot of energy and time. When processing carbohydrates, the body's metabolic rate increases by an average of 4%. However, within one hour of eating a lot of protein, the metabolic rate increases by 30%. To make matters worse, this situation may last as long as 3 to 12 hours. The faster the rate of metabolism, the faster the production of energy, which will eventually lead to a large amount of depletion of resources in the body, exhaustion of the functions of the internal organs and gradual loss of their functions.

Although protein can produce energy, in order to digest protein, the body must consume more energy and deal with the acidic substances left by protein. In other words, protein is negative energy, and the energy it creates is less than the energy consumed. The long-term high-protein and low-carbohydrate diet is extremely harmful to the human body. Therefore, adopting a diet with high protein and low carbon compounds is not a good way to control blood sugar.

Detoxification of the Body in Time Is very Important

Almost everyone has toxins in their bodies more or less, and these toxins seriously affect our health. There are two kinds of toxins, divided into exogenous toxins and endotoxins.

Exotic toxins such as: air pollution, pesticide residues in vegetables, automobile exhaust, industrial exhaust gas, chemicals, radiation, preservatives in food, excessive heavy metals in cosmetics, junk food and other toxic side effects brought about by modern civilization, pathogenic microorganisms.

Endogenous poison: the metabolic waste produced in the metabolism, the body will produce a kind of acid poison when angry, the toxins produced by the intestinal feces and sugar fat, protein metabolism disorder. Stool, turbid air, turbid water.

What are the sources of toxins around us?

Side effects caused by drugs, contamination of the food chain, agricultural products (residual pesticides), fish and animal husbandry products (hormones), processed foods (preservatives, pigments, additives, etc.).

There is also the pollution of drinking water, paper mills, chemical plants, mining, etc. Air pollution, cars, dust explosions, thermal power plants, etc.

If these toxins cannot be eliminated in time, they will directly interfere with the body's normal physiological activities and destroy the body's functions, causing great harm to our health. Detoxification should target different toxins and eat foods that clean up these toxins symptomatically. Detox foods must be eaten regularly, every day, in order to maintain a relatively clean environment in the body.

There are many ways to detox, drinking water to detox, exercise sweating to detox, soaking feet to detox, morning and evening abdominal massage to help detox, eat some detox foods, such as apples, kelp, black fungus, mung beans, bitter gourd, pig blood and so on.

Eliminate Turbid Qi, Turbid Water, and Stool in the Body in Time

The turbid air, turbid water, and feces in the human body are very harmful to human health.

Turbid water is the dampness in our body, that is, moisture. People who always spit, because there is too much water in the body. Turbid water is very harmful to the human body. If it rushes to the legs, it is edema. If it reaches the surface of the skin, it becomes eczema. If it runs into the blood, blood circulation is blocked, people are prone to get sleepy and cause cardiovascular and cerebrovascular diseases. If it reaches the head, it will cause dizziness. There are many causes of moisture in the body. (See the chapter 4 on removing dampness and detoxification)When there is turbid water in our body, it will be exposed through various phenomena, such as effusion, edema, eczema, abscess, congestion, etc. Diabetes patients should pay more attention to timely detoxification to eliminate hidden dangers of complications.

Adding a turbidity to the qi word means that the qi has changed its taste, from normal qi to turbid qi. Muddy qi is a variation of qi, and it is a destructive and unclean gas. The normal qi controls the blood flow in the body, pushing the blood vessels to work at a normal speed. Once the turbidity is generated, it will hinder the normal circulation of blood, just like a blocked road or a slow-moving car.

Muddy gas, to put it bluntly, it is the fart we let out. If the turbid qi stays in the body and is not discharged in time, it will be very harmful to the body if it goes up and down. If the turbid air is blocked in the heart, people will feel that the chest is stuffy, and they will feel flustered. When they go to the head, they will feel dizzy. When they go to the stomach, they will feel bloating, stomachache, nausea and vomiting.

So how is turbidity formed? After reading the expert's explanation, I realized that it was mainly caused by turbid qi staying in the body caused by anger. It is impossible to say that a person is not angry in his life. Everyone will always be angry with some big and small due to various reasons, and if these anger cannot be resolved in the form of farts and hiccups in time, it will be held in the heart and turned into turbid air, piled up to form a very destructive killer

Some scientists do experiments, put an experimental stick under the nose of an angry man, and then put it in the snow and put it in the snow, and the color of the snow will turn black after a while. This shows that the toxins released by people when they are angry are very large and are lethal toxins. People often say, " angry to death", "angry to heartache". That is to say, people will be killed by anger, and when people are angry, their hearts will also suffer. Our human body suffers from a variety of diseases, many of which are caused by anger, suffocation, and accumulation of toxins for a long time. When the turbid qi blocks the pores, it will cause dermatitis and eczema, and when the spleen is deficient, diarrhea will occur.

In addition, we also bring in some gas in the process of eating, which becomes turbid gas after it is not eliminated in time in the body.

Same, the internal organs of the human body will also produce some turbidity during operation. Muddy qi in the human body is often excreted in the form of hiccups and farts.

The human intestine is 5 to 6 meters long, and has thousands of folds, with an average of one bend every 3. 5 cm. Many residual wastes remain in the folds of the intestinal tract and cannot be discharged. Over time, these food residues can accumulate up to about 6. 5 catties. They dry, spoil, ferment under the action of bacteria, and it sticks firmly to the intestinal wall like rust, forming black, foul-smelling, and toxic substances that are stool.

Chinese medicine believes that the toxins contained in stool are the source of all diseases. Western medicine also believes that the body's body fat, sugar, protein and other substances produced by the metabolism of waste products and food residues in the intestines are the main sources of toxins in the body. Two-thirds of the human stool is a variety of miscellaneous bacteria and pathogenic bacteria. If it cannot be excreted within 24 hours, it can multiply more than 2 trillion bacteria. In particular, a large amount of acidic metabolites accumulate in the stool, and the toxins produced by it are absorbed into the blood by the intestinal villi, which makes the body fluids acidify and the body becomes acidic. It can be seen that stool is extremely harmful to human health.

Bad breath: The stool is corrupted and fermented under the action of bacteria, and constantly produces odorous gas. These odorous gases go up and exhale through the oral cavity to form bad breath.

Toxins: 22 kinds of toxins can be produced in the stool. These toxins are absorbed by the intestines and reach various parts of the human body through blood circulation, resulting in dull complexion, rough skin, and dilated pores.

Constipation: Too much stool accumulates in the human body, which compresses the intestinal wall, leading to intestinal dysfunction, slow intestinal peristalsis, and disorder of the excretory system, resulting in habitual and intractable constipation.

The reasons for the formation of stool: too much sugar, too much food, indigestion. The fundamental reason is that the human body does not get enough dietary fiber from food to inhibit the absorption of sugar, accelerate the decomposition of food, promote intestinal peristalsis, and help digestion. In the absence of dietary fiber, the "green scavenger" in the intestines, food residues cannot be cleaned up at any time, and stools will naturally form over time. Therefore, cleaning up the stool should start with supplementing dietary fiber

Keep bowel movements clear. Drink eight glasses of water during the day, and keep the same amount of urine excreted. Defecate every morning without staying overnight. Do not underestimate stool and urine, because normal stool and urine in diabetic patients is one of the signs that the body tends to be healthy.

Maintain the Balance of the Seven Nutrients in the Body

Food is the main source of our survival. People will feel hungry as long as they don't eat a meal. If we don't eat or drink for a few days, we will endanger our lives. Food not only provides our body with protein, fat, carbon compounds, dietary fiber and water, but also provides essential vitamins and minerals (including trace elements). Together, these are the seven nutrients that maintain our human life, provide energy, build body tissues, and regulate metabolism. Together, these seven nutrients are like a big family, with their own division of labor and the function of cooperating, all of which are indispensable. Once the balance is broken, the body will have problems, affecting the normal functioning of the body, and even serious diseases.

Although these 7 nutrients can be obtained in our daily diet, as time goes by, people slowly go from infancy to adolescence, to youth, to middle age, and to old age. Various external reasons have changed. The pure body of infancy has become impure over time, and the functions of the human body have gradually degraded. Our human body has begun to have a strong demand for vitamins, minerals, and trace elements. Especially for our diabetic patients, because the pancreatic islets lack minerals, the secretion of insulin is insufficient, and the lack of insulin regulation affects other parts of the body, resulting in the functional degradation of the entire body.

For example, the retina of diabetic patients is easily damaged, causing eye diseases such as dry eyes, glaucoma or blindness. In addition to taking medicine to lower blood sugar, adhere to exercise, scientific diet, but also take vitamin A to protect our eyes. Lack of vitamin A can also cause dry skin, scaling, goose bumps, easy colds, and poor body resistance.

For example, due to the erosion of diabetes, the body of our diabetic patients is more likely to accumulate free radicals and fats, which are extremely harmful to the formation of cardiovascular and cerebrovascular diseases and the five internal organs. This not only requires constant exercise, if we take vitamin B at the same time, it can effectively eliminate harmful substances in the body and increase the body's immunity, correct the body's fat metabolism disorder, and play a role in preventing and treating chronic complications of diabetes.

For example, people who work indoors all year round need to take vitamin D if they are less exposed to the sun. Merely taking calcium is not good, only the combination of calcium and vitamin D can have the best effect. Vitamin D also has the ability to fight cancer. For diabetics, it is not only necessary to increase vitamin D, but also to increase the minerals magnesium and zinc, both of which are part of the electrolytes in pancreatic islet cells.

For example, diabetics are afraid of body wounds. Some diabetics have to saw off a leg because the wounds on their legs or feet cannot heal for a long time. Vitamin C can prevent viral and bacterial infections, improve immunity, promote wound healing, and prevent infection. In addition, proper vitamin C supplementation can also effectively prevent colds, protect the liver, reduce fat accumulation in the liver, and improve liver function.

The guardian of vitality-vitamin B family. Vitamin B family is all coenzymes, and its important function is to participate in the metabolism of fat, sugar and protein in the body. The biggest obstacle for diabetic patients is the lack of insulin, poor glucose metabolism, and relatively weak fat metabolism and protein metabolism. Therefore, the vitamin B family is the best assistant for diabetics, because vitamin B is an indispensable substance for converting sugar, fat, and protein into calories.

We diabetics must maintain a balance of the 7 major nutrients and maintain a scientific proportion in the daily diet to meet the body's intake of protein, fat, carbohydrates, dietary fiber, water, minerals and vitamins, and supplement minerals and vitamins in appropriate amounts. Create a good material foundation for curing diseases.

Avoid Preservatives to Increase the Activity of Enzymes in the Body

Food preservatives are food additives that can prevent spoilage caused by microorganisms and extend the shelf life of food. It is also called antimicrobial agent because it has the function of preventing food poisoning caused by the reproduction of microorganisms. Preservatives restrict the activity of enzymes. Because if the food is not eaten in time, the activity of the enzymes contained in the food can easily cause food spoilage.

In the past, because there was no refrigerator to store food, people often went to the vegetable market every day to buy vegetables. What they bought was fresh vegetables and food. Later, with the refrigerator being able to store food, people went to the vegetable market and food store less and less, and the refrigerator became a cabinet for storing food. Modern people have a fast-paced life, and they often buy a lot of food, vegetables and meat at a time, in order to save time. Foods that can be preserved basically contain preservatives. Food preservatives and enzymes are a pair of contradictions. If food is not added preservatives, it is easy to spoil, but adding preservatives will inhibit the activity of enzymes and hinder the fine processing, meticulous classification and transportation of food by human chemical factories. Without enzyme activity, people are not only prone to indigestion, but also prone to metabolic diseases.

Therefore, we diabetics should try to eat fresh foods, generally fresh foods do not contain preservatives. When buying semi-finished or finished products, pay attention to the instructions on the label and choose foods with a short shelf life. Generally, the shorter the shelf life, the fewer preservatives in the food. There are also some foods that do not contain preservatives in accordance with the law, such as yogurt and milk. Natural foods such as beans, nuts, fruits and vegetables are also free of preservatives. Canned food, instant noodles and other processed foods that can be stored for a long time do not require preservatives. Only after manual processing, the moisture content is not low enough, and the processed food that needs to be stored at room temperature for a long time, it is possible to use preservatives, such as soy sauce, vinegar, sauces, pickles, jelly, preserved fruit, and certain some pastries, sweets, wet noodles, etc. Although the fresh-keeping wet noodles are sterilized and do not use preservatives, they can be kept for 10 months at room temperature. It is best that we buy the recently manufactured noodles when we buy them.

Try to choose fresh non-processed foods, avoid or eat less preserved products, such as sausages, bacon, cured fish, ham, canned food, pickles, etc. Because this kind of food contains nitrite, it is not good for the human body. If you must choose processed foods, try to choose products from big brands and choose products with fewer additives. I used to like to eat pickled products, because pickled products are appetizing, serve meals, and stimulate the appetite. Now I have changed my eating habits. I hardly eat bacon, sausages and other meats. Try to eat non-processed fresh or frozen meat, fish, chicken and other meats. If I want to eat side dishes, I also use fresh vegetables.

Generally speaking, I eat rice that I cook by myself, add very few seasonings to stir-fry, and do not buy processed foods from outside, so the chance of contact with preservatives is much smaller. Although there may be a bit of soy sauce and vinegar, after all, the amount used every day is small, and the preservative content is originally low, and the amount eaten is also very small, which will not cause major damage to the enzyme.

Eating fresh vegetables raw can keep the enzyme activity in the vegetables. If I eat raw vegetables, the stomach will be cold and difficult to digest. I use a mixture of fried dishes and cold dishes. Some dishes must be fried for easy absorption, so I will never eat them raw. Some dishes are suitable for cold dressing, taking into account the maintenance of fresh vegetable enzyme activity, without letting the stomach chill.

In short, keeping in good health is a daily homework. Doing a good job of this little thing will accumulate a good life habit. It can also be said that the purpose of health preservation is to cultivate good living habits.

Diabetics Can Live Beyond a Hundred Years

Speaking of Chen Lifu, people in the last century basically know that he is an important figure in the Chen family in the four major families of the Kuomintang period, "Jiang Song Kong Chen", and a politician of the Kuomintang; Mr. Chen Lifu has been in politics for most of his life. He has held various important positions such as Chiang Kai-shek's confidential secretary, Kuomintang secretary-general, education minister, and vice president of the Legislative Yuan. Mr. Chen Lifu also had a deep experience of raising chickens in the United States, and in his later years devoted himself to promoting the development of Chinese medicine.

Mr. Chen Lifu suffered from diabetes when he was 58 years old. He had undergone surgery for gallstones and bladder stones, as well as other diseases. He has gone through ups and downs in his life, right and wrong, but his body is healthy and long, and he can die of life, 103 years old. This is good news for the majority of diabetic patients. In other words, if we adhere to good living habits, we diabetic patients can live as long as normal people and live a hundred years.

Everyone who lives a long life must have its own way of health, and Mr. Chen Lifu's way of health is mainly to cultivate one's body and mind.

Health maintenance is to focus on physical exercise, keep exercising every day, and move our muscles and bones. The food we eat is mainly vegetarian, with meat and vegetables. Drink boiled water and insist on eating cooked food.

Nourishing the heart focuses on contentment and happiness, a clear heart and few desires, and not being moved by fame and fortune.

To cultivate one's body, one must move, but one's mind must be calm.

Chapter 9

The Nutrients Needed by the Human Body

The human body is a diverse family that requires many complex elements and nutrients to form, maintain and grow. These nutrients and minerals have different roles in the body, and each element has a different important mission to maintain life. These nutrients and minerals can be obtained from daily meals, and each food not only contains different nutrients and minerals, but also the content is quite different. Not a partial eclipse, not a picky eater, eating a variety of foods is the best way to balance nutrition, so that our body can get a full range of comprehensive nutrition.

Due to environmental factors, partial eclipse, self-immune system deficiency and many other factors, the nutrients and minerals in our body are insufficient, leading to discomfort and diseases of one kind or another. Especially for diabetic patients, due to lack of insulin, the gastrointestinal system cannot digest and absorb enough nutrients from food, which makes our weak body weaker, which seriously affects the therapeutic effect of diabetes. Therefore, to understand which important nutrients and minerals are involved in the human body, and which are the important elements that affect the glucose metabolism of diabetic patients, this is very beneficial to the auxiliary treatment of diabetes.

In the course of treatment, many diabetics have controlled their diet, exercise, and medication, but the effect is not very satisfactory after all, and complications have not been eliminated. Since I got diabetes , I have followed the guidance of the seven nutrients that the human body needs, balanced nutrition, drink plenty of water, a combination of meat and vegetables, and supplemented vitamins and minerals. Although I have diabetes for more than 20 years, there have been no complications. Blood sugar levels are often kept within the normal range. This has a lot to do with my adherence to the combination of meat and vegetables, a balanced diet, and taking a variety of vitamins and some minerals. These good eating habits have allowed my body to gradually return to a normal life track, and these small vitamins and minerals, it also plays an important role in the process of curing diabetes.

Every living cell is a life energy manufacturing plant. Each cell must have sufficient raw materials so that it can produce new cells and store a large amount of energy according to the needs of the body. Therefore, if vitamins and minerals have been digested by certain enzymes, cells will immediately manufacture them and supply them in time. If the body lacks vitamins and minerals, or lacks necessary enzymes, the cells will decline and the body will begin to age.

A healthy body must have proper nutrition in order to maintain its optimal working condition. Diabetes sufferers due to lack of insulin, impaired glucose metabolism, lack of nutrients such as fresh blood, oxygen, vitamins and minerals in the cells of the body, resulting in poor maintenance of physical condition.

Dear diabetic friends, if the blood sugar lowering effect is not very good after taking the medicine, look for the reason and see if you can regulate your body according to the seven nutrients that the human body needs, and if the body lacks certain vitamins and minerals. Diabetes is a metabolic disease in Western medicine. There is a problem with hormones that regulate sugar metabolism. Vitamins and minerals are mainly used to regulate physiological functions. Therefore, supplementing vitamins and minerals is necessary for people with diabetes, and it is also an important auxiliary way to cure diabetes.

Seven Nutrients Needed by the Human Body

Water: about 55%-65% of human body weight.

Protein: The basic substance that constitutes the human body needs about 70 grams per day, accounting for 20%

Fat: Provides essential fatty acids for the human body. accounting for 15%

Carbohydrates (sugars): One of the substances that provide calories. Accounted for 2%

Vitamins: Participate in the body's metabolism. Accounted for 1%

Minerals: The human body needs to grow and maintain a certain acid-base balance. Accounted for 5%

Fiber: One of the basic factors for maintaining health. Accounted for 0%

Macronutrients: protein, fat and carbohydrates. Mainly provide energy and tissue repair.

Micronutrients: Vitamins and minerals, which mainly regulate physiological functions.

1. Water-the Source of Life

People cannot do without water. Water accounts for 55%-65% of our human body weight, even 70% of the human body. Water can't provide heat, nor can water repair body tissues. It won't produce fat, just increase weight. When a person loses weight, the water in the body is lost, and when a person gets fat, the water in the body increases. Or as the saying goes, look at this man, dry thin. No one said that this person is watery skinny. People who are thin must have dry skin. Old people who are thin are like dead branches, their skin is bronzed, and their faces and hands are prominent. These are all caused by the loss of water in the body. The body's water content decreases with age.

"Drinking" is composed of "food" and "owing", which means that water cannot be lacking in food. "Diet",   drinking is first, but now we talk about "food" every day, but ignore "drinking". Water not only quenches thirst, it is also a structural nutrient, a carrier and medium. Biological macromolecules such as amino acids, glucose and nucleic acid in organisms participate in the life and metabolism activities of organisms through hydration. In other words, the fluid of life is composed of "solute" as the core, but it is inseparable from sufficient "solvent". Water is not only for quenching thirst, but mainly for its nutritional value and health functions in the human body.

Diabetic patients lack body fluids and cannot lock water, which can easily cause the loss of water in the body. Therefore, we are prone to thirst, so diabetic patients lose weight. Guaranteeing 8 glasses of water a day is not only the cheapest detox and beauty agent, but it is especially important for diabetics to ensure adequate water for the cells in the body. Water makes cell tissues fully moisturized, increases activity, facilitates the entry of insulin into cells, reduces diabetes complications, and provides good conditions for the ultimate cure of diabetes.

The role of water is to transport nutrients, excrete waste, regulate body temperature, maintain the body's pH and so on. 6-8 glasses of water per day, 2500---3000ml.

2. Protein - Ultimate Source of Life

The composition of the human body: human body-system-organ-cell-protein-amino acid.

Protein is the material basis of life. Without protein, there is no life. Therefore, it is closely connected with life and various forms of life activities.

Protein accounts for about 20% of the human body and is used to make muscle, blood, and skin together. Every cell and all important parts of the body have proteins involved.

There are many types of proteins in the human body, with different properties and functions, but they are all composed of more than 20 amino acids in different proportions, and they are constantly metabolized and renewed in the body.

The eight essential amino acids in the human body are: valine, methionine, isoleucine, phenylalanine, leucine, tryptophan, threonine, and lysine. For babies, histidine is also an essential amino acid.

Except for urine and bile, which have no protein, the rest of the human body is composed of protein. Cells need protein as their framework, and organisms cannot survive without protein, so protein is the source of life, and almost all nutrients help protein use.

Human body-system-organ-cell-protein-amino acid. Protein is made up of amino acids. Among the 22 known amino acids, 9 of them are "essential amino acids" that the human body cannot make on their own and can only be obtained from the outside world. The protein needed by the human body must be converted into amino acids before it can be absorbed and utilized by the body.

Function of protein:

1. The main components of organs and blood. Constructs and repairs body tissues and provides amino acids needed for body metabolism.

2. Construct and strengthen bones and teeth. The main raw material for the production of hormones and enzymes.

3. Regulate the body's water and electrolyte balance. Manufactures antibodies against bacteria and viruses for the immune system.

4. Help wound blood coagulation and promote wound healing

People who lack protein:

1. Weak resistance and get sick easily. Anemia, lower blood pressure. Indigestion, loss of appetite, constipation.

2. Poor thinking ability, thinking is not consecutive.

3. Hair is withered and yellow, nails are fragile, muscles are loose, loss of elasticity, and edema.

Proteins and Antibodies

"Antibodies" and "white blood cells" are the substances in the body that can resist virus infection. These two substances are produced and maintained by protein.

The liver produces antibodies, and the function of antibodies is to transform various viruses into harmless substances. With adequate nutrition, the body will produce various antibodies to resist the invasion of germs.

When a person changes from low-protein food to high-protein food, the antibodies produced in the body will double within a week.

The toughness of blood vessel wall tissue is composed of collagen (elastin).

The amount of blood is constant, and blood pressure will remain normal when the blood vessel wall tissue is tough. When the blood vessels are weak and relaxed, the pressure of the blood decreases, the nutrients carrie in the blood penetrate into the muscle tissues, and the amount of cells also decreases, resulting in fatigue.

Protein and Digestion

Enough enzymes are needed for good digestion, which can enter the blood after converting food into water. Only when food is rich in protein, digestive enzymes such as the stomach, small intestine, and pancreas will produce digestive enzymes.

3. Carbohydrates Account for 2% of the Human Body

Carbohydrates, protein, and fat are the three basic substances in the biological world, providing the main energy for the growth, movement and reproduction of organisms. It is one of the important substances necessary for human survival and development.

Carbohydrates should be called sugars, and they are a large family in nature. Its source is pure sugar, such as maltose, honey, brown sugar, white sugar and grains.

Carbohydrates are composed of three elements: carbon, hydrogen and oxygen. Since they contain two to one ratio of hydrogen to oxygen, which is the same as water, they are called carbohydrates. It is the cheapest nutrient among the three main nutrients that provide heat to the human body.

Carbohydrates in food are divided into two categories:effective carbohydrates that can be absorbed and utilized by humans, such as monosaccharides, disaccharides, and polysaccharides, and invalid carbohydrates that cannot be digested by humans, such as cellulose, are essential substances for the human body. Carbohydrate compounds are the main source of energy required by all organisms to maintain life activities. It is not only a nutrient substance, but some also have special physiological activities. For example, heparin in the liver has anticoagulant effect, and the sugar in blood type is related to immune activity. In addition, the composition of nucleic acids also contains sugar compounds-ribose and deoxyribose. Therefore, carbohydrate compounds are of more important significance to medicine.

Nutritional Supply of Carbohydrates:

(1) Energy supply: 16 kJ (4 kcal) of heat is produced per gram of glucose, and carbohydrates ingested by the human body are digested into glucose or other monosaccharides to participate in the body's metabolism.

(2) Constituent cells and tissues: Each cell has carbohydrates with a content of 2%-10%, mainly in the form of glycolipids, glycoproteins and proteoglycans, distributed in the meninges, organelle membranes, cytoplasm and in the intercellular substance.

(3) Save protein: The carbohydrates in food are insufficient, and the body has to use protein to meet the energy required for body activities, which will affect the body's use of protein to synthesize new protein and tissue renewal. Therefore, it is not suitable to not eat the staple food at all and only eat meat, because meat contains very few

carbohydrates, so the body tissues will use protein to produce heat, which is not good for the body. Therefore, the minimum intake of carbohydrates for weight loss patients or diabetic patients should not be less than 150 grams of staple food.

(4) Maintain the normal function of brain cells. Glucose is an essential nutrient for maintaining the normal function of the brain. When the blood sugar concentration drops, the brain tissue can impair the function of brain cells due to lack of energy, causing dysfunction, dizziness, palpitations, cold sweats, and even coma.

(5) Anti-ketone body formation. When the human body lacks carbohydrates, it can break down lipids for energy and at the same time produce ketones. Ketone bodies cause hyperketoacidemia.

(6) Carbohydrate metabolism can produce glucuronic acid, which is combined with toxins in the body (such as the drug bilirubin) to detoxify.

(7) Strengthen intestinal function. Related to dietary fiber. Such as: prevention and treatment of constipation, prevention of colon and rectal cancer, prevention and treatment of hemorrhoids, etc.

(8) The glycoprotein and proteoglycan in carbohydrates have a lubricating effect. It can control the permeability of the thin meninges.

9. The Main Physiological Functions of Carbohydrates:

1. An important substance that constitutes the body.

2. Store and provide thermal energy.

3. The energy necessary to maintain brain function.

4. Regulate fat metabolism.

5. Provide dietary fiber.

6. Save protein.

7. Anti-ketogenic effect.

8. Detoxification.

9. Enhance intestinal function.

Lack of carbohydrates in the diet will lead to general weakness, fatigue, lower blood sugar levels, dizziness, palpitations, and brain dysfunction. In severe cases, it can cause hypoglycemia and coma.

When there are too many carbohydrates in the diet, it will be converted into fat and stored in the body, making people too obese and leading to various diseases such as hyperlipidemia and diabetes.

The main food sources of carbohydrates are: sugars. Cereals: such as rice, wheat, corn, barley, oats, sorghum, etc. Fruits: such as sugar cane, melon, watermelon, bananas, grapes, etc. Dried fruits, dried beans, root vegetables: such as carrots. Sweet potatoes and so on.

As the carbohydrate content of food is different, we should choose our diet carefully.

For simple carbohydrates, it is very important to drink milk and fruit juices and eat moderate amounts of fruit. But edible sugar and other sweeteners can provide a lot of unnecessary calories in the body, which is harmful to health.

For complex carbohydrates, avoid only low-fiber carbohydrates, starches (such as potatoes) and refined grains (such as white rice, macaroni and white bread). The carbohydrates in these foods are quickly converted into simple sugars by the body.

Instead, try to eat as much carbohydrates that contain a lot of fiber. Especially beans and whole-grain foods are beneficial to human health.

Classification of sugar

Simple sugar (simple sugar: fast absorption)-directly feel the sweetness. Such as: white sugar, ice cream, chocolate.

Polysaccharides (complex sugars: slow absorption) --- Starches: rice, noodles, steamed bread.

The operation process of carbohydrates in the digestive system of the body:

Oral-esophagus-stomach-duodenum-pancreas-small intestine absorption-sugar enters cells-excess kidneys are excreted

Excessive carbohydrates cause - kidney failure - excessive insulin secretion - diabetes。

4. Fat Makes up 15% of the Body

Fat is a triglyceride composed of glycerol and three fatty acids. Fat is an important nutrient and a basic component of food. Excessive intake of saturated fatty acids can easily induce cardiovascular and cerebrovascular diseases, obesity, high blood pressure, diabetes, etc.

Lipids include phospholipids, lecithin, cephalin, and inositol phospholipids.

Glycolipids: cerebrosides, gangliolipids.

Lipoprotein: chylomicrons, very low density lipoprotein, low density lipoprotein, high density lipoprotein.

Steroids: cholesterol, ergoinol, corticosterol, cholic acid, vitamin D, androgens, estrogen progesterone.

All cells contain phospholipids, which are structures in cell membranes and blood. The content is particularly high in the brain, nerves, and liver. Lecithin is one of the most abundant phospholipids in the diet and in the body.

Triglycerides are an important form of energy storage and oxidation for the body.

Liver, adipose tissue, and small intestine are important places for synthesizing triglycerides, and the liver has the strongest synthesis ability. However, liver cells can synthesize fat but cannot store it. After fat synthesis, it must be combined with apolipoprotein, cholesterol, etc to form very low-density lipoprotein, which is transported into the blood to extrahepatic tissues for storage or utilization. If the triglycerides synthesized by the liver cannot be trans-ported in time, fatty liver will be formed. Adipocytes are the body's warehouses for synthesizing and storing fat.

Triglycerides composed of fatty acids and glycerin are also called neutral fats. Animal oils (such as lard, tallow, lanolin, cream and cod liver oil, etc.) and vegetable oils (such as sesame oil, peanut oil, soybean oil, rape oil, etc.) are mixtures of various triglycerides.

Both carbohydrates and protein can be converted into fat in the body.

Carbohydrates can be converted into energy, fat can be converted into energy, the difference between the two: explosive energy and lasting energy.

Essential Fatty Acids

Linoleic acid (mainly derived from terrestrial plants): It is transformed into blood coagulation substances in the body, and if too much, it is prone to cardiovascular disease and certain cancers.

Alpha-linoleic acid (there are more algae in the sea): It is transformed into fish oil in the body to produce antiblood coagulation substances, which can strengthen the brain, and if too much, cause bleeding.

The Physiological Functions of Fat:

1. Supply the necessary heat energy to maintain life, maintain body temperature and store heat energy.

2. It is one of the important components of body cells. Phospholipids and sterols in fat are indispensable substances for forming new tissues, repairing old tissues, regulating metabolism, and synthesizing hormones.

3. Fat is a solvent for fat-soluble vitamins A, D, E, K, etc.

4. Provide essential fatty acids to the human body.

5. Most aromatic substances are fat-soluble, and fat helps to improve the aroma and taste of foods to increase appetite.

6. It can prolong the staying time of food in the digestive tract and facilitate the digestion and absorption of various nutrients.

Fatty Food Sources:

1. Vegetable oil: peanut oil, rapeseed oil, soybean oil, sunflower oil, safflower oil, linseed oil, olive oil, fish oil, etc.

2. Animal meat and offal.

3. All kinds of nuts: such as walnut kernels, almonds, peanut kernels, decaihua seed kernels, etc

4. All kinds of beans: such as soybeans, red beans, black beans, etc.

5. Some grains: such as corn, sorghum, rice, red beans, millet, etc.

The Nutritional Value of Fat:

1. Essential fatty acid content. The content of linoleic acid and linolenic acid in vegetable oil is relatively high, and its nutritional value is higher than that of animal fat.

2. The content of essential fatty acids. The content of linoleic acid and linolenic acid in vegetable oil is relatively high, and the nutritional value is higher than that of animal fat. 3. Fat-soluble vitamin content. Animal storage fat contains almost no vitamins, but liver is rich in vitamins A and D, and milk and egg fats are also rich in vitamins A and D. Vegetable oil is rich in vitamin E. These fat-soluble vitamins are necessary to maintain human health.

Although fat has many functions and effects, its content in the body is limited. Too much will affect the body's metabolic activities and cause many diseases.

Fatty liver refers to the pathological changes of excessive accumulation of fat in liver cells due to various reasons. Fatty liver disease is seriously threatening people's health, becoming the second largest liver disease after viral hepatitis, and has been recognized as a common cause of hidden cirrhosis. The total fat in the liver of a normal person, which accounts for about 5% of the liver weight, contains phospholipids, triglycerides, fatty acids, cholesterol and cholesterol lipids. In patients with fatty liver, the total fat content can reach 40%-50%, mainly triglycerides and fatty acids, while phospholipids, cholesterol and cholesterol lipids only slightly increase.

In fact, the human body does not only rely on fiber to break down food fat. The digestion process also relies on the help of digestive enzymes to a large extent. In particular, the role of lipase in this process cannot be ignored. To be precise, without lipase, the body will have difficulty digesting the fat components of food.

The fat is hydrolyzed into glycerol and fatty acids. Lipase helps break down fat and help cell repair and regeneration. Pancrelipase is a lipase secreted by the pancreas and can catalyze the hydrolysis of fat into glycerol and fatty acids.

There is also a lipase used in the hydrolysis process to help break down fat molecules in the pancreas. It is also called pancreatic lipase. Insufficient pancreatic lipase can cause digestive system disorders and pancreatic diseases. However, when the amount is sufficient, the rate of fat decomposition can be accelerated, and excess fat can be removed more easily.

Since lipase is consumed by the body when it works, it is often in short supply. One of the ways to ensure adequate lipase in the body is to use nutritional supplements. It is best to drink some nutritional supplements before each greasy meal. They can help the body produce extra lipase for a long time.

The human body contains more lipases in the pancreas and adipose tissue. The intestinal juice contains a small amount of lipase, which is used to supplement the lack of pancreatic lipase for fat digestion. The gastric juice contains a small amount of butyric acid glyceryl esterase. Various lipases in the human body control the processes of digestion, absorption, fat reconstruction and lipoprotein metabolism. Bacteria, fungi and yeast are more abundant in lipase.

Fatty Acid Classification:

Saturated fatty acid, most animal and vegetable oils contain excessively high saturated fatty acids. Compared with natural unsaturated fatty acids, excessive intake is more likely to cause cardiovascular diseases.

Unsaturated fatty acids:

Cis fatty acid

Most of the natural unsaturated fatty acids are in cis, which are more common in vegetable oils. Because it is easy to deteriorate under high temperature, improper storage is also easy to rancidity, and its properties are unstable. But it is less likely to cause cardiovascular disease in the human body.

monounsaturated fat

It is relatively stable and is also beneficial to the prevention of cardiovascular diseases.

polyu aturated fatty acid

Among them, omega-3 fatty acids are easily deficient in modern diets. Adequate intake of omega-3 fatty acids can protect blood vessels, reduce the risk of cardiovascular disease, diabetes, cancer, and infertility. It can also help brain development. Most people take fish oil supplements, DHA and EPA are omega-3 fatty acids. Plant-based sources of omega-3 fatty acids include linseed oil, perilla and seaweed oil.

trans fatty acid

Trans fatty acids are more likely to cause cardiovascular diseases and are very harmful to the human body. It has become a consensus that reducing artificial trans fats in food is beneficial to health. Therefore, many oil processing industries switch to production that does not produce or only produce a small amount of trans fat. Many countries have formulated regulations and require that the fat label in food must be marked with saturated fatty acids and trans fatty acids that are likely to cause cardiovascular diseases.

5. Vitamins Account for 1% of the Human Body

1. Vitamins are water-soluble and fat-soluble, water-soluble: B, C, P---bioflavonoids; fat-soluble: A, D, E, K.
    Vitamins participate in the body's metabolism. Water-soluble vitamins cannot stored in the human body and

are easily lost. They must be replenished daily. Too much body can be excreted with urine and sweat. Will not cause poisoning.

2.   B vitamins: B1, B2, B6, B12, niacin, folic acid, pantothenic acid,

3.   Food sources of B vitamins: pork, green leafy vegetables (not high in content). Liver, beans, whole grains, dairy products.

Vitamin B1

Vitamin B1 is also known as thiamine. Its main function is to participate in sugar metabolism in the form of coenzymes, which can inhibit the activity of cholinesterase and reduce the hydrolysis of acetylcholine.

It is mainly used for the prevention and treatment of vitamin B1 deficiency (beriberi), for the auxiliary treatment of polyneuritis, polio sequelae, pediatric enuresis and myocarditis, and to eliminate fatigue after exercise.

Function: required to maintain a normal nervous system. Carbohydrate metabolism and energy production. Increase energy and reduce fatigue.

Vitamin B1 can maintain the normal function of the heart and nervous system. Vitamin B1 can reduce vomiting, especially those caused by motion sickness, motion sickness or seasickness.

Insufficiency symptoms: fatigue, beriberi, gastrointestinal disease, severe constipation, irritability and emotional instability, irregular heartbeat, shortness of breath, constipation depression, forgetfulness, slowed metabolism, lowered blood pressure.

Source of Vitamin B1: It is widely found in cereals, beans, nuts, yeast, pork, and liver. 80% of vitamin B1 in cereals is found in the outer skin and germ.

Riboflavin (Vitamin B2)

Riboflavin is an important prosthetic component of many enzyme systems in the body and participates in material and energy metabolism. It is one of the 13 essential vitamins for the human body.

The role of riboflavin:

1. Promote development and cell regeneration.
2. Promote the normal growth of skin, nails and hair.
3. Help eliminate inflammation in the mouth, lips, and tongue.
4. Improve eyesight and reduce eye fatigue.
5. Interact with other substances to help the metabolism of carbohydrates, fats, and proteins.

The new health benefits of riboflavin:

1. Diuresis to reduce swelling.
2. Prevent and treat tumors.
3. Reduce the occurrence of cardiovascular and cerebrovascular diseases.

Physiological Functions of Riboflavin

1. Participating in the metabolism of carbohydrates, protein, nucleic acid and fat can improve the body's utilization of protein and promote growth and development.
2. Participate in cell growth and metabolism, which is an essential nutrient for body tissue metabolism and repair.
3. Strengthen liver function and regulate the secretion of adrenaline.
4. Protect the function of skin, hair follicle, mucous membrane and sebaceous glands.

Deficiency symptoms: oral ulcers, angular cheilitis (rotten corners of the mouth), causing mucosal lesions.

1. Eye fatigue, discomfort, redness and swelling, photophobia.
2. Oily skin, prone to long face and acne.

3. Anemia affects development. Prone to hair loss and baldness.

4. Loss of libido, frigidity.

Foods rich in vitamin B2 include: lean meat, dairy products, animal liver and kidney, egg yolk, eel, carrots, mushrooms, seaweed, celery, cabbage, cauliflower, spinach, apple, citrus.

Niacin (Vitamin B3)

Niacin, also known as niacin, is an anti-mangie factor. It is one of the 13 essential vitamins for the human body. It is a water-soluble vitamin and belongs to the vitamin B family.

Niacin is produced mainly in the liver. Niacin is converted into nicotinamide in the human body. Niacinamide is a component of Coenzyme I and Coenzyme II, and participates in lipid metabolism in the body, the oxidation process of tissue respiration, and the process of anaerobic decomposition of sugars. Niacin is an important substance essential for the metabolism of protein, fat and carbohydrates in the body into usable energy.

Niacin plays a key role in the chemical processing of fat in the body. Fatty fatty acids usually require the presence of niacin in the structure of the body (such as cell membranes)to promote their synthesis. Like many fat hormones, steroid hormones, niacin is needed.

The cell genetic material of the human body is composed of deoxyribonucleic acid - DNA, whose production requires the participation of niacin. Niacin, like other complex B vitamins, is directly related to DNA damage defects. The special relationship between niacin and DNA damage can make niacin have the effect of preventing cancer.

Niacin can affect and regulate the function of the blood sugar hormone insulin. It has been proven many times to be an important substance for insulin metabolism and blood sugar regulation.

Niacin promotes the health of the digestive system and reduces gastrointestinal disorders, makes the skin healthier, prevents and relieves severe migraine, promotes blood circulation and lowers blood pressure; reduces diarrhea.

Niacin is one of the few vitamins that are relatively stable in food. Even after cooking and storage, it will not lose a lot and affect its effectiveness.

Deficiency symptoms: (leprosy) pellagra, dermatitis, diarrhea, dementia, glossitis, oropharynx, diarrhea and irritability, insomnia and paresthesia.

Niacin is widely found in animal and plant foods. The best source is animal food. The most abundant are liver, kidney, lean meat, and some fish and poultry eggs also contain niacin. In addition, plant foods such as yeast powder, whole grains, wheat germ, beans and nuts are also rich in niacin.

Pantothenic Acid (Vitamin B5)

Vitamin b5 is white powder, odorless, slightly bitter in taste, hygroscopic, and its aqueous solution shows neutral or weak alkaline reaction. It is one of the 13 essential vitamins for the human body. It is a water-soluble B vitamin. It is widely distributed in animals and plants, hence the name pantothenic acid.

The effect of vitamin B5 on the human body:

1. Manufacture and renew body tissues to help wound healing.

2. Produce antibodies, fight infectious diseases, prevent fatigue, and help fight stress.

3. Alleviate the side effects and toxins of various antibiotics and relieve nausea.

4. It plays an important role in maintaining the health of hair, skin and blood. When the hair lacks luster or becomes thinner, supplementing with pantothenic acid can be effective.

Deficiency Symptoms:

1. Fatigue, tiredness, headache, vomiting, back pain, weight loss.

2. Loss of appetite, glossitis, achlorhydria, symmetrical

dermatitis, neurological symptoms.

3. Easily cause blood and skin abnormalities, resulting in hypoglycemia.

4. Severe skin inflammation, diarrhea, and dementia appear at the end of lypiosis.

People who need vitamin B5:

1. People who often feel tingling in their feet need pantothenic acid.

2. Using pantothenic acid can provide resistance to upcoming tensions and existing tensions.

3. People with allergies, arthritis, antibiotics and women taking contraceptives should pay attention to supplementing pantothenic acid

Pantothenic acid is water-soluble, and excessive amounts are excreted in the urine. Overdose should not occur.

Foods rich in pantothenic acid (vitamin B5) include: meat, unrefined cereal products, malt and bran, animal kidney and heart, green leafy vegetables, brewer's yeast, nuts, chicken, unrefined molasses. Beef, beef heart, lamb heart, pork, pork heart, dried shrimp, turtle, mackerel, dried whitebait, chicken, lamb, tahini, peanuts, fried sunflower seeds, fresh mushrooms, seaweed, dried chili, sorghum rice, fried dough sticks ect.

Vitamin B6

Vitamin B6 is also called pyridoxine. It is a water-soluble vitamin, colorless crystal, easily soluble in water and ethanol, stable in acid solution, easy to be destroyed in lye, easy to damage when exposed to light or alkali, and not resistant to high temperature.

Vitamin B6 is the main coenzyme in glucose and lipid metabolism. Vitamin B6 deficiency is often accompanied by impaired glucose tolerance and impaired secretion of insulin and glucagon.

Vitamin B6 is a component of certain coenzymes in the human body and participates in a variety of metabolic reactions, especially closely related to amino acid metabolism.

Vitamin B6 is more abundant in yeast, liver, grains, meat, fish, eggs, beans and peanuts.

Vitamin B6 deficiency can cause:

Arteriosclerosis, baldness, high cholesterol, cystitis, greasy face, hypoglycemia, mental disorders, muscle disorders, neurological disorders, vomiting in early pregnancy, sensitivity to sunlight, etc.

Foods rich in vitamin B6: meat foods such as beef, chicken, fish and animal offal. Whole grain foods such as oats, wheat bran, malt, etc. Beans such as peas, soybeans, etc. Nuts such as peanuts, walnuts, etc. The highest vitamin B6 content is white meat (such as chicken and fish).

Biotin-Vitamin B7

Biotin is an indispensable coenzyme in the human body. Its properties are very stable and not easily damaged.

Where biotin acts on the body: hair, nails, skin, muscles.

The role of biotin also includes helping diabetic patients control blood sugar levels and preventing nerve damage caused by the disease.

Functions of Vitamin B7:

1. Cell growth.
2. The production of fatty acids.
3. Metabolism of protein, fat and carbohydrates.
4. Utilization of vitamin B family.

Deficiency symptoms: depression, dry skin, fatigue, gray skin, insomnia, pale muscles, loss of appetite.

Rich sources of vitamin B7: wheat, animal liver, nuts and soybeans.

Vitamin B12

Vitamin B12 is also called cobalamin. Vitamin B12 in nature is synthesized by microorganisms. Higher animals and plants cannot produce vitamin B12.

Vitamin B12 is the only vitamin that needs the help of intestinal secretions (endogenous factors) to be absorbed. Some people lack this endogenous factor due to gastrointestinal abnormalities, even if the source of the diet is sufficient, they will suffer from pernicious anemia.

There is basically no vitamin B12 in plant foods. It stays in the intestines for a long time, about three hours (most water-soluble vitamins only take a few seconds) to be absorbed.

Vitamin B12 participates in the production of bone marrow red blood cells, which makes the body's hematopoietic function in a normal state, prevents pernicious anemia, and prevents damage to the brain nerves. Vitamin B12 exists in the form of coenzyme, which can increase the utilization of folic acid and promote the metabolism of carbohydrates, fats and proteins. Vitamin B12 has the effect of activating amino acids and promoting the biosynthesis of nucleic acids, and can promote the synthesis of proteins. It plays an important role in the growth and development of infants and young children.

Vitamin B12 is an indispensable vitamin for the healthy function of the nervous system and participates in the formation of a lipoprotein in the nervous tissue. The lack of vitamin B12 can cause degeneration of the spinal cord, degeneration of nerves and peripheral nerves, and inflammation of the mucous membranes of the tongue, mouth, and digestive tract. Vitamin B12 deficiency is related to diabetic neuropathy, and vitamin B12 has been widely used in the treatment of diabetic neuropathy.

The main food sources of vitamin B12: Beef liver, beef kidney, pig liver, pig kidney, pig heart, beef, herring, shrimp, egg, lobster, flounder, crab, stinky tofu, tempeh, yellow sauce, soy sauce.

Folic Acid Vitamin B11

Folic acid function: participate in the production of red blood cells and hemoglobin together with vitamin C, prevent anemia, protect the liver and detoxify, provide energy to the body, improve immunity, and help depression and anxiety.

If folic acid is supplemented with vitamin C, minerals, and vitamin B12, the effect will be better. Studies by the Centers for Disease Control in the United States have shown that folic acid can reduce the incidence of cardiovascular disease. Together with vitamin B12, it can treat arthritis, strengthen the muscles of the hands and wrists, reduce pain and stiffness, and reduce the dosage of analgesics and anti-inflammatory drugs.

Deficiency: Macrocell anemia, cheilitis (such as painful and red tongue), apathy, fatigue, gray hair, insomnia, dizziness, shortness of breath, forgetfulness, paranoia, gastrointestinal dysfunction.

Food sources: egg yolk, green vegetables, milk, liver.

Choline

One of the B vitamins is a lipophilic vitamin (emulsifiable fat). It is an essential nutrient for humans and an important component of cell membranes. It is widely found in various foods.

Choline and inositol (another B vitamin) work together to utilize fat and cholesterol.

Choline is one of the few substances that can cross the "brain blood vessel barrier". This "barrier" protects the brain from changes in daily diet. But choline can enter brain cells through this "barrier" to produce chemicals that help memory. Choline is considered to aid in the development and memory of the human brain. Choline seems to emulsify cholesterol and prevent it from accumulating in arterial walls or gallbladder.

The effect of choline:

1. Helps transmit signals that stimulate nerves, especially the signals sent to the brain for the formation of memory.

2. Prevent the decline of old memory and help treat Alzheimer's disease (take 1~5g per day).

3. Because it has the effect of promoting liver function, it can help the body's tissues to eliminate toxins and drugs.

4. It has a calming effect and controls the accumulation of cholesterol. Helps treat Alzheimer's disease.
Adults should contain 500 to 900 mg of choline in their daily diet.

Symptoms of Choline Deficiency:

It may cause liver cirrhosis, liver fat degeneration, arteriosclerosis, and may also be the cause of Alzheimer's disease.

Food sources of choline:

Eggs, animal brain, animal heart and liver, green leafy vegetables, brewer's yeast, malt, soy lecithin.

Vitamin C

1. Vitamin C is a natural water-soluble antioxidant. It has the functions of scavenging free radicals, protecting endothelial cells, and preventing diabetes with neurological and vascular diseases.

2. Vitamin C helps the formation of collagen. The vitamin C level of diabetic patients is lower than 40-50% of normal people.

3. Vitamin C can reduce the content of sorbitol in the kidneys and nerve cells of diabetic patients, increase inositol, restore Na+-K+ATPase activity, remove free radicals, prevent capillary basement membrane lipid peroxidation, and protect the activity of superoxide dismutase and Notric Oxide, protect the endothelium, and prevent the formation of atherosclerosis.

4. Vitamin C can also improve diabetic carotid endothelial function and reduce cell apoptosis induced by high glucose.

5. Vitamin C promotes the absorption of calcium and iron, helps hematopoiesis, and bioflavonoids can help vitamin C exert greater efficacy.

The characteristics of vitamin C -- water-soluble, can not be stored, afraid of high temperature (above 60 degrees), afraid of oxygen, the color of the white vitamin C after oxidation will turn yellow.

Symptoms of vitamin C deficiency: easy bruising (black-green). Brushing your teeth will bleed easily, and your enamel and dentin will become weaker. The resistance to infectious diseases is weak and it is easy to catch colds. Wounds are not easy to heal, and fracture recovery is slow. Inflexible mobility, arthritis, rheumatism. Scurvy, low blood pressure. Uneven skin tone and lack of elasticity in muscles. Fatigue easily (under stress).

Calcium is an important component in the formation of human bones and teeth. Without vitamin C, calcium cannot function. For those who are sick to take medicine, the daily intake should not be less than 500 mg. Vitamin C can enhance the power of the medicine and reduce the toxicity.

Sources of Vitamin C: Fresh green vegetables and fruits，and vitamin C supplements

Vitamin A

Maintain normal vision, prevent night blindness and vision loss.

Strengthen the function of mucosal tissues, such as throat, sinuses, middle ear, lung, kidney, bladder and genitals where mucosal secretion is normal, and enhance resistance to infectious diseases.

Maintains the health of epithelial tissues, makes the skin smooth, and has a therapeutic effect on acne, acne and other symptoms.

Maintain the normal growth of the human body, improve the use of iron in the body, and promote hematopoiesis.

Many research results show that:lack of vitamin A can easily lead to lung cancer, gastric cancer, esophageal cancer, colon cancer, bladder cancer and laryngeal cancer.

Sources of Vitamin A:

Animals: such as liver, cod liver oil, egg yolk, cream.

Plants: β-carotene is found in carrots, apricots, green vegetables, seaweed, yellow fruits (such as mango, papaya), tomatoes, etc.

Vitamin E King of Vitamins

The main effects of vitamin E:

1. Prevent vascular diseases and delay aging

2. Prevent neonatal jaundice and anemia.

3. In an environment with high oxide concentration, some abnormal cells in the blood divide too much. Vitamin E will reduce the body's need for oxygen, thereby producing anti-cancer effects.

4. Male: Improve sperm count and motility. Women: According to information, if pregnant women can absorb enough vitamin E, they will not give birth to deformed children or mentally retarded children.

5. Vitamin E is anti-oxidant and can strengthen liver cells and improve liver function.

6. Vitamin E helps blood circulation and is an essential nutrient for tissue repair. It can also promote normal blood coagulation to help wound healing and reduce wound scars.

7. Regulate endocrine.

When vitamin E is deficient, intracellular creatine and amino acids easily disappear with urine, leading to muscle weakness. Insufficient vitamin E in pregnant women, children are prone to strabismus, crawling, sitting, and standing slowly

The blood clot attaches to the wall of the vein, and the blood vessel swells, preventing the return of blood. Timely supplementation of vitamin E, blood vessels will straighten, blood clots will dissolve, and blood will flow back smoothly.

After vitamin E is absorbed, it not only reduces the peroxidation of lipids and lipoproteins on cell membranes, protects the normal function of cells, but also locks moisture, so it is called the "natural moisturizer" of the skin. When the skin is affected by ultraviolet rays and induces the generation of free radicals, vitamin E can be absorbed through the skin and has the effects of delaying skin aging, sun protection, and inhibiting sun erythema.

Vitamin E deficiency symptoms:

Endocrine disorders, aging of the human body, precipitation of skin stains, infertility, muscle weakness, difficulty in healing wounds, and varicose veins.

When vitamin E is lacking, unsaturated fatty acids are mixed with oxygen, and the cells rupture to produce pigment spots.

Vitamin E can also prevent the oxidation of vitamin A, C and carotene in the body and increase their activity.

Source of Vitamin E: Natural Vitamin E is widely found in various oil seeds and vegetable oils. Cereals, nuts and green leafy vegetables contain a certain amount of natural Vitamin E. Especially in the germ of the seed. Corn, brown rice, nuts, beans, wheat germ oil, soybean oil, sesame, sunflower oil, rapeseed oil, peanut oil and cottonseed oil are also rich in vitamin E.

Vitamin D

Vitamin D is a sterol derivative with anti-rickets effect, also known as anti-rickets vitamin. The most important members of the vitamin D family are D2 and D3. Vitamin D is the derivative of different pro-vitamin D after ultraviolet irradiation. Plants do not contain vitamin D, but vitamin D precursors (provitamind, the raw material for producing vitamin D) exist in animals and plants.

Vitamin D is a fat-soluble vitamin with five compounds. The more closely related to health are vitamin D2 and vitamin D3. The precursors of vitamin D exist in the skin. When exposed to direct sunlight, it will react and transform into vitamin D3，and this part of vitamin D accounts for 90% of the body's vitamin D supply.

The relationship between vitamin D and pancreas:

1. Vitamin D supplementation reduces the risk of developing type 1 diabetes. There are vitamin D receptors and

2. vitamin D-dependent calcium-binding proteins in the pancreas.

3. Vitamin D receptor gene polymorphism is related to type 1 diabetes.

4. Vitamin D can reduce the resistance to insulin, and insulin resistance is one of the main factors leading to heart disease.

5. Vitamin D can inhibit the autoimmune response against pancreatic β cells to a certain extent and reduce insulin resistance. Vitamin D deficiency can easily lead to decreased insulin secretion.

6. Vitamin D or the like can increase insulin secretion in type 2 diabetic patients and prevent bone loss in newly-onset type 2 diabetic patients.

Other symptoms caused by vitamin D deficiency:

Vitamin D deficiency can cause rickets in children and rickets in adults. Symptoms include bone and joint pain, muscle wasting, insomnia, nervousness, and dysentery and diarrhea.

Vitamin D is used by the parathyroid on the neck thyroid gland. These glands secrete a hormone that regulates calcium levels in the body, and calcium helps regulate blood pressure.

Lung tissue undergoes repair during a person's life. Vitamin D affects the growth of a variety of cells, and it may play a role in the repair process of the lung.

Vitamin D is mainly used to form and maintain strong bones. It is used to prevent and treat children's rickets and adult's rickets, arthralgias and so on. People suffering from osteoporosis can effectively increase the absorption of calcium ions by adding appropriate vitamin D and magnesium. In addition, vitamin D is also used to reduce the risk of colon cancer, breast cancer and prostate cancer, and it also has a boosting effect on the immune system.

β-Carotene

Beta-carotene is one of the carotenoids and is also an orange-yellow fat-soluble compound. It is the most ubiquitous and most stable natural pigment in nature.

β-carotene has a good effect in promoting the reproduction and growth of animals.

Beta-carotene is an antioxidant with detoxification effect and an indispensable nutrient for maintaining human health. It has significant functions in anti-cancer, prevention of cardiovascular disease, cataract and antioxidant. And thus prevent aging and various degenerative diseases caused by aging.

Excessive intake of vitamin A in the human body can cause poisoning. The human body will convert β-carotene into vitamin A only when it is needed. This feature makes β-carotene a safe source of vitamin A, and there will be no accumulation of vitamin A poisoning caused by excessive intake.

Carrots also contain hypoglycemic substances, which is a good food for diabetic patients. Some of the ingredients contained in it, such as laxenin and kaempferol, can increase coronary blood flow, reduce blood lipids, promote the synthesis of adrenaline, and lower blood pressure, heart strengthening effect, it is a good food therapy for patients with hypertension and coronary heart disease.

Beta-carotene is an antioxidant. Eating foods rich in β-carotene can resist oxidation and prevent the body from contacting free radicals.

Many natural foods, such as green vegetables, sweet potatoes, carrots, spinach, papaya, mango, etc. , are rich in β-carotene.

6. Mineral Substance

Minerals are the tissue components of the human body, accounting for 5% of the human body. There are about 55 kinds of minerals needed by the human body. According to the amount of minerals in the body, minerals can be divided into two categories: those with a content greater than 0. 01% of body weight are called "major elements" or "macro elements, such as Calcium, phosphorus, potassium, sodium, magnesium, chlorine, sulfur, etc, are all essential elements for the human body, and the daily requirement is more than 100 mg. Those whose content is less than 0. 01% of body weight a re called "trace elements", such as iron, Iodine, copper, zinc, selenium, molybdenum, etc.

Human tissues contain almost all the elements that exist in nature. Carbon, hydrogen, oxygen, and nitrogen mainly exist in the form of organic compounds, and other elements are called "minerals" or "inorganic salts".

The human body has found that there are more than 20 kinds of essential minerals, namely inorganic salts, which account for about 4-5% of the human body. Inorganic salts cannot be synthesized in the body and must be taken from food.

Minerals cannot produce energy. A very important function of minerals is to regulate the physiological functions of the human body.

The physiological functions of minerals include:

1. Participate in the formation of bones, teeth, muscles, glands, blood, enzymes, hair and other human tissues, such as calcium, phosphorus, and magnesium are the main components of bones and teeth.

2. Regulate the physiological functions of the human body, maintain the normal distribution of body water, acid-base balance and neuromuscular excitability.

3. Maintain the normal beating of the heart.

4. Minerals are the activators and constituents of some enzymes.

Minerals are extremely important nutrients for the human body. For example, the lack of certain trace elements can lead to the decline of the body's immunity and induce related diseases. Due to metabolism, a certain amount of minerals are excreted from the body through urine, sweat, hair, nails, skin, etc, so they must be supplemented by diet.

Calcium

Calcium is a metal element, symbol Ca, silver-white crystal. Animal bones, clam shells, and egg shells all contain calcium carbonate.

The role of calcium:

1. Form strong bones and teeth, effectively reduce bone loss caused by aging, and relieve osteoporosis.

2. It has a certain degree of effect on lowering blood pressure.

3. Reducing the accumulation of aluminum in the body can help lower cholesterol levels. Calcium can regulate the heartbeat and keep the heart contracting and expanding alternately. It has a preventive effect on senile dementia, hypertension and other cardiovascular diseases.

4. Calcium can maintain muscle contraction and the transmission of nerve impulses, so that nerves and muscles maintain normal responses. Calcium stimulates platelets and promotes blood clotting after injury. Help muscle contraction and expansion, and help regulate heartbeat

5. It can reduce the proliferation of intestinal mucosal cells, thereby reducing the risk of colon cancer.

6. In the body, there are many enzymes that require calcium activation to show their activity. Calcium is very important for diabetic patients.

The human body needs vitamin D to absorb calcium. Without enough vitamin D, the human body cannot produce enough synthetic calcitriol hormone (also known as active vitamin D). If the active vitamin D is not produced enough, the body cannot get enough calcium from the diet. In this case, the body has to consume the calcium stored in its own bones to obtain enough calcium. This depletion can make bones fragile and prevent the formation of healthy new bones.

Magnesium is also an important part of promoting bone growth and synthesis. The lack of magnesium will affect the absorption and metabolism of calcium. Especially for diabetics, calcium supplementation must supplement magnesium and vitamin D.

The combination of calcium, magnesium and vitamin D can promote the growth of healthy bones. It is the best combination of three elements to maintain good bone function.

Magnesium

The original name of magnesium is taken from the Greek place name magnesia.

Magnesium is the main cation in human cells. It is concentrated in the glands, second only to potassium and phosphorus, and third only to sodium and calcium in the extracellular fluid. It is an essential substance for the basic biochemical reactions of many cells in the body. Magnesium is an essential substance in the metabolism of calcium, vitamin C, phosphorus, sodium, potassium, etc. It participates in protein synthesis and muscle contraction, and plays an important role in the normal operation of neuromuscular functions and the conversion of blood sugar.

Magnesium plays a very important role in human motor function activities. The reason why people live depends on a series of complex biochemical reactions in the human body to maintain life activities, and catalyzing these biochemical reactions requires thousands of enzymes. There are metabolic systems that use magnesium as a catalyst everywhere in the human body. Magnesium can activate about 325 enzymes in the body. Magnesium particiates in almost all metabolic processes in the body. Magnesium can be called an activator of life activities.

In recent years, foreign scientists have pointed out that people need "magnesium" food after middle age. That is, eat more foods rich in magnesium. Cardiovascular diseases, such as coronary heart disease, high blood pressure, hyperlipidemia, myocardial infarction, diabetes, etc, mostly occur after middle age, which is related to the decrease of magnesium content in the body.

The role of magnesium:

1. Activate the activity of multiple enzymes Magnesium acts as an activator of multiple enzymes and participates in more than 300 enzymatic reactions.

2. Prevents calcium from depositing in tissues and blood vessel walls,

3. preventing the formation of kidney and gallstones.

4. Maintain bone growth and neuromuscular excitability.

5. Maintain the function of the gastrointestinal tract and hormones.

6. Maintain the function of the gastrointestinal tract and hormones.

7. Promotes heart and blood vessel health and prevents heart attacks

8. Helps fight depression and acts as a natural sedative in combination with calcium.

Magnesium deficiency can lead to muscle weakness and reduced endurance. Due to exercise, especially long-term high-intensity exercise, a large amount of magnesium is consumed in the body, thereby reducing the activity function of muscles, and even convulsions, spasms, etc, will occur.

Some studies have shown that magnesium depletion can lead to insulin resistance.

Food sources of magnesium:

Magnesium is commonly found in food. Magnesium is the core atom of the chlorophyll molecule, so green leafy vegetables are rich in magnesium. People usually think that bananas are high in magnesium. In fact, they are just the champion of magnesium in fruits. Almost all dark green leafy vegetables are good sources of magnesium, and the content can reach or exceed the level in bananas. Because every chlorophyll molecule contains a magnesium ion, the greener the color, the more magnesium it contains.

Foods such as coarse grains and nuts are also rich in magnesium, while the magnesium content in meat, starchy foods and milk is moderate. Tofu also contains a high content of magnesium, often eat some brine tofu, can solve the "convulsions" caused by magnesium deficiency.

In addition to food, a small amount of magnesium can also be obtained from drinking water. However, the content of magnesium in drinking water varies greatly. For example, hard water contains high magnesium salt, while soft water contains relatively low content. The utilization rate of magnesium in animal foods is higher, reaching 30%- 40%, and the utilization rate of magnesium in plant foods is low.

Another best source of magnesium is nuts and seeds.

The appropriate intake (AI)for adults is set at 350 mg/d, and the tolerable maximum intake (UL) is set at 700 mg/d.

Diabetics need to supplement magnesium.

Phosphorus

Phosphorus is an essential mineral nutrient for the human body.

Phosphorus accounts for a quarter of the total minerals in the human body. In other words, one percent of the human body's weight is phosphorus. An adult weighing 70 kg contains about 560 grams to 850 grams of phosphorus, and the pure weight of phosphorus in the cell accounts for 2%-4%, of which 85% is combined with calcium in the state of inorganic salts to form bones. Of the insoluble apatite in teeth, 1% is in blood and body fluids, and the remaining 14% is in soft tissues such as muscles and internal organs. The ratio of calcium to phosphorus in bones is 2:1. The content of phosphorus in soft tissues is far more than that of calcium, and the phosphorus in this tissue is mostly organic compounds.

Phosphorus in the blood is divided into two categories: 70% organic and 30% inorganic:

70% organic state: mainly phospholipids, they are the components of the cell membrane, regulating the entry and exit of solutes between cells, and the phosphorus-containing lipoproteins can help the absorption of fat.

30% inorganic state: inorganic phosphorus and sodium, calcium, magnesium phosphate compounds.

The main function of phosphorus in the human body is to constitute the structure of cells, regulate biological activity and participate in energy metabolism.

Phospholipids are the main component of cell membranes, phosphate is an important component of bones and teeth, and light apatite is the mineral component of bones.

Lack of phosphorus will slow down growth, increase the loss of potassium, magnesium, and nitrogen in cells, thereby affecting cell function. Whether the absorption of phosphorus is good or not directly affects bone calcification. Vitamin D can promote the absorption of phosphorus.

Phosphorus is widely present in food. Different types of foods have different levels of phosphorus. The rich sources of phosphorus are cocoa powder, fish meal, peanut powder, zucchini seeds, pumpkin seeds, rice bran, soybean meal, sunflower, and wheat bran. Good sources are beef, cheese, fish, seafood, lamb, liver, nuts, peanut butter, pork, poultry and whole grain flour. Common sources are bread, cereals, dried fruits, eggs, ice cream, milk, most vegetables and white flour.

Molybdenum

Molybdenum is an essential trace element for the human body, animals and plants. It is silver-white metal, hard and tough. Various tissues of the human body contain molybdenum. The total amount in an adult's body is 9mg, with the highest content in the liver and kidney.

Molybdenum is mainly stored in the liver, kidneys, adrenal glands and bones. Molybdenum is a cofactor of a variety of enzymes, which can help human nucleic acid metabolize urea, remove excessive purine derivatives in the body, and help the body's metabolism. Lack of molybdenum leads to mental illness and damage to the crystals.

The physiological function of molybdenum is realized by the activity of various molybdenum enzymes, and molybdenum is an essential component in the enzymes that help digestion, generate energy and remove waste in the human body. All molybdenum enzymes contain molybdenum cofactors and actively participate in the catalytic reactions of various molybdenum enzymes. Molybdenum is required for the production and activity of several enzymes in the body upon which various vital body functions depend.

Molybdenum is indispensable in enabling the body to utilize biosulfur compounds, which are essential for connective tissue, which depends on molybdenum for optimal function, as active sulfite oxidase cannot do without molybdenum. The enzyme converts toxic sulfites into sulfates, the stage where sulfur in the body performs its function through a reaction called sulfation. In addition, if is too much accumulation of sulfites and sulfates, the human liver will not function properly. As such, molybdenum helps detoxify the liver, promotes connective tissue development, and contributes to sulfur balance throughout the body.

Molybdenum is also required for the function of xanthine oxidase, which converts hypoxanthine and xanthine into uric acid, which contributes to the enhancement of plasma antioxidant capacity in the blood. Molybdenum is a vital mineral nutrient without which humans, animals and plants would not be able to survive. Organisms cannot manufacture molybdenum compounds, so they must be obtained from external sources, including food.

Food sources of molybdenum: Meat: animal liver, animal kidney, etc. Green leafy vegetables. Cereals: whole grains, brown rice. Legumes: lentils, red beans, etc.

Many over-the-counter multivitamin and mineral dietary supplements also contain molybdenum, usually about 50 micrograms per unit dose.

Sodium

The total amount of sodium in the body of a normal adult is generally considered to be about 1 gram per kilogram of body weight, of which 44% is in the extracellular fluid, 9% is in the intracellular fluid, and 47% is in the bones.

Sodium and potassium are elements found at the same time, and both are indispensable substances for normal growth and development. Sodium can dissolve calcium and other minerals in the blood, which is closely related to metabolism.

Sodium efficacy: Prevent dehydration, maintain the balance of water in the body, contribute to the activity of the nervous system, used for muscle contraction, including the contraction of the heart muscle; also used for the production of energy in the body, and help transport nutrients to the cells.

Sodium deficiency: dizziness, lack of energy, loss of appetite, muscle cramps, nausea, vomiting, low blood pressure, rapid pulse, weight loss, and headache.

Food sources of sodium: salt, kimchi, ham, celery, crab, etc.

Potassium

Potassium is one of the important components in human muscle tissue and nerve tissue.

Potassium can regulate the appropriate osmotic pressure in the cell and the acid-base balance of body fluids, and participate in the metabolism of sugar and protein in the cell. Helps maintain nerve health, has a normal heartbeat, prevents strokes, and assists in normal muscle contraction. When high sodium intake causes high blood pressure, potassium has the effect of lowering blood pressure.

Lack of potassium in the body can cause irregular and fast heartbeat, abnormal electrocardiogram, muscle weakness and irritability, and finally lead to cardiac arrest. In general, healthy people will automatically excrete excess potassium out of the body. However, people with kidney disease should pay special attention to avoid excessive potassium intake.

The functional role of potassium

Involved in sugar, protein and energy metabolism. When glycogen is synthesized, it needs to enter the cell together with potassium, and when glycogen is decomposed, potassium is released from the cell. Protein synthesis requires about 3 mmol potassium concentration per gram of nitrogen, and potassium is released when it is decomposed.

Participate in maintaining the osmotic pressure and acid-base balance of the intracellular and external fluids. Potassium is the main cation in the cell, so it can maintain the osmotic pressure of the intracellular fluid. In acidosis, due to the decrease in the amount of potassium excreted by the kidneys and the movement of potassium from the inside of the cells, the blood potassium tends to rise at the same time. In the case of alkalosis, the situation is the opposite.

Maintain neuromuscular excitability.

Maintain myocardial function. One of the main driving forces of the potential changes of the myocardial cell membrane is due to the intracellular and extracellular transfer of potassium ions.

Potassium is an indispensable substance for life. It works with sodium to regulate the balance of water in the body and regularize the heartbeat. Potassium is very important to the chemical reactions in cells, and it plays a very important role in helping to maintain a stable blood pressure and the conduction of nerve activity.

Potassium deficiency will reduce the excitability of the muscles, so that the contraction and relaxation of the mus-cles cannot proceed smoothly, and it is easy to get tired. In addition, it can hinder intestinal peristalsis, cause constipation, cause edema, hemiplegia, and heart attack. When the body's potassium intake is insufficient, sodium will carry a lot of water into the cells, causing the cells to rupture and cause edema. A lack of potassium in the blood can increase blood sugar, leading to hyperglycemia. In addition, potassium deficiency causes the most serious damage to the heart, and potassium deficiency may be the main cause of death due to heart disease in humans.

The main symptoms of potassium deficiency in the human body are: fast heartbeat and irregular heart rate, muscle weakness, numbness, irritability, nausea, vomiting, diarrhea, low blood pressure, confusion and mental apathy.

Magnesium helps maintain potassium in cells, while excessive intake of sodium, alcohol, carbohydrates, diuretics, light doses, corticosteroids, and excessiv psychological stress can hinder the absorption of potassium.

Food sources of potassium:

Dairy products, fish, fruits, vegetables, legumes, meat, poultry, unprocessed grains, various fruit juices, especially orange juice, are also rich in potassium, and can replenish water and energy.

Chlorine

Chlorine is one of the essential macroelements of the human body. It is necessary to maintain the balance of body fluids and electrolytes, and it is also an essential component of gastric juice.

It often exists in the form of chloride in nature, and the most common form is table salt. The average content of chlorine in the human body is 1. 17g/kg, the total amount is about 82-100g, accounting for 0. 15% of body weight, and it is widely distributed throughout the body. It is mainly compounded with sodium and potassium in the form of chloride ions. Among them, potassium chloride is mainly in the intracellular fluid, while sodium chloride is mainly in the extracellular fluid. Sodium and potassium form compounds.

Chloride ions can regulate and maintain the acid-base balance of the blood. Chlorine can kill bacteria in the intestines and assist the liver to help remove toxins from the body. Chlorine is also one of the main components of gastric juice.

Efficacy and physiological function:

1. Maintain the acid-base balance of body fluids.

2. Maintain the flexibility of the body.

3. Chloride ions and sodium ions are the main ions that maintain osmotic pressure in the extracellular fluid, and they account for about 80% of the total ions, which

regulate and control the volume and osmotic pressure of the extracellular fluid.

4. Chloride ions are also involved in the formation of gastric acid in gastric juice. Gastric acid promotes the absorption of vitamin B12 and iron, activates salivary amylase to break down starch, and promotes food digestion.

5. Stimulate liver function and promote the excretion of metabolic waste in the liver.

6. Chlorine also stabilizes the membrane potential of nerve cells.

Chlorine deficiency: Insufficient blood chlorine can cause muscle cramps, and lack of chlorine can cause hair loss.

Food sources: salt, kelp and other seaweeds, and processed foods such as soy sauce, cured meat or smoked foods, pickles and savory foods are all rich in chloride. Almost all natural water also contains chlorine.

Sulfur

Sulfur exists in every cell. It is not only a relatively large element required by the human body, but also one of the constituents of amino acids. It also helps maintain the health and luster of the skin, hair and nails, maintain oxygen balance, and help the normal operation of brain functions.

Sulfur and B vitamins play an important role in helping the body's basic metabolism.

Effect:

1. Make the skin healthy and the hair shiny.

2. Help maintain the basic metabolism of the human body and benefit the brain function.

3. Promote bile secretion and help digestion.

4. Helps fight bacterial infections.

Food source:

Dried beans, fish, milk, lean meat, wheat germ, shellfish and other protein-rich foods, as well as onions, radishes, dried fruits, cabbage, etc. When you eat enough protein, you have enough sulfur.

Iron

Iron is the main substance that sustains life; it is the main substance in the production of heme (pigment in red blood cells) and myoglobin (pigment in muscle).

About 8% of the iron ingested by the human body is actually absorbed into the blood. An adult weighing 70 kg has about 4 grams of iron in the body, most of which is used to make heme. Heme is recycled and reused when blood cells are replaced with new cells every 120 days. The iron bound to protein is stored in the body.

Copper, cobalt, manganese, and vitamin C are needed to absorb iron.

Iron is an essential substance to promote the metabolism of the B vitamins. Vitamin B is an indispensable participant in the body's metabolism.

The utility of iron:

1. Promote development, increase resistance to diseases, and prevent fatigue.

2. It can prevent and treat anemia caused by iron deficiency and restore a good blood color to the skin.

Rich sources of food are animal liver, kidney, and animal blood. Followed by lean meat, egg yolk, chicken, fish, shrimp and beans. Green leafy vegetables contain more iron in alfalfa (alfalfa clover) spinach, celery, rape, amaranth, shepherd's purse, day lily, tomato and so on. Among the fruits, apricots, peaches, plums, raisins, dates, cherries, etc. contain more iron. Dried fruits include walnuts. Others such as kelp, brown sugar, and sesame paste also contain iron.

The absorption rate of iron in food ranges from 1% to 22%. Iron in animal foods is easier to absorb and utilize than plant foods. The absorption rate of iron in animal blood is the highest, between 10%

and 76%, the absorption rate of iron in liver and lean meat is 7%. Plant foods also contain a lot of phytic acid and polyphenols. These substances can form insoluble compounds with iron, which will affect the absorption of iron.

Zinc

Zinc is one of the 25 essential elements in the human body and a trace element in the body, but it cannot be synthesized in the body and can only be provided by external food.

Zinc is a component of many important enzymes in the human body and an essential element for the synthesis of insulin. It plays an important role in the synthesis of protein and nucleic acid, maintaining the integrity of red blood cells, and in the process of hematopoiesis. It is a key element to promote growth and development, especially for the development of children's brain and nervous system. If we want to maintain the vitality of the human body, we should take in enough zinc.

Physiological regulation: Zinc is not only a component of many enzymes, but also an activator of certain enzymes. For example, zinc is involved in sugar metabolism. Each insulin molecule contains two zinc atoms. Zinc is closely related to the production, secretion, storage and activity of insulin. Zinc is also involved in the enzymes involved in red blood cells transporting oxygen and carbon dioxide.

Zinc is closely related to the synthesis of nucleic acid and protein and to the growth of cells. Zinc-containing enzymes are involved in bone growth and nutrient metabolism. Zinc is also an essential element to maintain normal skin growth.

Zinc is a key element to promote the development of sexual organs. Promote wound healing. Zinc is related to the synthesis of vitamin A reductase and the metabolism of vitamin A. Zinc can improve dark vision and night vision. There is a salivary protein in saliva, called taste element, which contains two ions in its molecule. Zinc affects taste and appetite through taste hormone, which is also a nutrient for oral mucosal epithelial cells. Zinc can improve immunity. Zinc deficiency can reduce some immune functions in the body. For example, the respiratory tract is prone to repeated infections and the skin is prone to lichen.

The rich sources of zinc are gluten, sesame, mushroom, beef, liver, condiments and wheat bran.

Good sources are egg yolk powder, watermelon seeds, scallops, scented tea, shrimp, peanut butter, peanuts, pork and poultry. Common sources are squid, pea yellow, dried sea rice, shiitake mushrooms, white fungus, black rice, green tea, black tea, beef tongue, pork liver, beef liver, beans, golden needles, eggs, fish, sausages and whole grain products.

Drinking water in most areas also contains a small amount of zinc.

Selenium

Selenium is an essential micronutrient element for the human body, which can significantly improve the immune function of the human body. The total amount of selenium in the human body is only 3-20 mg. Selenium is found in various tissues, organs and body fluids. The concentration of selenium is highest in the kidneys. Most of it exists in the eyes, liver, pancreas, and kidneys of the human body, with the eyes having the highest selenium content.

Scientific research has found that the level of blood selenium is closely related to the occurrence of cancer. A large number of survey data show that the level of selenium in food and soil in a region is directly related to the incidence of cancer. Scientists call selenium the "anti-cancer king" of human trace elements.

Anti-oxidize effect:

Selenium is a component of glutathione peroxidase (GSH-Px), containing 4 grams of atomic selenium per mole of GSH-Px. The role of this enzyme is to catalyze the redox reaction of reduced glutathione (GSH) with peroxide, Therefore, it can play an antioxidant role and is an important free radical scavenger. In vivo, GSH-Px and vitamin E have different antioxidant mechanisms, and the two can complement each other and have a synergistic effect.

Organic selenium can scavenge free radicals in the body, eliminate toxins in the body, and resist oxidation. It can effectively inhibit the production of lipid peroxides, prevent blood clots, remove cholesterol, and enhance the body's immune function.

Prevent diabetes: Selenium is an active ingredient that constitutes glutathione peroxidase. It can prevent the oxidative destruction of pancreatic β cells, make them function normally, promote sugar metabolism, reduce blood sugar and urine sugar, and improve the symptoms of diabetic patients.

Selenium can protect the retina, enhance the smoothness of the vitreous body, improve vision, and prevent cataracts.

Selenium is an important element to maintain the normal function of the heart, and has the effect of protecting and repairing the heart body. The decrease in the blood selenium level of the human body will lead to a decline in the function of scavenging free radicals in the body, resulting in an increase in the deposition of harmful substances, an increase in blood pressure, a thickening of the blood vessel wall, a decrease in blood vessel elasticity, a slowdown in blood flow, and a decrease in the oxygen supply function. This leads to an increased incidence of cardiovascular and cerebrovascular diseases. A moderate amount of selenium supplementation can destroy the cholesterol deposited on the arterial wall, and has a good effect on preventing cardiovascular and cerebrovascular diseases, hypertension, arteriosclerosis and controlling the development of cancer cells.

Selenium supplementation can prevent bone marrow end lesions, promote repair, and have a good preventive and therapeutic effect on arthritis patients

Detoxification : selenium has a strong binding force with metals, and it can resist the toxic effects of cadmium on the kidneys, gonads and central nervous system. Selenium combines with mercury, tin, thallium, lead and other heavy metals in the body to form a metal selenoprotein complex to detoxify.

Selenium can prevent liver disease and protect the liver. The best sources of selenium: mushrooms, cod, shrimp, salmon, flounder, beef liver, mustard seeds, garlic, onions, pork. Eggs contain more selenium than meat.

The selenium content of plant foods is determined by the selenium content in the local soil and water. The soils in the United States and Canada contain enough selenium. Many foods contain selenium, but Brazil nuts are brazil nut, whole grains (whole wheat bread, oatmeal, barley).), white rice and beans are particularly high in content.

Vitamins that help selenium absorption:Vitamin A, Vitamin C, Vitamin E. Do not take inorganic selenium together with vitamin C. Do not take too much selenium supplementation, do not exceed 450 mg per day.

Chromium

Chromium is one of the essential trace elements for the human body. Normal human body only contains 6-7 mg, mainly in bone, skin, fat, adrenal gland, brain and muscle. Chromium is very important to the human body. As long as 1 microgram of chromium per kilogram of body weight is given, it is enough to show its biological function. Although the amount required is so small, the problem of chromium deficiency still exists. This is mainly because people take chromium from food, and a large number of refined foods lose a lot of quality during processing.

The main function of chromium is to play a special role in the body's glucose metabolism and lipid metabolism. Chromium is involved in sugar and glucose tolerance, the oxidation of glucose to carbon dioxide and the conversion of glucose to fat. When sugar is used, chromium is consumed. When sugar is used in large quantities, it may cause a lack of chromium, and when chromium is insufficient, it will affect the use of sugar. Chromium is the only metal element whose body levels decrease with age. While chromium decreases with age, glucose tolerance also decreases with age. The susceptibility of the elderly to diabetes may be related to this.

Chromium and insulin: The body's tolerance to glucose is regulated by glucose tolerance factors, and chromium is an indispensable factor for the stability of glucose tolerance factors. Glucose tolerance factor can promote the action of insulin, and can increase insulin activity, thereby reducing the dosage of insulin and helping to control blood sugar. It should be said that the function of chromium is achieved through insulin. The role of chromium is the insulin receptor on the cell membrane. Chromium is not a substitute for insulin, but promotes the action of insulin. The trace element chromium has the effects of hematopoiesis, weight loss, and blood sugar regulation.

Chromium deficiency reduces the sensitivity of tissues to insulin, and chromium is closely related to diabetes and cardiovascular disease and atherosclerosis. The incidence of diabetes is high in areas with severe chromium deficiency, and there is very s ufficient evidence to prove that chromium deficiency causes abnormal glucose tolerance. The vast majority of people who eventually develop diabetes begin with impaired glucose tolerance, so chromium plays a role in preventing diabetes in preventing impaired glucose tolerance. Such as timely intake of adequate chromium, can normalize glucose tolerance and prevent the occurrence of diabetes. Type II diabetics produce a lot of insulin, but blood sugar is not well controlled. With chromium supplementation, endogenous insulin is reduced and glucose tolerance can be improved.

Chromium deficiency is a common link between diabetes and atherosclerosis. Low-chromium foods can reduce glucose tolerance and can also cause arteriosclerosis. Adding chromium-containing compounds to food can restore glucose tolerance, and prevent and control the occurrence of atherosclerosis. The blood chromium content of patients with coronary heart disease is significantly lower than that of normal people. The content of chromium in the aorta tissue of people who died of coronary heart disease was significantly lower than that of those who died from sudden accidents. Animal experiments have also shown that increasing chromium can prevent the formation of atherosclerosis. Chromium deficiency can cause disorders of fat metabolism and promote atherosclerosis. Chromium supplementation can reduce serum total cholesterol and increase high-density lipid cholesterol.

People get a small amount of chromium mainly from food, drinking water and air.

The best source of chromium is meat, especially liver and other internal organs.

The rich sources of chromium are beef, pepper, wheat, brown sugar, brown rice, whole grains, corn, brown rice, dairy products, tea, ginseng, Ganoderma lucidum, astragalus, softshell turtle, Polygonum multiflorum, seaweed, beer, yeast, mushroom, bran and so on. There are also some sources such as potatoes, apple peels, eggs, cheese and so on.

After the grain is processed and refined, the chromium content is significantly reduced. The content of chromium in natural foods is low. High-chromium yeast can improve glucose tolerance and is effective for non-insulin- dependent diabetic patients.

Iodine

Iodine is an essential element for the human body. It is used to produce thyroxine to regulate cell metabolism and neuromuscular tissue development and growth. Adults contain 20-50 mg of iodine, and most of the iodine is present in the thyroid. The thyroid gland can control metabolism, and the thyroid gland is affected by iodine.

The iodine needed by the body can be obtained from drinking water, food and salt. Iodine ions in food and drinking water are easily absorbed by the digestive tract and transported to the plasma. Part of the absorbed iodine is taken up by thyroid epithelial cells, and the amount depends on the activity of the thyroid. The ingested iodide ions will be oxidized by peroxidase into elemental iodine, and then combined with thyroxin by the action of iodination enzyme and then stored. If iodine is insufficient, it will cause mental retardation, obesity and lack of energy.

Human body effects of iodine:

1. Dissolve excess fat and help reduce weight.

2. Properly develop and give vitality.

3. Improve response agility.

4. Promote the health of hair, nails, skin and teeth.

Food sources of iodine: kelp and other seaweeds, onions and seafood, vegetables produced in iodine-rich soil.

Deficiency: thyroid hypertrophy, hypothyroidism.

Copper

Copper is an essential trace mineral for the human body. It plays an irreplaceable role in the body's hematopoiesis, metabolism, growth and reproduction, and enhancing the body's resistance. Copper deficiency can cause a variety of animal diseases. One of the most important physiological roles of copper is cofactor for ferrous oxidase, cytochrome C oxidase, copper-zinc superoxide dismutase, tyrosinase cofactor for lysyl oxidase and dopamine-beta-hydroxylase as a key enzyme in the body. Copper is also a component of coagulation factor V and metallothionein.

Copper participates in oxidative phosphorylation, free radical detoxification, melanin synthesis, catechol ammonia metabolism, connective tissue cross-linking, iron and ammonia oxidation, uric acid metabolism, blood coagulation and hair formation in the form of enzyme cofactors. In addition, copper is necessary for the metabolism of glucose metabolism, cholesterol metabolism, bone mineralization, immune function, myelin formation, heat regulation, red blood cell production and heart function.

Copper can enter the blood 15 minutes after ingestion, and it can also exist inside and outside the red blood cells. It can help the transferrin and play an important role in the formation of heme. Moreover, the copper element is not easily destroyed during the food cooking process.

The efficacy of copper:

Helps the absorption of iron, helps the formation of heme, improves vitality, and is conducive to the absorption of vitamin C. Promote the use of tyrosine, one of the amino acids, and become an element of hair and skin pigment.

Food sources of copper: beans, whole wheat, straw mushrooms, peanuts, olives, honey, organ meats, shellfish, shrimps, crabs, etc.

Deficiency: A lack of copper in the body can cause anemia, edema, bone disease, and possibly rheumatoid arthritis.

Overdose manifestations: liver cirrhosis, poisoning, zinc reduction or even deficiency.

Manganese

Manganese participates in the composition of various enzymes and affects the activity of enzymes. Manganese can activate hundreds of enzymes in the body.

Manganese is a necessary trace mineral element, a necessary substance for normal bones, and has many functions.

Manganese may be closely related to the maintenance of normal brain function, and has a curative effect on Alzheimer's disease

Manganese can activate the necessary enzymes so that vitamins H, B, and C can be used by the body smoothly. Manganese is also indispensable in the manufacture of thyroxine.

Manganese has many functions and can help regulate the blood sugar concentration in the body. Lack of this trace mineral may have a negative impact on blood sugar control. After manganese deficiency, the stem cells of insulin may be destroyed, and the utilization rate of glucose will decrease, which will reduce the synthesis and secretion of insulin, thereby affecting the body's glucose metabolism.

When manganese is deficient, the activity of manganese-containing enzymes in the body decreases, which can cause the activity of bone cells to be restricted, the bone holes enlarge and it is easy to get osteoporosis, bone deformities, and cartilage damage.

Thyroxine secreted by the human thyroid gland is a hormone that regulates the metabolism of vital substances in the body, but it must be involved in manganese to perform its normal functions.

The normal division and proliferation of human cells, as well as the synthesis of proteins, require the participation of manganese.

When there is a lack of manganese in the body, the body's functions will be degraded, which will accelerate the aging process of the elderly.

The efficacy of manganese:

1. Make the skin healthy and the hair shiny.
2. Help maintain the basic metabolism of the human body and benefit the brain function.
3. Promote bile secretion and help digestion.
4. Helps fight bacterial infections.

Food sources of manganese: brown rice, rice bran, spices, walnuts, dried beans, fish, milk, lean meat, wheat germ, whole grains, peanuts, shellfish and other protein-rich foods, as well as onions, potatoes, radishes, dried fruits , Cabbage and so on.

In daily life, if you eat enough protein, you will also get enough manganese.

Lack of crowds, diabetics, cancer patients.

Cellulose

Dietary cellulose is what we often call crude fiber, which refers to food nutrients that are generally not easily decomposed by human digestive enzymes. It mainly comes from the cell walls of plants, including cellulose, hemicellulose, resin, pectin, and lignin. Cellulose is rich in a variety of minerals, cellulose and oligosaccharides, it is a natural food for humans to lose weight and reduce fat.

Dietary fiber is indispensable for a healthy diet. Fiber plays an important role in keeping the digestive system healthy. At the same time, getting enough fiber can also prevent cardiovascular disease, cancer, diabetes and other diseases. Fiber can slow down the speed of digestion and excrete cholesterol most quickly, so blood sugar and cholesterol in the blood can be controlled at the optimal level.

Fiber can clean the digestive wall and enhance digestive function. Fiber can also dilute the concentration of harmful substances in the intestinal tract and reduce the retention time of harmful substances such as aflatoxins, nitrosamines, phenols, polycyclic aromatic hydrocarbons, etc in the intestinal tract, thereby reducing the body's absorption of them, accelerates the removal of carcinogens and toxins from food, protects the delicate digestive tract and prevents colon cancer.

The large intestine is considered the most filthy place among the human organs. The human body absorbs the nutrients needed in food, and the unnecessary substances are formed into feces and discharged from the large intestine. The role of cellulose in the intestine is like a scavenger, it can be diluted the toxins in the feces can also promote intestinal peristalsis, so that the feces will not stay in the intestines for too long.

Food sources of dietary fiber:

Insoluble dietary fiber: peels of fruits and vegetables, whole grains and seeds.

Water-soluble dietary fiber: fruits, vegetables, oats, oat bran, barley, peas, dried beans.

Dietary fiber can increase the sensitivity of insulin receptors and increase the utilization of insulin. Dietary fiber can wrap the sugar of food, make it gradually absorbed, have the effect of balancing blood sugar after meal, so as to achieve the effect of regulating the blood sugar level of diabetic patients and curing diabetes.

Elevated serum cholesterol levels can cause coronary heart disease. The excretion of cholesterol and bile acid is closely related to dietary fiber. Dietary fiber can be combined with bile acid to quickly excrete bile acid from the body. At the same time, the combination of dietary fiber and bile acid will promote the conversion of cholesterol to bile acid, thereby reducing cholesterol levels.

Dietary fiber can absorb ions and exchange with sodium ions and potassium ions in the intestinal tract, thereby reducing the ratio of sodium to potassium in the blood, thereby lowering blood pressure.

The effect of dietary fiber on diabetes:

Regulate blood sugar, prevent diabetes, lower blood cholesterol, prevent high blood pressure, cardiovascular and cerebrovascular diseases, increase the feeling of fullness, help control body weight, prevent constipation, dilute carcinogens in the large intestine, shorten the passage time of the intestine, and prevent colorectal cancer. Dietary fiber can improve the sensitivity of insulin receptors and improve the utilization rate of insulin, dietary fiber can wrap the sugar in food so that it can be gradually absorbed, which has the effect of balancing postprandial blood sugar, so as to regulate the blood sugar level of diabetic patients. The role of the treatment of diabetes.

Dietary fiber can improve the sensitivity of insulin receptors and improve the utilization rate of insulin. Dietary fiber can wrap the sugar in food so that it can be gradually absorbed, which has the effect of balancing postprandial blood sugar, so as to regulate the blood sugar level of diabetic patients, the role of the treatment of diabetes.

Many studies have shown that certain water-soluble fibers can reduce postprandial blood glucose and blood insulin elevation response. This is because the fruit acid in dietary fiber can prolong the residence time of food in the gastrointestinal tract, prolong gastric emptying time, slow down the body's absorption of glucose, and prevent the body's blood sugar level from rising sharply after a meal. And reduce the body's demand for insulin, which is conducive to the improvement of diabetes.

Dietary fiber has the effect of lowering blood sugar. Experiments have shown that 26 grams of edible corn bran (91. 2% fiber) or soybean hulls (86. 7% fiber) are added to the diet every day. As a result, after 28-30 days, glucose tolerance improved significantly. Therefore, the long-term increase of dietary fiber in the diabetic diet can reduce the amount of insulin required and control the metabolism after a meal. It should be used as an auxiliary measure for the treatment of diabetes.

Food sources of dietary fiber. Brown rice and germ-polished rice, as well as coarse grains such as corn, millet, barley, wheat husk (rice bran) and wheat flour (the material of black bread). Root vegetables and seaweeds also contain more dietary fiber, such as burdock, carrots, green beans, red beans, peas, potatoes and wakame.

Our bodies are very faithful responders, and she will honestly reward you with whatever you eat, as long as we meet the needs of the body to increase the necessary nutrition, repair and restore physical strength, and develop good living habits, our body will rebalance various functions in the body, we diabetics can also live healthy and happy lives.

Love life, cherish yourself, and maintain a healthy body and mind.